Parental Influences
In Health and Disease

Parental Influences
In Health and Disease

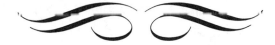

Edited by

E. James Anthony, M.D., F.R.C.Psy.
Professor of Child Psychiatry,
Washington University School of Medicine;
Training and Supervisory Psychoanalyst
and Director, Division of Child and
Adolescent Psychoanalysis,
St. Louis Psychoanalytic Institute,
St. Louis, Missouri

George H. Pollock, M.D., Ph.D.
President,
The Institute for Psychoanalysis;
Professor of Psychiatry,
Northwestern University;
President, Center for Psychosocial Studies,
Chicago, Illinois

Little, Brown and Company
Boston/Toronto

*Our gratitude to
Anna Freud and Therese Benedek
for sharing with us their
abundantly rich professional lives
and for leaving us a legacy of
new understanding*

Contents

III. *The Abandoning Parent*

IV. *Specific Influences*

Preface

Although this book represents a completely new contribution, it can also be regarded as a continuation of *Parenthood: Its Psychology and Psychopathology*, put together by E. James Anthony and Therese Benedek in 1970, which has become a resource book in many university departments responsible for the dynamic training of mental health professionals. The present work is different in its overall emphasis on the clinical aspects of parenting, although it continues to explore further aspects of parenting's multifarious normalcy.

Two of the authors in the earlier volume have been cited frequently for the originality of their conceptualizations in this area: Therese Benedek and Anna Freud. First a few words about Dr. Benedek.

Therese would certainly have approved of this extension of our knowledge to an even wider variety of parental dysfunction. She had a special capacity for picking out what was most worthwhile in the work of others rather than confining her attention to criticism. Because of the breadth and depth of her unusual mind, she was able to range comfortably from the biological to the psychoanalytical and to extract theoretical nuggets from the most unpromising morass of material. Within this comprehensive framework, she could write a paper on the relevance of molecular biology to psychoanalysis, on the relationship of the internal hormonal milieu to the fantasies of women, on the complex intergenerational transactions that led to the formation of a "depressive constellation," on the influence of culture on the developing psyche, and on the "developmental phases" of parenthood. What she tried to do and succeeded in doing was to take a closer and more psychoanalytic look at the Eriksonian life cycle, adding new and deeper dimensions to the interplay between the various stages. Without being overly concerned with the controversial issues regarding developmental continuity, she encouraged us in her writings to consider the manifold ways in which nature interacts with nurture and to take careful note of both in the ontogenesis from infancy to old age. She illuminated for us the singular truth that parenthood, like every mature component of life, is built up, step-by-step, from the beginning of life. The way in which the child is parented relates closely to how he or she parents his or her own children. Such apparent truisms are deeply rooted in the less accessible parts of the personality and are therefore often taken for granted without being further explored.

Therese followed the commonplace inwardly and brought its unconscious meaning to light. A number of the contributors to this book have been researching this intergenerational transmission.

Anna Freud did so much to further our understanding of children that one tends to forget that parenthood also profited from her astute psychoanalytic insights. A fine example of this, which had immediate and continued repercussions in the field, was her reappraisal of the concept of rejection. At a time when many investigators were engaged in establishing the consequences of such monolithic constructs as the "rejecting mother," Anna's firsthand experience with developing children and their parents led her to discount such simplistic connections. Her focus was not on the vicissitudes of parental development, but with its variability during any period of time. She concluded that even normal "good-enough" mothers habitually rejected their children at certain times of the day, certain weeks of the month, or when preoccupied with their own lives and interests, and that they could be accepting and caring during one stage of development and less so at another. It is quite normal for mothers to become gradually less intensely preoccupied with their children from infancy onward into adult life. Thus, the "goodness" or "badness" of the average mother at any given point in time is relative to the endless circumstances that determined and over-determined her behavior. This lucidly stated viewpoint helped to abate the torrent of "clinical abuse" leveled at mothers during Anna Freud's era. The "witch-hunt" was over and, thankfully, the mothers of today are not for burning.

It is, therefore, with a sense of privilege and gratitude, that we dedicate this book to the monumental accomplishments of these two great pioneers.

E. J. A.
G. H. P.

Contributing authors

E. James Anthony, M.D., F.R.C.Psy.
Professor of Child Psychiatry, Washington University School of Medicine; Training and Supervisory Psychoanalyst and Director, Division of Child and Adolescent Psychoanalysis, St. Louis Psychoanalytic Institute, St. Louis, Missouri

Anni Bergman, Ph.D.
Clinical Associate Professor, The City University of New York; Senior Research Scientist, The Margaret S. Mahler Psychiatric Research Foundation, New York, New York

George L. Engel, M.D.
Professor Emeritus of Psychiatry and Professor Emeritus of Medicine, University of Rochester School of Medicine and Dentistry, Rochester, New York

Vivian T. Harway, Ph.D.
Associate Professor of Child Psychiatry, University of Pittsburgh School of Medicine; President, Psychological Consultation Associates, P.C., Pittsburgh, Pennsylvania

James M. Herzog, M.D.
Assistant Professor of Psychiatry, Harvard Medical School; Director of Training, Psychiatry, The Children's Hospital and Judge Baker Guidance Center, Boston, Massachusetts

D. Wilson Hess, Ph.D.
Associate Professor of Pediatrics, University of Rochester School of Medicine and Dentistry, Rochester, New York

Judith S. Kestenberg, M.D.
Clinical Professor of Psychiatry, New York University School of Medicine; Pediatric Research Psychiatrist, L.I.J.-Hillside Medical Center, New Hyde Park, New York

Anna Ornstein, M.D.
Professor of Child Psychiatry, University of Cincinnati College of Medicine;
Attending Psychiatrist, University Hospital, Cincinnati, Ohio

Paul H. Ornstein, M.D.
Professor of Psychiatry, University of Cincinnati College of Medicine; Attending Psychiatrist, University Hospital, Cincinnati, Ohio

George H. Pollock, M.D., Ph.D.
President, The Institute for Psychoanalysis; Professor of Psychiatry, Northwestern University; President, Center for Psychosocial Studies, Chicago, Illinois

Franz K. Reichsman, M.D.
Professor Emeritus of Medicine and Psychiatry, State University of New York Downstate Medical Center College of Medicine, Brooklyn, New York

John Munder Ross, Ph.D.
Adjunct Associate Professor of Psychology in Psychiatry, Cornell University Medical College; Associate Attending Psychologist, The New York Hospital, New York, New York

H. David Sackin, M.D.
Associate Professor, Department of Psychiatry, University of Toronto Faculty of Medicine; Senior Staff Psychiatrist, The Hospital for Sick Children, Toronto, Ontario, Canada

Brandt F. Steele, M.D.
Professor Emeritus of Psychiatry, The University of Colorado Health Sciences Center; Psychiatrist, Kempe National Center for Prevention and Treatment of Child Abuse and Neglect, Denver, Colorado

Robert J. Stoller, M.D.
Professor of Psychiatry, University of California, Los Angeles, School of Medicine, Los Angeles, California

Judith S. Wallerstein, Ph.D.
Executive Director, Center for the Family in Transition, Corte Madera; Senior Lecturer, School of Social Welfare and School of Law, University of California at Berkeley, California; Principal Investigator, California Children of Divorce Study

Parental Influences
In Health and Disease

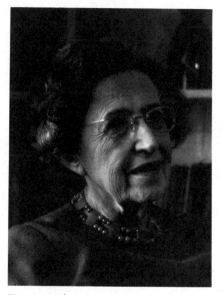

Fig. I-1. *Therese Benedek, M.D.*
(Photo by Samuel Weiss, M.D.)

Introduction

E. James Anthony and George H. Pollock

WE CARRY WITHIN US THE WONDERS WE SEEK WITHOUT US.
THERE IS ALL AFRICA, AND HER PRODIGIES IN US.

Sir Thomas Browne

Parental Influences: In Health and Disease is about the process of parenting and is written by psychoanalysts. It presupposes a special view that focuses chiefly on the interior of the individual and yet is sensitive to specific influences from the outside. It tries to understand the complex interplay between factuality as it exists externally and "psychic" or inner reality that is fashioned within the mind of the individual and is shaped idiosyncratically by experience, particularly early experience associated with parenting. This postulate somewhat simplifies the concept of reality by regarding it as bifurcated, whereas a more authentic viewpoint conceives of it as a many-layered formation with different strata that closely interact with one another. Such a schema renders disorders of reality more intelligible. For example, the surface layers of outer reality may undergo changes in normal people from time to time; the basic layers can be distorted by psychotic processes; the testing of inner reality is frequently deranged by neurosis. It is a matter of gradation.

Applying this schema to the process of parenting, the parent and child are in a closely reciprocating relationship at all levels of reality. Psychoanalysis has attempted to trace the various effects of the relationship in order to present a more comprehensive picture of the mutuality. A transacting system such as this involves interactions between the participants in addition to reactions of one to the other. When Winnicott [33] asserted, perhaps too categorically, that there was no such disorder in childhood as "reactive," he was both overstating the case and, at the same time, making an important point. Parents and children manifestly react to one another and can be described as reactively disturbed when they do so. The reaction may remain on the surface layers of reality with very little if any lasting effect on the individual concerned. In the case of a neurotic parent or neurotic child, the reactive disturbance is internalized into the inner realms of reality and is transformed in the process by

1

additions from the psychic life of the child or parent. This means that the reactive disturbance is overlaid with memories, fantasies, and feelings, thereby becoming the individual's own disorder. What started as interpersonal becomes personal and gradually, if the situation is repeated often enough, a part of the personality.

In 1950, Kris [26] called for a "new consideration of the environment" in approaching the problem of the child's interaction with his parents in terms of such undeniable realities as permissiveness, indulgence, frustration, and rejection in an effort to link together internal and external danger situations. Some studies have affirmed the relevance of the parent's conflicts in the shaping of the child's characterological attitudes and defenses [23], although for this to be demonstrated with any degree of conviction, it would require both parent and child to illuminate the giving and receiving end of the parenting process in analysis. Much of the earlier work on parenthood had stemmed either from direct observation of parent-child interactions or from reconstructions made during the analysis of adults. Gaps in our knowledge could be closed, although not completely, by the simultaneous analysis of parents and children, and this has been done by Anna Freud and her colleagues in London.

In summary, a comprehensive psychoanalytic picture of parenthood can be derived from a number of converging sources.

1. The direct longitudinal observation of parents and their children from infancy onward.
2. Reconstruction of the early parent-child relationship from the analysis of the parent. This furnishes us with the antecedent factor of the "depressive constellation" [2], vis-à-vis the mother's own experience of being mothered. Such cross-generational information helps in the understanding of how parental influences are transmitted.
3. The analysis of adult parents who are in the throes of parenting furnishes us with more detailed knowledge of the impact of parenthood on certain personality characteristics of the parent such as masochism, narcissism, and passivity. Some psychoanalysts might well question the introduction of this parameter into the classical transference analysis and would be more inclined to analyze these derivatives as they appear spontaneously in the transference. Child analysts, who analyze adult patients who are parents, may be more alert to the parenting factors in their patients without actively calling attention to them. Under such conditions, the "developmental stages of parenthood" [3] may be fully delineated.
4. Child analysis may disclose in depth and detail the ups and downs of

preparatory parenting as they appear in the child. As treatment intensifies and defenses are analyzed and weakened, the adult as parent to the child may be better understood.

5. Child analysis furnishes us with the childhood antecedents of adults' parental behavior and traces these to their very earliest sources.

All these approaches, as Hartmann [21] reminded us, have only been made possible through the systematic analytic study of the ego and its related structures, providing an "indispensable frame of reference" that enables us to understand both satisfactory and unsatisfactory structural articulations between corresponding minds. The impact on ego development of incomplete or empty relationships with the mother received a special emphasis in the work of Spitz [28] and Ribble [27]; Hartmann felt the structural viewpoint was overlooked and that consequently, the theory presented was simplistic. To quote his words [22], "the fact that the mother has 'rejected' her child in one way or another is frequently, in unilinear causal relation and rather indiscriminately, made responsible for nearly all varieties of later pathological developments and particularly of ego disturbances. That the ego needs, in order properly to function and to develop, a secure relation not only to the drives but also to the objects is obviously true. But ego development and object relationships are correlated in more complex ways than some recent work would lead us to believe." In this same context, both Therese Benedek and Anna Freud were fully aware of the hazards of "unilinear causal relations," having both been brought up analytically in the complex culture of overdeterminism.

The advance of psychoanalytic knowledge of parenting would imply structural articulations between parent and child that, in turn, would require the simultaneous analysis of mother and child. Sigmund Freud was excited by the opportunities that were opened up when the day-to-day living experiences of parent and child were seen in parallel with day-to-day analytic experiences. Such analytic "experiments" would allow the psychoanalytic investigation of the mysterious leaps of thought from one mind to another. In the context of parenthood, Freud could have added that the dual situation would permit us to follow the parenting process as it crossed generational lines and to examine how the parental image constructed in one generation could become the dominant parental image in the subsequent generation. Such transfers are all too easily and glibly explained in terms of limitations, identifications, incorporations, introjections, and empathies that describe but still fail to explain the cross-internalizations. In his new introductory lectures [16],

Freud reported on a case of simultaneous analysis of mother and child by Burlingham [6].

One day the mother spoke during her analytic session of a gold coin that had played a part in one of the scenes of her childhood. Immediately afterwards, after she had returned home, her little boy, about 10 years old, came to her room and brought her a gold coin which he asked her to keep for him. She asked him in astonishment where he had got it from. He had been given it on his birthday; but his birthday had been several months earlier and there was no reason why the child should have remembered the gold coin precisely then. The mother reported the occurrence to the child's analyst and asked her to find out from the child the reason for his action. But the child's analyst threw no light on the matter; the action had forced its way that day into the child's life like a foreign body. A few weeks later the mother was sitting at her writing desk to write down, as she had been told to do, an account of the experience, when in came the boy and asked for the gold coin back, and he wanted to take it with him to show in his analytic session. Once again the child's analyst could discover no explanation of his wish. (P. 56)

What one can observe here is the uncanny way in which the mother's thoughts, reaching back into her own childhood, are reflected, without any apparent connection, in the behavior of her child, almost as if a hypnotic suggestion had been made to him and had resulted in a posthypnotic act. The mother's curiosity led her to inject herself into her child's analysis, recruiting the child's analyst for this purpose. Unfortunately, the analyst is unable to make any link between the mother's memory and the child's wish. We are not told what part the gold coin played in the mother's childhood, nor why it had seemed fit to give the boy a gold coin as a birthday present during his childhood. Are we to be put off by this failure to elucidate the transmission? Are we to assume that the uncovering capacity of child analysis is less effective than in adult analysis? Or can we simply say that a significant early memory of the mother reappears in the transference relationship of the son to the mother-analyst and might well constitute a nuclear fantasy in the pregenital or genital yearnings of the child that would come gradually to light as the transference relationship was systematically explored.

This little vignette helps to clarify the ways in which the process of parenting and being parented are reciprocally related. Had the mother's and child's analysts collaborated with this particular psychological area in mind, we might have learned much more about the dynamics of parenthood. Fortunately for the analytic process and its preservation, but unfortunately for our understanding of the parenting process, the analysts in question failed to share their private knowledge in any depth.

There is another good reason why psychoanalysis provides such pertinent information about parenting: In many of its aspects, the analytic situation seems to be modeled on the parental relationship. The first phase of treatment was referred to by Spitz [28] as *diatrophic,* signifying a dependent relationship similar to that found in the first years of life. Gitelson [18] concurred with this viewpoint. In the first phase of treatment, the patient appears to regard the analyst as a nurturing parent, and later, with the full development of transference, the analyst becomes the oedipal parent. This indicates that psychoanalysis replicates the many vicissitudes of the parent-child relationship, and for this powerful reason, offers a splendid laboratory for a detailed inquiry into the original process of parenting and the child's response to it. The picture is of course overlaid with fantasy and distorted by retrospection so that reconstruction can only be approximate.

Once the "tilted" relationship is established, the basic paradigm gradually unfolds through the mechanism of transference and the countertransference in response to the parental feelings evoked in the therapist. The analytic office has many features corresponding to a nursery setting: The recumbency, quietness, comfort, subdued lighting, and analyst's preoccupation with his patient are all in the direction of good parental care. Winnicott [31] has compared the functions of the analyst and parent. There is a "thereness" about the analyst. He is there but not obtrusively so; he is often silent, frequently in a state of free-floating consciousness, but his slight movements and breathing will indicate, even when he is silent, that the patient is not alone. The mother exists and is there "to be sensed in all possible ways." The "thereness" of the analyst is therefore comparable to that of the parent in that both convey a presence that is pervasive of the situation and the psyche.

Bowlby [5] has criticized the notion that the child's tie to the mother stemmed from the gratification of need and suggested instead that it was based on a phylogenetically derived set of instincts. If this is true for the infant's tie to the mother, what governs the mother's tie to the infant? Is there a parallel set of instincts? During the last two decades, the idea of mother and infant as a reciprocating unity has become a familiar and accepted dynamism in psychoanalysis, and it is not surprising that a similar concept of mutuality [7] has been recognized as an integral part of the analytic situation. Earlier, Glover [19] had pointed out that most descriptions of psychoanalytic treatment referred to only one-half of the treatment unit, that is, what is taking place in the patient, and he pointed to the need for an "analytic toilet." In these days, the analyst and patient are recognized as enmeshed in a "holding environment," in a special kind of "intimate separation," in an endless curiosity about each other, and in a transference-countertransference matrix. As a result of these considerations, a greater emphasis is being placed on what takes place in the mind of the analyst.

The same peculiar problem had haunted the area of parenthood, and once again, Winnicott [31] provided the welcome balance when he wrote that "one half of the theory of the parent-infant relationship concerns the infant, and is the theory of the infant's journey from absolute dependence through relative dependence to independence . . . (the other) half of the theory of the parent-infant relationship concerns maternal care, that is to say the qualities and changes in the mother that meet the specific and developing needs of the infant." What this means is that for a total portrayal of parenting, one needs to know as much about the parents and what is going on inside them as they go about the work of parenting as one knows about the child who is being parented.

According to Winnicott, "good enough parenting" by normal, devoted parents brings about a continuity of being in the children that is the hallmark of successful child development. Here, once again, we have the close correlation between the parenting response and the response to being parented. The latter is reflected in the ego strength, ego competence, and ego confidence; the former can be observed in the caring qualities that show themselves like a new personality development in the mother. One can almost observe the two egos growing harmoniously side by side, with the infant's ego increasing its active demands and the mother's ego surrendering to this or at times battling in a rear-guard action against the thrust for autonomy. Greenacre's "fighting" infant [20] protests actively against unwanted procedures and throws away objects not acceptable as substitutes. One has to bear in mind that acceptances and rejections are built into the parent-infant pair from the very beginning and that the "fight" can begin before there is any organized or organizing ego or even an awareness of a separate body ego.

Winnicott [1] drew on his psychoanalytic data on parenting from the analysis of adult parents, the analysis of children, and the observation of parent-child interactions. He also created, single-mindedly, a lexicon of parenthood, the idiosyncrasies of which seem so peculiar to his way of thinking that it came as a surprise when many of his key, homespun phrases were adopted into the language of everyday parlance. Speaking of mothers, it was his inner conviction that women are "likely" to make the best mothers because of their greater "female element potential" to identify with the female element in the infant, to preoccupy themselves with interchanging with the externalized baby, to "handle" the baby in such a way as to put their body parts together, and to "facilitate" the baby's "continuity of being" and subsequent sense of identity. These functions are "natural" since they stem from the woman's nature and from the nature of her body. Because the mother was a baby once, she has memories buried within herself of having once been a baby and of having been cared for, and these can help or hinder her own experience as a mother. These "hidden memories" are part of the intergenerational transmission of parental attitudes and behavior.

If a small child is well mothered, a fantasy (to create a living child) begins to germinate within and this fantasy is then played out in countless rehearsals throughout childhood. As an integral part of development, there is a constant observation of the parents parenting or an active caretaking of younger siblings. Thus, the potential for parenthood exists at the beginning of life and is elaborated through experience.

The birth of a baby can be therapeutic for parents. They have been struggling with anxieties, depressions, guilt, and shame regarding the act of procreation and are frequently inundated with good and bad fantasies. The baby comes along and its very aliveness relieves the anxious oppressions in the parents and their sense of unworthiness. Winnicott makes the important point that parents need children in order to become better spouses to each other. Parenting is both a natural and very complicated process. It involves loving and hating, caring and, at times, rejecting, and increasing identification with the infant. This increasing identification characterizes the state of "primary maternal preoccupation" [30], the brief period of heightened sensitivity that appears toward the end of pregnancy and is then repressed by the mother. It is "almost an illness" but paradoxically, a woman must be healthy enough in order to develop it as well as to recover from it. It is this state that gives the mother "her special ability to do the right thing." Women with a strong male identification are not likely to develop it, whereas those who become pathologically preoccupied and overidentified with the baby do so because of schizoid or depressive tendencies.

If the child is held and handled reasonably well, his or her development becomes "personalized," which implies that the psyche has come to rest comfortably within the soma. Personalization is an important task for the mother and if she fails in this, psyche and soma go their own ways and the disconnection conduces to various forms of psychopathology. When a mother succeeds, she derives pleasure from her efficient management and the infant, in turn, learns to inhabit the body he or she has and to enjoy its many functions. Not only does the mother help to relate the child's psyche to his or her soma, but she also presents the world to her infant in a steady and consistent way that is part of the process of child management.

Winnicott brings together, in different ways, the analytic and parental situations. He speaks, for instance, of the "holding environment" created by the mother and the holding environment evolving in psychoanalysis; he speaks of the environment structured by the mother that preserves the infant from "infinite falling" and of the analytic patient who experiences "infinite falling," which is preventable by the analyst [30]; he speaks of the child playing in the presence of the mother and of the patient playing with words and ideas in analysis; he speaks of the capacity to be alone with mother and the ability to be by oneself in the analytic situation without feeling abandoned; he speaks of the mother mirroring the baby's reactions and of the analyst similarly reflecting the thoughts and feelings of the patient [35]. The two different kinds of care (i.e., the mother and the analyst) show the common paradigm, thus allowing for illuminating extrapolations.

Winnicott also had a great deal to say about the "ordinary devoted mother" to whom he was so extraordinarily dedicated that some critics considered him mawkish. "There are many who assume that I am sentimental about mothers and that I idealize them, and that I leave out fathers, and that I can't see that some mothers are pretty awful, if not in fact impossible [34]." However, he denied that he was sentimental about mothers since he was also able to recognize that a mother's love was "a pretty crude affair," often characterized by possessiveness, greed, irritability, omnipotence, and inconsistency. In a much quoted statement, he declared that there were many reasons why an ordinary devoted mother sometimes hated her baby: because the baby interfered with her private life, treated her like a servant, exploited her and then discarded her "like an orange peel," refused her food, made her doubt herself, and then, "after an awful morning with him" she would go out, and he would smile at a stranger who would remark, "Isn't he sweet?" [29]. How can a mother not be at times enraged when she is "a free-house to her children," when she has no secrets from them, and when she has to put up with the infinite claims made on her at all times of the day and night? Fortunately, the rewards of motherhood are much greater than the evils. Just as a writer is surprised by the wealth of ideas that turns up when he puts pen to paper, so the mother is constantly surprised by what she finds in the richness of her minute-to-minute contact with her own baby [32]. It is not surprising that for the baby, the mother's pleasure is "like the sun coming out" [32]. But clouds can also overcast the sky and the infant soon comes to recognize that there is also a great deal to fear in the mother. He or she gradually learns to deal with this through identification with her angry reactions.

All these empathies create the conviction that Winnicott's own primary identification was with the mother, and it does not come as a surprise to learn that he has been accused of neglecting fathers and the father's role and of not giving fathers equal time and consideration. However, he was too shrewd an observer of the total family scene to be utterly oblivious to the male parent. In fact, he recognized that there are husbands who make better mothers than their wives [32]. Nevertheless, he insisted that when fathers become mothers, this interfered with their function as fathers. He wanted fathers to be fathers and not surrogate mothers, which was what present-day Western culture was forcing on them. At the end of pregnancy and in the first months of life, the father supplies a "protective covering" to permit the mother to carry out her mothering activities at a time when she is particularly vulnerable to impingements and interferences from the outside [31]. The mother, in turn, later paves the way toward the emergence of the father as a father. Her maternal punctuality, strictness, and sternness are forerunners of the cluster of feelings usually associated with the responses of the father. However, the mother also needs to convey that she can hold up both ends of the parental dimension when the father is not actually there.

One advantage of having two parents is that one can remain loving while the other is being hated, and having a parent to fall back on is a stabilizing influence [32]. For good results, the parenting couple has to work together in complementary fashion, and as Winnicott put it, the mother represents "the stability of the house," and the father represents "the liveliness of the street" [32].

Winnicott was a major contributor to our understanding of parenthood from a psychoanalytic point of view, but it is important to recognize that his intuitions were derived from a much wider sphere of experience than is usually the case with the psychoanalyst. He came into working contact with parents in clinics, hospitals, private practice, pediatric work, referrals from the juvenile courts, and consultation, but wherever he saw patients, he looked at them from the same psychoanalytic penetrating perspective that absorbed so much so quickly. His aim was not only to reach psychoanalysts and other clinicians, but also parents; thus, he became, in the service of prevention, a popularizer.

In contrast, Benedek was a seminal contributor to this field whose goals and achievements were quite different from Winnicott and whose personal style had far less flamboyance. Her work was guided from the beginning by a scientific attitude that set out to observe facts and to draw predictions from them that were verifiable by other facts. She represented a marked contrast to Winnicott for whom facts were at times almost indistinguishable from fantasy and who played with facts in the creative way that a child plays with toys. Benedek's psychoanalytic approach generated two kinds of data: the primary data of observation and the secondary data arrived at by the interpretative process. In contrast to Winnicott, she was always careful to distinguish assumptions from facts. For her [4], the "fundamental facts" of psychoanalysis were affects to which the analyst responded with an empathy that constituted the "basic fact of psychoanalytic communication and experience" [25]. She recognized that the problem with the psychoanalytic fact is that it has a once-only occurrence and is not susceptible to replication. For this reason, the psychoanalytic investigator must eschew the usual scientific approach and turn instead to a search for patterns that have repeated themselves with sufficient consistency so that reasonably sound conclusions can be drawn from them. Her data were essentially "soft" when compared with the usual scientific data and included such intangibles as wishes, fantasies, and dreams. Her psychoanalytic method, covering long periods of time, furnishes two views of phenomena: the long view, which follows the personality as it was put together and consolidated; and the short view, which examines the diurnal variations of psychic equilibrium.

With this scientific equipment in hand, Benedek proceeded to research the organization of the reproductive drive and the mental and physical correlations associated with particular phases of the ovarian cycle. She laid the foundation of her theories of parenthood on a firm biological and psychoanalytic basis, moving steadily from primary data to primary hunches and then to secondary data derived from interpretations and finally, to secondary theories. In the 1950s, her efforts were unique and extraordinary and have remained so to this day.

What Benedek found was startling in its simplicity and rang true to the clinician's experience. The estrogenic phase of the menstrual cycle was correlated with an active, object-directed sexual drive that was expressed in wishes, fantasies, and dreams, while the progesterone phase corresponded with a passive-receptive tendency. For the first time, hormone production was linked to the psychodynamic state and suggested how important it is for the analyst analyzing a woman during her reproductive years to be constantly aware of the continued impact of her menstrual rhythm on her psychosexual life. Not only does a mother undergo fundamental shifts in her psychic life every month, but her children respond in complex ways to her active outer-directed and passive inner-directed phases in specific and nonspecific emotional ways. Theoretically, at least, it should be possible for the child analyst treating a child to discern the cyclical responses of his or her patient to these changes, but this represents research work for the future.

Next Benedek [2] looked at the intergenerational relationships, beginning with the mother's mother in relation to the mother as a baby and moving to the mother as she related to her baby. This concept of sequential transmission was based on her belief that the infant incorporates memory traces of positive and negative experiences into his or her primary mental structures during the oral phase of development. Thus, the memory of gratified needs is integrated with a developing confidence in the mother, in his or her own well-being, and in his or her thriving, good self; the memory of frustrated needs becomes associated with an unsatisfying mother, a lack of confidence in her, and in an unhappy, bad self. This sets up an internal "core of ambivalence" that Benedek termed the "depressive constellation" and saw as a powerful influence on the ongoing mother-child relationship and on the further personality development of the child [2]. These influences persist over time and across generations so that even a generation later, these primary ego structures can be recognized as motivating factors in parental attitudes [4].

For the first time in psychoanalytic literature, attention was called to the evolving experience of parenthood both across generations and across the human life cycle, and it was this aspect that made Benedek much more sympathetic to Erikson's views than was usual in psychoanalytic circles, particularly with his concept of generativity in the making of parents. Erikson had pointed out that the making of a baby did not necessarily imply the emergence of a parent [7]: It was the attribute of generativity that established and guided the next generation. The stages of childhood and adulthood can be regarded as a system of generation and regeneration, and as these are institutionalized by tradition, each generation is enabled to meet the needs of the next in conformity with community expectations independent of personal differences and changing conditions. The same driving power of generativity can motivate the couple to look beyond the sexual act to the offspring that ensues and to the creativity that enhances the culture. When generativity fails, parenthood fails, and stagnation results. Concern becomes self-concern that inhibits the development of true care. The failure can often be traced to early childhood impressions (e.g., a faulty identification with parents, a persistence of infantile narcissism, and a lack of faith in the future of the species). In the absence of generativity, the offspring are vulnerable to a variety of estrangements from themselves and their surroundings [7].

It should be noted that all three psychoanalytic investigators — Winnicott, Benedek, and Erikson — were concerned with the failure of "true care" but regarded it from different perspectives. Winnicott perceived it in relation to mothers with schizoid or depressive dispositions who were unable to preoccupy themselves with their infant, meet his or her total needs, or help the infant to put his or her psyche and soma together in a workable integration; Benedek ascribed the failure to a "core of ambivalence" that was transmitted from generation to generation; and Erikson, while noting problems with identification and narcissism, made greater use of a wide-angle lens to include the social, cultural, and historical factors that contributed to the shaping of the parent. It says a great deal about the flexibility of the psychoanalytic approach that each of these authors could range comfortably across the spectrum of understanding from the biological to the intrapsychic with intermediate references to the interpersonal, the psychosocial environment, and the historical moment.

Benedek then turned her attention to another set of transformations. Psychoanalysts, since S. Freud, had been aware of the many meanings that the fetus acquired at the different trimesters of pregnancy, but it was Benedek who stressed that many women, in addition to other unconscious equivalents, have a tendency to identify the fetus with feces and thus to relive the ambivalent feelings and mysteries of the infantile sexual fantasy of the "anal child." This interferes with the pleasure of pregnancy because the object relation to the unborn child becomes so intensely hostile or ambivalent that motherhood is feared as menacing. This is only one example of the unconscious equivalents that may affect the smooth evolution of pregnancy; other representations are also projected onto the unborn child and help to determine subsequently what the child means to the mother.

Another innovative idea put forward by Benedek was in relation to the drive organization of motherhood and motherliness that is concerned with the interaction of the two types of cycles involved in the reproductive function: the short cycle (from menstruation to menstruation) and the long cycle (from conception to the care of the infant, in which progesterone is dominant and stimulates psychodynamic retentiveness). In fact, it can be said that the whole pregenital and genital psychosexual experience is transformed during the course of development to motivate the reproductive functioning of the woman.

These two interactive arcs of the reproductive cycle are also recognizable in men. There is a short cycle from one sexual urge to the next brought about by a gradually intensifying state that is narcissistic, extraverted, object-directed, and goal-reaching until it culminates in penetration, orgasm, and relaxation; there is a long cycle from conception to the attainment of sexual maturity in procreativeness. Generally speaking, a man's sexual apparatus is more influenced by psychological than hormonal factors, but the cycles are more evident when bisexuality is present.

In a less striking way, fatherliness can also be considered as biologically based for two reasons: (1) man's intrinsic bisexuality and his long period of biological dependency on the mother and (2) nature, it seems, recognized the father's role and endowed him with hormones (i.e., androgens, estrogens, and progesterone) with as much chemical input as given to women. Hormonal fathering is further strengthened by an identification with the protecting and nurturing mother and the providing father. In this way, the secondary manifestations of fatherliness are in continual transaction with the primary manifestations of motherliness so that both motherly and fatherly qualities are integrated in the final manifestation of parental behavior. In both sexes, for the generative impulse to emerge at the right time, maturational factors must be intricately interwoven with psychosexual development, hormonal activity, and cultural shaping. When this occurs, parental behavior, parental ideation, parental fantasies, and intropsychic parental processes produce an operational move to intrapsychic processes.

Following the admonitions of Hartmann cited earlier, Benedek did not omit structural theory from her general thesis on parenting; but neither did she leave out the important influence of family dynamics, relating it, as Flugel [8] first did, to the interplay of oedipal factors between family members.

Parenthood evolves almost imperceptibly into grandparenthood. In this passage, a curious reversal of generations takes place as first described by Ernest Jones [24], when the parent as a need-fulfilling object for the child gradually gives place to the child as a need-fulfilling object for the parent, and the child becomes identified with the grandparent. Jones developed the concept of intergenerational transferences or the transmission of tradition as early as 1913 and long prior to Flugel's and Benedek's work.

It is no exaggeration to say that, to a greater or lesser extent, there always takes place some transference from a person's parent to the child of the corresponding sex . . . It is quite common to find a mother trying to mould a boy along her father's lines, or a father trying to mould a girl along his mother's — i.e., *making the child incorporate in itself the grandparent's character.* The child's own personality is thus moulded, or distorted, not only by the effort to imitate its parents but by its effort to imitate its parents' ideals, which are mostly taken from the grandparent of the corresponding sex . . . We doubtless have here the deepest reason for the constant identification of grandson with grandfather; both are equally feared by the father, who has reason to dread their relationship for his guilty wishes against them. (Pp. 411–412)

Grandparenthood is the penultimate developmental phase of parenthood that terminates in the "childless parenthood" of old age. Benedek made a number of psychodynamic observations on the psychology of the grandparent [1]. As with parenthood before the present insurgence of interest, the role of grandparents had also been taken for granted. In some cultures they are much revered as part of the ancestral connection, while in others they are grossly neglected and overlooked as unproductive and therefore superfluous in the case of serious food shortages. Most extended family groups regard them not only as heads of the clan but also as ancillary parents with an available fount of experience when some predicament overtakes the family. As a grandparent herself, Benedek became aware of the emotional significance of this status for the elderly. She came to understand why it was popularly referred to as a "new lease on life": but the "new lease" was also a matter of timing. The age at which grandparenthood occurred determined its degree of vitality. If the grandparents are still within the procreative period, their attitudes and behavior are not unlike those of the parents themselves and they seem to treat their grandchildren like their children. If, on the other hand, they are old, ailing, and postclimacteric, their emotional investment in grandchildren tends to become less with each passing year until they began to react to the nuisance value of noisy and mobile youngsters.

The stages of grandparenthood simulate to some extent the developmental stages of parenthood. For example, "expectant grandmothers" relive their own pregnancies with their daughter's pregnancy and tend to transmit their reactivated anxieties. They are often apt to take over the care of the baby and set their homespun wisdom in opposition to modern "highfalutin" ideas. As with parents, however, there inevitably comes a time when their grandchildren grow up and away from them, and some measure of depression often follows. They begin to feel unwanted and unneeded by the grandchildren at a time when these feelings are what they are experiencing from the world at large. The grandchildren in turn, are likely to become disillusioned with the outdated outlook of the grandparents and to view them as even more antediluvian than their parents.

From a psychosexual point of view, the grandparent situation is generally much less conflicted than the parent situation. This is parenthood "one step removed." The relationship with grandchildren is altogether less stressful, less demanding, less responsible, and less burdened by anxieties with every passing developmental event. More crucially, it is not exposed to the devastating ambivalences that typify the parent-child relationship. The intermittent nature of the contact is also less fraying to the nerves on both sides. Grandparents are able to give less conditionally and expectantly, contented with affection and remembrance. From the intrapsychic point of view, the classical intrafamilial conflicts are not there to threaten the relationship and generate unmanageable guilt and shame from unconscious wishes and thoughts.

Unlike Benedek, Anna Freud was never herself a parent and her concentration on the parent in her studies was never as total as Benedek's. Winnicott, too, was childless but had the experience of foster parenting and learned to respect the emotional complexity of the job, especially in terms of negative feeling. Anna Freud's intuitive and empathic capacities in the area of parenthood were derived from the fact that she had been brought up in an integrated family and had been well mothered and fathered. She was apt to quote her father's remark, apropos himself, that the loved son of a young adoring mother was likely to remain confident and optimistic all his life, and, at the same time, to point out that the opposite was equally true: that the rejected son of a neglectful mother might well be pessimistic. What she might have added (which she did not), was that the beloved daughter of an adoring and appreciative father could end up becoming his "son" and successor. What she had, therefore, in lieu of a parenting experience, was a first-hand knowledge of the proclivity of parental influence.

The way in which Anna Freud's close friend, Lou Andreas-Salomé, once referred to Sigmund Freud with regard to herself also was true for Anna: "He was the father-face that has presided over my life."[17] How closely did this model daughter follow in the footsteps of her father, and not only in the area of psychoanalysis? In one of his letters, Sigmund Freud wrote: "My one source of satisfaction is Anna. It is remarkable how much influence and authority she has gained among the general run of analysts . . . it is surprising, too, how sharp, clear and unflinching she is in her mastery of the subject. Moreover, she is truly independent of me; *at the most I serve as a catalyst* . . . Of course, there are certain worries; she takes things too seriously. What will she do when she has lost me? Will she lead a life of ascetic austerity?" [17].

A good parent is an effective catalyst of a child's development who helps the child to become increasingly independent from the parent. In the light of the very close relationship between Sigmund and Anna Freud, one wonders how truly independent she was of her father, as expressed in his own doubts: "What will she do when she has lost me?" To paraphrase this question, would one anticipate that she would take herself to a nunnery? She did set up an order of lay analysts at Hampstead, but she did not mourn him to a degree of melancholia, and she did not retreat from the world. She continued her own extraordinary work with children and created an unsurpassed center for the study of children and their parents. However, the presence of her father was never absent from Hampstead.

Anna Freud pointed to the importance of the analytic situation as a laboratory for parenthood. Even when the child reacts to her parents with rejection and resentment, it is easy to demonstrate in the analytic transference that this is by no means the case. For example, she tells of one girl who came with a "I couldn't care less" attitude toward her parents [14].

In the analysis . . . she was extremely eager for her hours, extremely upset whenever an hour was called off, either by her or by me; and the more upset she was the less she cared. Her "I couldn't care less" was an external portmanteau reaction which was believed by her and was ego-syntonic, but which suddenly revealed itself in the transference as an insatiable hunger for attention, for being looked after . . . . (P. 228)

This little vignette tells us, so clearly and simply, that what the child feels for the parent may be completely masked by habitual defenses and may only come to light in transference. It was not surprising that Anna Freud interpreted the analyst's task as not too different from that of the parent [14].

What we call the good or helpful parent in these years is the parent who can give the child unobtrusive but steady assistance in overcoming one anxiety after another, one crisis after another, one conflict after another, so that he is not arrested at any stage of development but can pass on to the next—sometimes only from one problem to the next, and from one conflict to the next. But, after all, that is life. (P. 231)

Anna Freud thought that the elements of need fulfillment in the parent-infant relationship [9] reappeared in the analysis of adult patients as a wish for help, but that this anaclitic phase can act as a resistance and lead to a backing off of treatment since the analyst has to refuse to be a need-fulfilling object. However, she did not see earliest object relations being carried into the therapeutic alliance, which was derived from the later stages. Transference crisis and suggestibility seemed to her to be a direct outcome of early infantile compliance to the mother.

The psychoanalyst has, as his long-term aim, the prevention of arrests and inhibitions by crippling regression, conflicts, and compromise formations. Both parent and psychoanalyst are therefore engaged in setting free the child's spontaneous energies that are needed for the completion of his or her development. In addition to this problem-resolution, the good parent meets the child's needs for continuity, stimulation, mutuality, and affection.

From 1941 to 1945 in her Hampstead War Nursery, Anna Freud tried to provide surrogate parents for children who had lost their parents in the war. In order that her institution would not create the very problem that it was trying to solve, she also arranged for mothers who worked in the nursery to keep their infants with them. She organized small "artificial families" and found that this prevented many of the institutional reactions that occurred in ordinary residential units. Furthermore, the emotional reactions of the children in these "artificial families" were not unlike those seen in natural family settings with typical displays of envy, jealousy, and possessiveness. The children treated their "artificial parents" differently from the way in which they reacted to teachers and other grown-ups. The artificial parents experienced all the conflicts, disappointments, and frustrations familiar to the natural parents. Basic care factors (i.e., feeding, dressing and undressing, bathing, toileting, tending to all physical needs, and putting to bed) elicited child-to-parent responses. Whoever cared for a child in this way became a parent-figure for the child and was imbued with parental reactions toward the child [12].

Anna Freud's observations of the mothering process were full of sharp details and she assessed attitudes to motherhood and fatherhood in her developmental profile for adults [10]. She observed the behaviors that took place in the playground of the mother's lap. She noted that an infant treats parts of the mother's body as if they were his or her own and plays with the mother in the same way as he or she plays with him- or herself; they appear to share one body. A mother's interest brings out a primitive exhibitionism in a child and the child's behavior elicits profound narcissistic responses in the mother, who constantly overestimates the child's capacity. In these ways, mother and child gratify each other constantly; it is a golden age when the baby can do no wrong. These exhibitionist transactions between child and mother do not take place in institutions unless the child has formed a close relationship with the mother substitute. There is another interesting contrast between home and institution; whereas sexual curiosity and questioning are common in normal homes, in institutions, this insatiable inquisitiveness is often displaced onto details of everyday routine such as medical examinations and staff meetings behind closed doors [12].

A. Freud's prototype of the father is clearly different from that of the mother. He is strong, powerful, and only intermittently present; but what impresses both boys and girls is his "bigness." In the absence of parents, as in residential settings, the intrapsychic developments with parents in the form of oedipal configurations are conspicuous by their absence as if the basic issues of development cannot be worked out without the actual parents [12].

Lucid though she was, and incomparably shrewd in her observations, there is very clearly a difference between Anna Freud's approach to parents from that of Benedek's. One gets the impression that she saw them objectively from the outside, whereas Benedek experienced them as an insider and brought a new depth to the understanding of the parenting process. Winnicott, with the assistance of an exquisite feminine sensibility and a strong maternal identification, tried to bridge the gap between outsider and insider and frequently succeeded in becoming the mother in fantasy. He always seemed to inhabit that "intermediate area" between outside and inside, and between the boundaries of the mother and those of the infant. When he came out with his striking comment that "there is no such thing as a baby" [29] he was occupying this transitional zone, this potential space, when one is neither one thing nor the other.

Because of her "outsider" position, Anna Freud's writings in this area are characterized by common sense and practicality. She did not produce any innovative theories—only illuminating comments based on sound observations. For example, she pointed out that the rejecting mother [13], long regarded as causative in the psychopathology of her children, is far from rejecting all the time, and that the ordinary devoted mother rejects her children on many occasions during the day, the week, or the month when she becomes preoccupied with her own thoughts, interests, emotional needs, and bodily wants. There are also mothers, more mothers than wives, who give themselves so unreservedly to the child that they cannot separate from him or her at all; but even they can be perceived by the offspring as "rejecting." In spite of such mild criticism, she was always ready to exonerate the parent. In contrast, Winnicott was quite ready to blame the mother for failing the child and thus generating a lot of "deficiency" diseases [32]. Anna Freud would frequently come to the defense of the parents and see them much less as villains in the drama of the child's psychopathology. "In the analysis of adults as well as children, it is one of our tasks to disentangle the real personality of the parents from the projections and fantastic additions with which their image is overlaid in the child's mind, so that they are turned into frightening and threatening figures." Having said this, she also warned us not to forget that transmogrifications were not all products of the child's fantasy [14].

Anna Freud's experience told her that there are actual mothers with compulsions to throw their children out of windows, to put poison in their food, to exhibit their own naked bodies for the child's curiosity, and to elevate the child to the role of a substitute sexual partner. She tried to differentiate between the parent's disturbance as directly responsible for the child's pathology through identification and excitation and indirectly responsible through her incapacity for the task of mothering.

A. Freud described how psychoanalysis had brought about radical changes in the work she did with parents in clinics. Parents were now no longer taught facts on an intellectual and authoritarian basis because "analytic discoveries have laid bare the intricate emotional relationships between child and parent; the role of internalization of the parent's personality traits and attitudes, and identification with their qualities; the constancies of love and hate; the subtle or crude forms of seduction; the overriding importance of any one of the developmental phases, whether libidinal or aggressive, being acceptable or repulsive to the parent. Once the parent-child relationship is seen in this light, work with the parents ceases to imply a teacher-pupil attitude and takes on the aspect of a therapeutic relationship" [12]. However, she questioned whether such work with parents is effective *only* if directed toward changes in their personalities, and felt that she was "a heretic in some of these respects." For her, the therapeutic approach to parents was no more than one among a whole series of possible approaches, all of them serving the same ultimate purposes of beneficial change, prevention, and enlightenment. She was aware that this view of her's was "rather unpopular" [11].

From a psychoanalytic point of view, Anna Freud came to two important conclusions. If the pathogenic agents on the mother's side remain internal, the effective treatment of the child by analysis is possible; but if the mother's pathology is reinforced by action that uses the child as an object of pleasurable or painful stimulation, then only simultaneous analysis of both mother and child can change the situation. A mother needs to be approached therapeutically when she is depressed or when her mothering functions are interfered with by a pathogenic masculinity complex. Mothers also need to be helped when their children pose special problems due to handicaps.

A. Freud's lifelong interest in the parent-child relationship took on still another aspect when, along with Solnit and Goldstein, she became the international advocate for the "psychological" mother, which was a logical development from her earlier work on setting up "psychological" mothering in residential centers. The point that she makes is that the biological mother is of no consequence or may even be a detriment to the child's emotional development unless she develops a capacity for psychological mothering or unless a "psychological" mother takes over the job. Benedek would argue this point since, for her, mothering is rooted in biology and there is a long psychobiological preparation that culminates in conception, pregnancy, birth, and early care. Benedek would not deny that a "psychological" mother could take up the job with a particular baby, but she believed that the mother would be coming in on the drama at some time in the "third act," at which point she would need to develop a mothering stance toward the baby.

It is probably simplistic to presume that the two theoretical positions reflect two different life experiences of a parent and a nonparent. Interestingly enough, the nonparent Winnicott had the additional difference of being a man, and he chose to speak a great deal about mothering, but very little about fathering.

This trio of brilliant analytic observers and theoreticians went their different ways into the field of parenthood, while maintaining their common psychoanalytic heritage and perspective. Should one be surprised by this, or grateful that the psychoanalytic mind has so much diversity at its command? We are reminded here of the story told by Anna Freud when she received a doctoral award in 1964 [12a].

When I was a young girl and dissatisfied with my appearance—as girls often are—I felt comforted by a saying then popular in Vienna: "After a certain age every woman gets the face she deserves," i.e., the face she creates for herself. Today I want to apply this assertion to the work of every psychoanalyst: I think it is true that after a certain age and point of his career, every psychoanalyst creates for himself the type of work that he deserves. (P. 515)

She went on to talk about how fortunate she was to fulfill herself in so many different ways within the field of psychoanalysis, adding that "there is no better life for the analyst than to be able to be in constant contact with all the facets of human behavior, from childhood to adulthood and from normality to the severest forms of pathology." We would take the liberty of adding: "and from the life of 'single blessedness' to all the diverse aspects, normal and abnormal, or parenthood."

Winnicott, Anna Freud, and Therese Benedek were the three major contributors to the psychoanalytic observation and theory of parenthood. We shall sadly miss their ongoing inquiries into this field, especially since they focused, unlike other psychoanalysts involved in this area, *on the process of parenting* rather than on the outcome in the child. They did not neglect the mutuality and reciprocal influences, but they demonstrated an extra concern for what was taking place in the mind of the parent. What each of them brought to the task was their own individual perspective, basically psychoanalytic, but with a characteristic focus: Winnicott, from the angle of object-relations; Benedek, from an existential, transactional, and psychobiological standpoint; and Anna Freud, from the position of classical structural theory leavened by an understanding of and experiences with children, both with and without parents.

In this introduction, we have been speaking of parenthood as a desirable state that adds to the personality, enhances one's experience of life, and rounds off the human life cycle. Without being too aware of it, we may have been idealizing a process that has been good for us and therefore assuming its universal goodness. Might it not be better, as Oscar Wilde suggested cynically, to have one's origins anonymously in the lost property office of a railway station? The leading French writers of our time, Sartre and Gide, have raised the same question. Sartre thought that because his father had died before he was born, he had not been compelled, like Aeneas, to carry him on his shoulders through life, weighed down by imitations, identifications, and passive submissions; he could be free to be his own man. Gide, in his play, *Oedipus,* has his hero make the following comment: "So long as I thought I was the son of Polybus, I applied myself to mimicking his virtues. Listening to the lesson of the past, I looked only to yesteryear for my so-be-it, my prophecies. Then suddenly the thread is broken. Springing from the unknown, no more past, no more model, nothing on which to base myself, everything to create, country, ancestors, to invent, to discover. No one to resent but myself . . . it is a call to valor not to know one's parents."

These are the responses of gifted children to parenting and its limitations. The psychoanalyst can also turn a shrewd, cynical eye on parental virtues much applauded by the world in general. S. Freud [15], with his usual ruthless honesty, attributed all these admirable attitudes and behaviors to the workings of narcissism.

If we look at the attitude of affectionate parents towards their children, we have to recognize that it is a revival and reproduction of their own narcissism, which they have long since abandoned . . . . They are under a compulsion to ascribe every perfection to the child—which super observation would find no occasion to do—and to conceal and forget all his shortcomings. . . . The child shall have a better time than his parents; he shall not be subject to the necessities which they have recognized as paramount in life. Illness, death, renunciation of enjoyment, restrictions of his own will, shall not touch him; the laws of nature and of society shall be abrogated in his favor; he shall once more really be the center and core of creation—"His Majesty the Baby" as we once fancied ourselves. The child shall fulfill those wishful dreams of the parents which they never carried out—the boy shall become a great man and a hero in his father's place, and the girl shall marry a prince as a tardy compensation for her mother. At the most touching point in *the narcissistic system,* the immortality of the ego, which is so hard pressed by reality, is achieved by taking refuge in the child. Parental love, which is so moving and at the bottom so childish, is nothing but the parents' narcissism born again. (Pp. 90–91)

Freud, in his study of genius, pointed out that psychoanalysis did not explain the phenomenon but illuminated it. The same would be true of parenthood: It is *not* explained by narcissism, and psychoanalysis in no way claims to have written the last word on it. Psychoanalysis has, however, thrown new light on a very ancient profession.

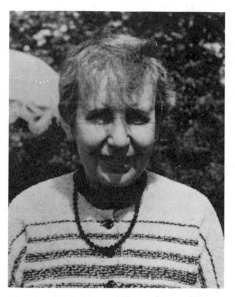

Fig. I-2. *Anna Freud.*
(Portrait by Allan Chappelow, M.A. [Psych], F.R.S.A.)

References

1. Anthony, E. J., and Benedek, T. B. *Parenthood: Its Psychology and Psychopathology.* Boston: Little, Brown, 1970.
2. Benedek, T. B. Toward the biology of the depressive constellation. *J. Am. Psychoanal. Assoc.* 4:389, 1956.
3. Benedek, T. B. Parenthood as a developmental phase. *J. Am. Psychoanal. Assoc.* 7:389, 1959.
4. Benedek, T. B. The organization of the reproductive drive. *Int. J. Psychoanal.* 41:1, 1960.
5. Bowlby, J. *Attachment and Loss.* London: Hogarth Press, 1969. Vol. 1.
6. Burlingham, D. Child analysis and the mother. *Psychoanal. Q.* 4:69, 1935.
7. Erikson, E. H. *Identity: Youth and Crisis.* New York: Norton, 1968.
8. Flugel, J. D. *The Psycho-Analytic Study of the Family.* London: Hogarth, 1921.
9. Freud, A. The theory of the parent-infant relationship. *Int. J. Psychoanal.* 43:240, 1962.
10. Freud, A. Metapsychological assessment of the adult personality. *Psychoanal. Study Child* 20:9, 1965.
11. Freud, A. *Writings of Anna Freud.* New York: International Universities, 1965. Vol. 6.
12. Freud, A. *Writings of Anna Freud.* New York: International Universities, 1968. Vol. 4.
12a. Freud, A. *Writings of Anna Freud.* New York: International Universities 1969. Vol. 5 (1956–65).
13. Freud, A. The Concept of the Rejecting Mother. In E. J. Anthony and T. B. Benedek (Eds.), *Parenthood: Its Psychology and Psychopathology.* Boston: Little, Brown, 1970.
14. Freud, A. *Writings of Anna Freud.* New York: International Universities 1971. Vol. 4.
15. Freud, S. On Narcissism: An Introduction. In J. Strachey (Ed.), *The Standard Edition of the Complete Psychological Works of Sigmund Freud.* London: Hogarth, 1914. Vol. 14, pp. 90–91.
16. Freud, S. New introductory lectures on psychoanalysis. *Standard Edition.* 1933. Vol. 22, p. 56.
17. Freud, S. Letter to Lou Andreas-Salomé June 1, 1935. E. Pfeiffer (Ed.), *Sigmund Freud and Lou Andreas-Salomé Letters.* New York: Harcourt Brace Jovanovich, 1935.
18. Gitelson, M. Curative factors in psychoanalysis. *Int. J. Psychoanal.* 43:194, 1962.
19. Glover, E. *Technique of Psychoanalysis.* New York: Basic Books, 1952.
20. Greenacre, P. Considerations regarding the parent-infant relationship. *Int. J. Psychoanal.* 41:571, 1960.
21. Hartmann, H. Comments on the psychoanalytic theory of the ego. *Psychoanal. Study Child* 5:74, 1950.
22. Hartmann, H. The mutual influences in the development of ego and id.

Reprinted in Essays on Ego Psychology. New York: International Universities, 1964.

23. Jackson, E. B., and Klatskin, E. H. Rooming-in research project: Development and methodology of parent-child relationship study in a clinical setting. *Psychoanal. Study Child* 5:236, 1950.

24. Jones, E. The Phantasy of the Reversal of Generations. In *Papers on Psychoanalysis*. London: Bailliere, Tindall and Co., 1948.

25. Kohut, H. Introspection, empathy and psychoanalysis. *J. Am. Psychoanal. Assoc.* 7:459, 1959.

26. Kris, E. Notes on the development and on some current problems of psychoanalytic child psychology. *Psychoanal. Study Child* 5:24, 1950.

27. Ribble, M. *The Rights of Infants*. New York: Columbia University Press, 1943.

28. Spitz, R. Hospitalism: An inquiry into the genesis of psychiatric conditions in early childhood. *Psychoanal. Study Child* 1:53, 1945.

29. Winnicott, D. W. (1947) Hate in the Countertransference. In *Collected Papers Through Paediatrics to Psychoanalysis*. New York: Basic Books, 1958.

30. Winnicott, D. W. Primary Maternal Preoccupation. In Collected Papers Through Paediatrics to Psychoanalysis. London: Tavistock Press, 1958.

31. Winnicott, D. W. The Theory of the Parent-Infant Relationship. In *The Maturational Processes and the Facilitating Environment: Studies in the Theory of Emotional Development*. London: Hogarth Press, 1960.

32. Winnicott, D. W. The Baby as a Going Concern. In *The Child, the Family and the Outside World*. New York: Penguin Books, 1964.

33. Winnicott, D. W. The Affect of Psychotic Parents on the Emotional Development of the Child. In *The Family and Individual Development*. London: Tavistock, 1965.

34. Winnicott, D. W. The ordinary devoted mother. Talk given to Nursery School Association of Great Britain and Northern Ireland, London Branch, 1966.

35. Winnicott, D. W. Minor-Role of Mother and Family in Child Development. In P. Lomas (Ed.), *The Predicament of the Family: A Psychoanalytic Symposium*. London: Hogarth Press, 1967.

I
Cross-generational influences

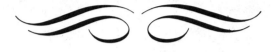

1

Monica: infant-feeding behavior of a mother gastric fistula-fed as an infant: a 30-year longitudinal study of enduring effects

George L. Engel, Franz Reichsman, Vivian T. Harway, and D. Wilson Hess

Monica,[1] the subject of this report, and her family have been under uninterrupted study since October 1953 [6, 7, 8, 9, 10, 11, 14]. Monica was born July 16, 1952 with congenital atresia of the esophagus and was fed by gastric fistula until 2 years of age when surgical repair of the atresia finally enabled her to eat normally by mouth. She is now 30 years old, married, and the mother of four daughters aged 2, 5½, 8, and 10. A longitudinal case study of such detail as this one, which spans four generations (i.e., grandparents, parents, siblings, and children), provides a unique opportunity to explore many aspects of human development not otherwise readily accessible for investigation.

In this paper we report on the striking correspondence between how Monica was handled as an infant during fistula-feeding and how she herself handled her own infants during bottle-feeding when she became a mother, behavior already evident during Monica's doll-feeding play as a child and baby-sitting as an adolescent. Neither her mother, sisters, nor husband has exhibited bottle-feeding behavior comparable to Monica's, the salient difference being that Monica, never held in arms during fistula-feeding, does not hold her babies during bottle-feeding; the others regularly do. Her three daughters old enough for doll play, all of whom were bottle-fed in arms by their father but not by Monica, show increasing preference to hold their dolls in their arms while bottle-feeding.

[1] Except for Monica, whose identity as a fistula-fed infant is too well known, all names in this report are pseudonyms.

Such cross-generational data documenting developmental continuity of infant- and maternal-feeding behaviors are submitted as a contribution to an understanding of the determinants of human maternal behavior and are recorded here in detail for the first time.

The Nature and Handling of the Data

Formal study began at the age of 15 months when Monica was admitted to The Strong Memorial Hospital in Rochester, New York for the third time, a stay that extended from October 12, 1953 to July 3, 1954. Retrospective reports from family, visiting nurses, and social workers, plus the hospital records from her first two admissions, at 3 days old for esophagostomy and gastrostomy (July 19–31, 1952) and at 11 months old because of "failure to thrive" and "depression of infancy" (June 19–July 31, 1953), provided the principal sources of information about her first 15 months of life. During the nine months of the third hospitalization, which culminated in the successful surgical correction of the esophageal defect and the beginning of normal feeding, Monica was observed virtually daily on the ward or in the laboratory. During a fourth hospitalization for closure of the fistula (May 11–June 23, 1955), similar detailed observations were carried out.

Over the 28 years (1954–1982) since restoration of esophageal function, there has been a total of 104 day-long study periods, 97 in the laboratory and 7 at home or in school. The typical study period involved Monica interacting in several one-hour long sessions (e.g., play sessions, interviews, and/or psychological testing) with each of two or three different investigators. Until her marriage at 19, Monica's mother was usually interviewed on each visit, and her father, stepfather, and grandmother were interviewed occasionally. A sibling also undergoing interviewing and psychological testing commonly accompanied the group. Once married, Monica's husband and subsequently each of their four children became regular subjects of study, alone and as a family. Since July 1981 when her husband moved the family to the deep South for better employment opportunities, we have kept in touch periodically by telephone. In May 1982 we traveled south for a home visit.

All the sessions in the laboratory were observed through a one-way vision mirror, and notes were made by the observers as well as by those working with the subjects. All proceedings have been audiotaped (since 1955) or videotaped (since 1972) and transcribed. Periodically sessions were filmed as well. The raw data include the following eight items.

308 hours of minute-by-minute observations of Monica's spontaneous behavior during two periods of hospitalization (aged 15–22 months and 35–36 months).

321 tapes, transcribed verbatim, of play sessions, interviews, and/or psychological testing sessions of Monica from ages 3 to 29 and of family members.

140 reports of minute-by-minute observations of Monica and of her siblings during play sessions, interviewing, and psychological testing sessions in the laboratory or at home or school.

115 summarizing notes by study members of their interactions with Monica and family members during play sessions, interviewing, and psychological testing sessions in the laboratory or at home or school.

224 psychological test procedures on Monica and members of her family with corresponding raw test protocols and reports.

90 miscellaneous items (e.g., hospital records; pediatric, medical, and surgical notes; letters, phone messages).

22,600 feet of 16 mm silent color film taken between 1953 and 1978 in the laboratory and at home; 2,550 feet of super-8 mm movies taken at home from 1972–1974 by Monica and her husband: each with detailed written descriptions of the filmed behavior.

40 hours of videotapes (¾-inch color videocassettes) taken between 1972 and 1982 with detailed written descriptions of the recorded behavior.

The range of information accumulated about Monica since 1953 thus includes:

1. Information *about* Monica reported by family members, physicians, nurses, social workers, teachers, and others.
2. Information *from* Monica about herself and about others.
3. Information *from* family members about themselves and others.
4. Observations of Monica's behavior alone and/or interacting with staff, family members, and others on the hospital ward, in the laboratory, at home, at school, and on trips into town.
5. Observations of the behavior of Monica's siblings and her children in the laboratory or at home or school.
6. Psychological test data on Monica and family members.

This mass of material has now been classified and filed chronologically according to 216 categories, a task that required two years to complete. It involved reading through the more than one thousand typed protocols (i.e., the raw data listed above) and writing in the margins of each page the numbers of the categories (001–216) that appeared on that page. This could range from one to more than 20 different categories per page. Each page on which each category number appeared was photocopied and filed separately and chronologically. Each category thus has a chronological file of its own.

For this report we have reviewed the files of all categories containing information about gastric fistula-feeding by mother and grandmother at home and by nursing staff in the hospital; infant-care practices of mother, father, and grandmother at home and by medical and nursing staffs during Monica's three hospitalizations; infant-care practices of Monica during doll play as a child, baby-sitting as an adolescent, and mother-hood; infant care practices of Monica's husband; and doll-feeding play of Monica's three older daughters. This material was drawn from a total of 17 of the 216 categories.

Category 022 (child-rearing, Monica) may be used to illustrate the procedure. "022" was written in the margin of each page whenever any of the following items of information was noted, whether it appeared as behavior actually observed or as statements by or about Monica.

Doll play involving child care

Baby-sitting

References to, attitudes about, reactions to, and descriptions of babies and children and their care

Child-rearing practices and child-care activities with Monica's own or others' children

Monica's views and theories about mother-child relationships and child-rearing practices

Such citations may refer to an entire page or to only a sentence or two. Some idea of the amount of information available in this category is indicated by the fact that "022" appears in the margins of an estimated 1,400 pages of typed protocols. The earliest citation is on May 12, 1955 (age 2 years, 11 months), and the most recent citation is on May 8, 1982. Since this report concerns only Monica's feeding of infants and not all of her parenting behaviors, only those items of category 022 having specifically to do with infant-feeding are discussed in this chapter.

How Monica Was Fistula-Fed

For 23½ months, from her birth until recovery from the surgical repair of the esophageal atresia, Monica was totally dependent on the gastric fistula for feeding. Thus, during a period in which oral-feeding activities are thought to play a prominent role in development, Monica not only was deprived of many experiences ordinarily associated with nursing and feeding, but she also was subject to experiences quite different from what normal infants ordinarily encounter. However, this does not mean that she had no oral experience. She could and did put a variety of objects into her mouth. She chewed on crackers and potato chips, and she licked lollipops, all of which, along with saliva, drained from the esophageal fistula surgically produced in her neck for that purpose. But until after reconstructive surgery, she had never chewed and swallowed a bolus of food into the stomach. She never had the opportunity to relate such oral experiences as sucking, tasting, swallowing, and biting with cycles of hunger and satiation or with the person feeding her. She never participated actively in her own feeding and hence was deprived of many of the developmental sequences relating feeding and oral experience with sensorimotor development and self-object differentiation. It was in such respects that deprivation of oral-feeding was total and curtailment of other oral experiences was considerable.

For presentation, the fistula-feeding period is divided into three periods based on different life circumstances for Monica.

Period 1: Home with mother and grandmother (birth–5 months)
Period 2: Alone with a depressed mother (5–11 months)
Period 3: In hospital (11–12½ months and 15–23½ months)

PERIOD 1: HOME WITH MOTHER AND GRANDMOTHER (BIRTH–5 MONTHS)

Joanne (born November 5, 1932), Monica's mother, had breast-fed Tommy (born November 26, 1950), her first child, for eight months. She had planned to breast-feed Monica but had to give that up when the first feedings were regurgitated and Monica choked and became severely cyanotic. Joanne was never to forget the terror she experienced; she was certain her baby would die. And indeed she might have, had not an esophageal fistula promptly been established in the neck to provide for drainage of saliva and prevent aspiration. This was done on Monica's third day of life. Two days later, a gastric fistula was established for feeding purposes. Fistula-feeding was begun by the nursing staff on the sixth day and was designated in nursing notes as "well tolerated." Nursing notes record that Monica cried as though hungry if not fed within two hours and that she quieted down with the feeding.

Before hospital discharge when Monica was 2 weeks old, the nurses instructed her mother in the gastric fistula-feeding procedure. The formula was poured into a funnel and allowed to flow into the stomach by gravity. If the flow was sluggish, a rubber bulb could be attached to the tubing and compressed to force through the formula. Administration of the formula required the use of both hands: one to hold the funnel, the other to pour. *For this reason, Monica never was held or cradled while being fed.* Instead, her mother laid Monica on her lap crosswise or with the baby's head extended toward her knees. Otherwise, she placed Monica on a crib or sofa and poured the formula while she sat or stood next to her. This feeding situation clearly increased the physical distance between mother and baby and reduced the opportunity for social interaction during feeding.

Monica often cried before feeding time, indicating hunger. She often fell asleep while still being fed or soon afterward. Joanne soon realized that neither Monica's falling asleep nor her crying interfered with going ahead with the feeding, even though the crying increased intraabdominal pressure and sometimes slowed or even reversed the flow of the formula in the tubing. In order to provide some oral activity, the doctors instructed Joanne to give Monica a nipple to suck during the feeding. She insists she did so, but with what consistency we do not know.

On completion of a feeding, the tubing regularly had to be removed, flushed, and cleaned and then reinserted and left protruding through the fistula in the abdominal wall, covered by gauze padding. Usually there was some drainage around the tube that required frequent cleanups and changes of dressing. In addition, the esophageal fistula in the neck drained saliva continuously, also necessitating frequent changes. Sometimes there were difficulties in reinserting the tube into the fistula. For Joanne, this was very frightening, especially when Monica screamed and struggled. On several occasions, Joanne became faint and nauseated and had to bring the baby to the local hospital for help to get the tube back in place. Despite reassurance, she never could overcome the fear that she might somehow injure Monica in the process. For a long time, she also could not overcome her fear that Monica might choke if given anything by mouth. "I had my hands full feeding her and wouldn't have been able to do anything if she choked," she reported later.

The constant presence of the tube protruding through the abdominal wall also served to limit how Monica was held, even when not being fed. Concerned that the tube could poke into and injure Monica, Joanne learned how to maneuver Monica so as not to apply pressure on it. In particular, Monica was not hugged closely face-to-face, nor held over the shoulder without care being taken so that the tubing was not pressed. (Of course, Monica was never burped, an unnecessary procedure since the esophagus was not patent.) All in all, it was frustrating and disappointing for Joanne to have to be so careful about how she fed and handled her new baby.

During this five-month period, Joanne, her common-law husband Harold, Monica, and her 16-month older brother Tommy were living with the maternal grandparents. When Monica was about 2 months old, Joanne took a factory job. Mrs. Woods, the maternal grandmother, then did the tube feeding, but only when Joanne was at work. When difficulties arose, she took the baby to the factory to have Joanne handle the problem. Harold never fed Monica, but on at least one occasion, he was the one to reinsert the tube. Mrs. Woods characterized herself as an "old-fashioned mother." Joanne reported that between feedings Mrs. Woods would "sit and hold her on her lap all day if you let her." Certainly she provided Monica with a great deal of nurturing during those critical first few months. Joanne, in contrast, felt "You can get them into bad habits if you hold them all the time." Harold occasionally held Monica on his lap when he was home between long-distance truck hauls. So too did the grandfather and the great-grandmother, a feeble old lady in her nineties living with the family at that time.

Neither mother nor grandmother considered anything about Monica's development during this early period to be unusual. They described her as a content baby who hardly ever cried. Mrs. Woods, herself a nurturing and caring woman who had raised several foster children in addition to her own five, seemed a reliable witness in this regard. By the age of 2 months, Monica had gained almost 2 pounds (910 gm) from her birth weight of 6 pounds (2,700 gm). Beyond that, we only have Joanne's report that Monica "gained fine" until December 1952.

PERIOD 2: ALONE WITH A DEPRESSED MOTHER (5–11 MONTHS)

As Monica approached 5 months of age (December 16, 1952), a series of untoward events served to disrupt her relationship with her mother and grandmother. First, Joanne realized that she was pregnant again. This upset her because she felt unprepared to care for another child and was afraid that it might also be defective. In addition, escalating conflict between Harold and her parents caused him, shortly after Christmas, to abruptly move his family to a small run-down farmhouse in a remote area. Separated from her parents, isolated from neighbors, cut off by heavy snows, alone with two small children for days or weeks at a time while her long-distance truck driver husband was on his hauls, Joanne became depressed; Monica responded to her mother's depression by withdrawing.

Joanne felt ashamed about this period and would have preferred to forget it altogether, especially because the social worker and visiting nurse charged her with neglect of her children, based mainly on the finding that Monica was several times left soaked in malodorous drainage from the esophageal and gastric fistulas. Despite years of our working closely with Joanne, she never has been able to talk about this dark period of her life. Nonetheless, it is clear that although both children indeed were relatively neglected during that winter, Joanne by no means can be characterized as a basically neglectful mother in the sense that such a characterization is ordinarily applied. As we watched her raise five children to adulthood over the years, she emerged as a competent and committed parent for whom the period in the farmhouse was an aberration. Even so, there is considerable evidence that Joanne was never able to bond fully with Monica, the baby with whom the alimentary-symbiotic relationship could not be established. And when Joanne became depressed and Monica in turn began to go into decline, further barriers between mother and infant developed.

Details of the fistula-feeding itself during this period are few, but we do know that the depressed mother found it increasingly difficult to mobilize herself when Monica cried. Even when she had been in good spirits, fistula-feeding Monica was never a gratifying experience for her. When she became depressed, it became a burden; Monica's crying would no longer elicit the usual response from her mother. As a result, Monica first became more and more fretful and cranky, and then withdrawn and increasingly unresponsive, "as though discouraged." This behavior we originally designated as a "depression of infancy," but later conceptualized it as an expression of conservation-withdrawal, a biological regulatory system to protect her from depleting reserves with fruitless crying and motor activity [12].

Thus began a vicious cycle in which mother and child progressively disengaged from each other, a development further accentuated by the impersonal nature of fistula-feeding, which allowed Joanne to administer the feedings in keeping with her own moods rather than with Monica's needs. For example, Monica could be fed while fussing and crying or asleep, if that suited Joanne at the moment. Little Tommy was more persistent in his demands, so by default, it became simpler for Joanne to leave Monica unattended for long periods.

With grandma no longer at hand to hold and cuddle her and with mother depressed and withdrawn, the net effect for Monica over those five months was a major reduction in the mothering she had previously known. She did not experience her share of the mother-child interactions that ordinarily occur during the second six months of infancy, neither comforting nor playing. Conspicuously missing was learning how to feed herself — an important step in achieving autonomy at this age. Monica spent most of her time alone lying on her back. She could not yet turn over or sit up. In addition, her frequently invoked conservation-withdrawal response served further to reduce opportunities for stimulation and human transactions.

Toward the end of this period, Joanne began to overcome her depression and became alarmed about Monica's failing condition. When Monica contracted chicken pox, her general condition worsened and the doctor recommended she be sent to Rochester for hospital care. She was admitted to the hospital on June 23, 1953, three weeks before her first birthday. She weighed 10 pounds, 10 ounces (4,830 gm), only two pounds, 12 ounces (1,250 gm) more than when she was 2 months old.

PERIOD 3: IN HOSPITAL (11–12½ MONTHS AND 15–23½ MONTHS)

Whatever stability in fistula-feeding may have been achieved during the first eleven months by virtue of her mother's being the only one to feed her was disrupted when Monica entered the hospital. During the first six-week hospitalization, nursing notes indicate that she was fed by no less than 32 different nurses, probably many of them students taking advantage of the opportunity to learn the procedure. Other than nursing notes commenting on occasional difficulty in forcing formula of too thick consistency through the tubing, there are no descriptions of how the feedings were actually carried out by these different people or how Monica behaved during the feedings. The hospital record does not reveal whether she was given a nipple to suck or food to ingest during or between feedings.

Only one nurse (K.D.) was involved in Monica's feedings with any consistency over this six-week period. In fact, K.D. took Monica under her wing and came to be one of the more stable mothering figures for her during this period and again during the subsequent nine-month hospital stay that began when Monica was 15 months old. She often held Monica in her arms while attending to her other nursing tasks.

At the end of six weeks (July 31, 1953), Monica was ready to go home. She had gained 1 pound, 5 ounces (600 gm) and nursing notes reported her generally to be more outgoing and cheerful. Joanne was in the last month of her pregnancy and was no longer depressed. She actively attempted to make up for her earlier neglect of Monica, holding her on her lap a good deal, including when the family was at meals. Monica now behaved as though hungry all the time, getting excited even when hearing the table being set and grabbing for food as she sat on her mother's lap. In one month, she gained another 1 pound, 8 ounces (700 gm). She was fistula-fed lying in the crib, but it is not known whether or how often she was given anything by mouth. She no longer showed interest in the pacifier.

On August 30, 1953 Joanne gave birth to Doris, and Monica stayed with her grandmother for a week. Mrs. Woods had not seen Monica in eight months and was shocked by her underdeveloped and malnourished appearance. During the week alone with grandma, she was held and cuddled a great deal.

On return home, Monica acted glad to see her parents but wanted to be held all the time. She seemed jealous of the new baby, crying and fussing whenever Doris was held or fed. Monica's teeth were coming in and Joanne thought she seemed to bite more than suck. She avidly reached for lollipops, which seemed to serve as effective pacifiers. After a few weeks, Monica became increasingly irritable and then withdrawn, lapsing once again into the conservation-withdrawal pattern of the previous winter. She again began to lose weight rapidly despite regular fistula-feedings. On readmission to the hospital on October 12, 1953, she weighed only 10 pounds (4,560 gm). Thus, at 15 months, she weighed 10 ounces (270 gm) less than when she entered the hospital at 11 months the previous June. The admitting pediatrician described her as "very depressed" (Fig. 1-1A).

The nine-month hospitalization from October 12, 1953 to July 3, 1954 began the period of Monica's intensive study and culminated in the surgical reconstruction of a functioning esophagus and the beginning of regular oral-feeding. During this prolonged hospital stay, her parents only visited her twice during the first month, and then not again until surgery was imminent when she was 21 months old. They ascribed their failure to visit more often to the harsh winter and the poor condition of their car.

By the time of the operation, Monica had long since recovered from the "depression" and had gained much strength and more than 6½ pounds (3 kg). However, although she could turn from side to side, she still could not sit up by herself. She never rolled from supine to prone, possibly because of the tubing that protruded from her abdomen. Thus, during this entire period, how she saw her surroundings and how she organized her experience was influenced by the fact that most of her time was spent lying flat on her back or propped up in a hospital crib. From that perspective she took in the sights and sounds of a busy pediatric ward as they swirled about her. Only for relatively brief periods each day did anyone hold or carry her. In this regard, being fistula-fed while lying on her back was only a continuation of her everyday supine existence.

The most complete information about the fistula-feeding during this period comes from the fourteen occasions when a feeding took place during one of the hour-long observation periods when an unobtrusive observer was seated behind Monica's crib making detailed notes. In addition, one fistula-feeding was filmed. Random reports and notes, including nursing notes from the hospital chart and data on seven sham feeding[2] experiments in the laboratory round out the fistula-feeding data (Figs. 1-1B, 1-1C, and 1-1D).

Between the ages of 15 and 20 months, Monica clearly showed signs of anticipation and pleasure at the sight and sounds of preparation for a feeding. She reached, vocalized, opened her mouth, protruded her tongue, smacked, chewed, swallowed, and put her finger, hand, clamps, tubing, and other items to or in her mouth. If given the formula bottle, she would bring it to her mouth and attempt to take off the paper cap with her fingers and teeth even though, as far as we know, she never in fact actually tasted or swallowed any of the formula. In the laboratory we established that copious secretion of gastric juice occurred during such anticipation of feeding, including even the crackling sound of unwrapping the cellophane wrappers of lollipops, and of course, during sham feeding [11].

During most of the fistula-feedings of this period, Monica was given crackers, zwieback, and potato chips to chew or suck. Sometimes she was noted to be carefully retrieving and refeeding herself the morsels that drained from the esophageal fistula in her neck. At times she dozed off during the feeding, holding a cracker in her hand. At other times, she cried and resisted the feeding, as though in pain. On such occasions, the increased intraabdominal pressure sometimes forced the formula up the tube even to the point of its overflowing and spilling over the bed.

A multitude of nurses administered the feedings. Though nursing orders directed that Monica be held on the lap during feeding, this in fact

---

[2] Sham feeding involved either letting Monica chew and swallow food that then drained from the esophageal fistula in the neck or merely letting her see the formula being poured into tubing that, in fact, drained into a bottle under her crib.

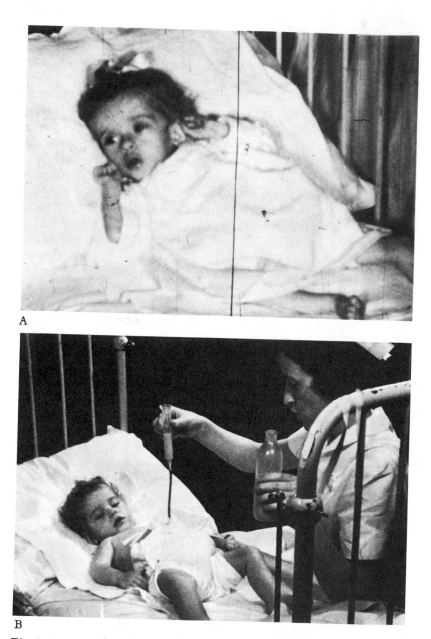

A

B

Fig. 1-1. Monica (A) on hospital entry (15 mo); (B) fistula-feeding, unengaged (20 mo); (C) fistula-feeding, playing by herself (20 mo); and (D) fistula-feeding, engaging with nurse (20 mo).

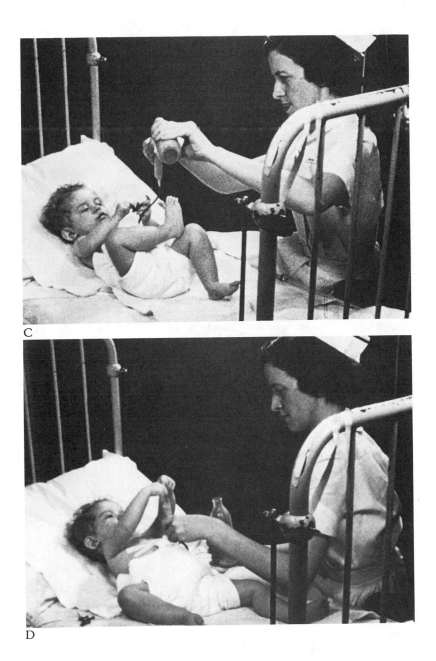

C

D

rarely, if ever, was done. Nurses varied greatly in how they administered the formula. Some were all business — the preparation and feeding occupying no more than 5 to 10 minutes with the nurse standing up and impassively pouring the formula — almost like a gas station attendant filling the tank. Such nurses were likely to ignore any overtures Monica might make such as reaching, touching, or smiling, and interdicted any attempt on her part to touch or play with the feeding paraphernalia. Others, K.D. in particular, sat down alongside the crib and engaged Monica actively and affectionately before and during the feeding, often extending the process for as long as 20 to 30 minutes as they alternated between playing and pouring. Unless there were mechanical difficulties, these were obviously enjoyable periods for both the nurse and the child. While some let Monica finger or play with the funnel and tubing and even made a game of it, we never observed a nurse trying to involve Monica in feeding herself (e.g., letting her hold the funnel or even pour the formula). Sometimes Monica's mood changed abruptly in the middle of a feeding, from cheerful and outgoing to cranky and irritable, not always for any obvious reason. At such times, some nurses continued to pour while others stopped to investigate or try to cheer her up. More often than not, if their efforts to palliate her did not succeed rather quickly, they were likely to resume the feeding regardless of Monica's mood. For a nurse to persist in the feeding even in the face of screaming and kicking or whimpering and withdrawal was not unusual. There was no way Monica could refuse the proffered food as children this age ordinarily do when they do not want to eat.

At times Monica simply ignored the feeder, especially if she were a stranger to her. Instead, she played with a clamp, pulled apart a piece of tissue, or even fell asleep, sometimes with a cracker or lollipop in her hand.

During her long stay on the pediatric floor Monica daily saw infants being bottle- or spoon-fed or feeding themselves. Early in her stay she paid little attention, but later she was more often noted to be watching, occasionally intently. At times she even seemed to become upset. Once a nurse described her "as fit to be tied when the other children are being fed." While watching the feedings or preparations for feeding, she was likely to put her finger or some other object to or in her mouth; this sometimes also occurred simply when she saw a nurse merely holding a baby.

Overall, Monica's nine-month hospital stay was characterized by a degree of enforced passivity as well as a lack of meaningful human contacts and stimulation usual for a child in her second year. Only two people, Dr. Reichsman and K.D., sustained a relationship with her throughout her stay. This undoubtedly was a significant factor in Monica's transition from her initial withdrawn, marantic state to one of relative contentment and more active engagement with her environment, as well as her weight gain and general physical improvement.

At age 21 months, surgery (intrathoracic transplantation of the right colon) finally established continuity between Monica's mouth and stomach [3]. Postoperative surgical complications made for a slow recovery and it was just before her second birthday that she finally went home. By that point, she was taking all her nutrition by mouth and, for the first time, beginning to feed herself. She still weighed only 16 pounds (7,300 gm), which is at the third percentile of expected weight for a 2-year-old child, but she finally was at least able to sit up by herself. It was to be more than another year before she could stand by herself.

Fistula-feeding had become a thing of the past. Monica remembers nothing about the fistula-feeding period other than what she was later told by her mother. She knows that she was fed by a tube through a hole in her stomach (the abdominal scar of which she can identify) but has no reportable recollection of the actual experience. Her mother has shown her photographs taken in the hospital of a smiling Monica of 20 months lying on her back in a crib, but without the fistula or tubing visible. These photographs constitute the only record she has of herself as an infant during the fistula-feeding period. As recently as our last visit with Monica (May 1982), she showed us these photographs.

SUMMARY. During almost two years of fistula-feeding, Monica was never held in arms during a feeding. When small, she was laid crosswise or lengthwise on the lap by the person administering the formula. Later she was placed on some convenient surface with the feeder sitting or standing next to her. Pouring the formula occupied a good deal of the attention of the person doing the feeding and also made him or her physically more distant. Monica in no way participated in her own feeding and indeed could be and often was fed while crying, fussing, playing, or sleeping. The many persons feeding her during the two years differed greatly with regard to the extent to which they engaged with her during feedings.

Monica often was provided edibles such as lollipops, crackers, and potato chips to suck or chew, but not in any consistent relationship with hunger or feedings. Swallowed saliva and morsels of food drained out through the esophageal fistula in her neck.

How Monica Feeds Her Own Babies: Comparison with Her Husband, Sisters, and Mother

Monica was married in 1971 and between 1972 and 1980 had four babies, all girls. All were bottle-fed; breast-feeding was not seriously considered. Her older brother had been breast-fed, but none of her four younger siblings had been. Hence, while growing up Monica did not ever see her mother nursing an infant at the breast.

We will first summarize the salient findings and then present the detailed protocols on the feeding of each of the four babies in succession. The data include reports by and observations of Monica and Dan feeding each of the babies, as well as reports on the bottle-feeding behavior of Monica's mother (Joanne) and Monica's two sisters. The five bottle-feeding positions identified, listed in order of decreasing support and physical closeness, are as follows.

En face: The baby is held fully enfolded in the arm close against the breast in a face-to-face position (see Figs. 1-7, 1-11, 1-13).

Lap, fully supported: The baby rests on the lap with head supported on the forearm and torso firmly grasped by the hand (see Fig. 1-2).

Lap, partially supported: The baby rests on the lap with head on the forearm or grasped by the hand, torso unsupported (see Figs. 1-3, 1-9).

Lap, unsupported: The baby lies free on the lap with no support from arm or hand (see Figs. 1-4, 1-8, 1-10, 1-12).

Propped: The baby, lying by herself on crib or sofa, is supported on her side by a pillow, and the bottle is propped (see Fig. 1-5).

Monica's techniques of bottle-feeding her babies during their first four months of life were observed a total of 32 times (Table 1-1). All four babies were handled in the same way. At no time were any held in the en face position. All observed feedings were on the lap (25 episodes) or alone with the bottle propped (7 episodes). Bottle-propping began as early as 2 weeks. On only three occasions, all in the hospital nursery on the first or second day, was the baby fully supported on the lap, and then only briefly. Eleven times the baby was partially supported, 11 times unsupported. Support usually was relinquished within a minute or two with Monica complaining that the weight of the baby fatigued her arm. She often used her free hand to gesture, to smoke, or sip coffee while feeding the baby. Quickly bored when bottle-feeding by herself, she watched television. When with someone, her attention often was more on that person than on the baby. Once the baby was able to hold the bottle by herself, Monica rarely held it during feeding.

Table 1-1. *Infant-feeding positions with mother and father during first four months*

Infant-feeding position	Mother (Monica)				Father (Dan)			
	Hospital nursery	Home	Laboratory	Total	Hospital nursery	Home	Laboratory	Total
Infant-feeding episodes	4	12	16	32	3	3	4	10
To left	4	12	16	32	0	2	2	4
To right	0	0	0	0	3	1	2	6
En face	0	0	0	0	3	3	4	10
Lap, fully supported	3	0	0	3	0	0	0	0
Lap, partially supported	0	2	9	11	0	0	0	0
Lap, unsupported	1	5	5	11	0	0	0	0
Propped	0	5	2	7	0	0	0	0

In sum, *Monica's manner of handling her babies during bottle-feeding closely resembled how she herself was handled while being fistula-fed.* Body contact was minimal or nonexistent, and the face-to-face distance between mother and baby increased.

Under circumstances other than feeding, Monica also never held the baby close to her, but she did engage more actively with the baby and maintain more eye contact than while feeding. Such nonfeeding behaviors have yet to be fully analyzed.

In contrast, Dan, her husband, on the ten occasions documented, fed the baby exclusively in the en face position (see Figs. 1-7, 1-11, 1-13; Table 1-1).

Monica's mother and two younger sisters were reported to consistently bottle-feed babies held firmly in their arms. Joanne, once observed feeding Adele in the laboratory, held her close to her with her arms encircling the baby even though she was 8 months old and already holding the bottle herself (see Fig. 1-6).

Data are now presented chronologically and in sequence for each of Monica's four daughters.

ADELE (BORN SEPTEMBER 19, 1972)

1 Day Old (September 20, 1972)
Adele is 12 hours old and this is the first time Monica has held her and will be her first effort to feed her (Fig. 1-2). A nurse has just instructed Monica in the proper procedure. The super-8 mm film taken in the hospital nursery shows Monica seated semiupright in her hospital bed with the 1-day-old Adele lying across her lap. She has rested the baby's head on her left forearm and is grasping her thigh. As Monica holds the bottle to the baby's mouth, she tilts her head forward and gazes into her face with a faint smile. The scene ends as she abruptly takes the nipple from the baby's mouth. Next Monica is seen gently wiping the baby's mouth with a diaper. She briefly lifts the baby up en face, smiles and murmurs to her and then brings the baby over her right shoulder to burp, supporting Adele on her right forearm without using her hand to hold her. During the burping, Monica tilts her head back to see Adele's face. The film ends with Monica again placing the baby on her lap with the baby's head on her left arm. She is picking up the bottle to resume nursing when the scene ends. Later Monica reported this first effort to feed Adele to have been unsuccessful. "She wouldn't eat for me *at all!*" The nurse quickly took the baby away.

Dan, in a hospital gown, is feeding Adele later the same day. He is

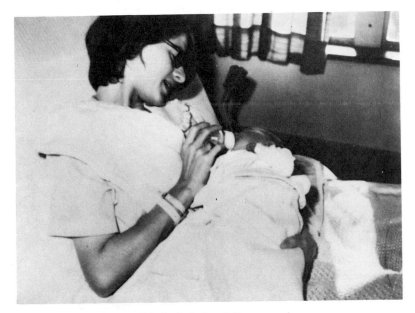

Fig. 1-2. *Monica feeding Adele (1 day): lap, fully supported.*

seated supporting her fully enfolded by his right arm, with his right hand firmly grasping her thigh as he presents the bottle with his left hand. His head is held forward and he gazes intently in her face as she suckles (the en face position). Only fleetingly does he glance up to say something to the photographer. When Adele stops sucking, he removes the nipple and with both hands firmly encircling her chest, he brings her over his shoulder to burp. His right arm and hand fully support her under the buttocks as he gently pats her back with his left hand. After a couple of minutes he returns her to the same position as before to resume nursing her. When the bottle is emptied, he continues to hold her in his arms and gently finger her lips and cheek.

COMMENT. Even though Monica has her left arm around the baby during the feeding, Adele still is resting on her lap; Dan supports the baby fully in his arm (the en face position).

3½ Weeks Old (September 13, 1972)
This videotape taken in the laboratory shows Dan seated feeding Adele, who is held snugly in his arms en face. After burping her over his

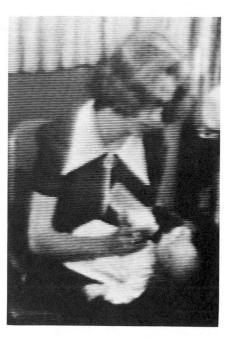

Fig. 1-3. *Monica feeding Adele (3½ wk): lap, partially supported.*

shoulder, he hands her to Monica, who places the baby flat across her lap (Fig. 1-3). Adele's head extends somewhat beyond Monica's thigh. Monica is not actually supporting the baby's head other than by grasping her neck from behind between her thumb and forefingers. When she reaches down with her right hand to pick up the bottle from the floor, the baby's head wobbles. As the baby begins to suck, Monica brings her face closer, briefly smiling and murmuring to Adele. Her hand holding the bottle is resting on the baby's abdomen. As the feeding continues, Monica looks alternately to Dr. Vivian Harway (V.H.), with whom she is talking, and to the baby, with an occasional side glance toward Dan.

After a few minutes, Monica puts a diaper over her shoulder and lifts Adele up to be burped. In effect, she seats the baby over her right forearm, leaving her right hand extended and does not support the baby as she pats her back with her left hand. Again she lays the baby down across her thighs with Adele's head extending beyond her thigh and grasped from behind with her left hand so that her fingers actually are covering the baby's ear. The nipple is inserted into the baby's mouth; the bottle is now in effect being propped by Monica resting her wrist on the baby's chest while her fingers tilt it to the proper position. For several minutes the feeding continues uninterruptedly; most of the time Monica has her head tilted slightly forward as she looks into the baby's eyes.

Monica interrupts the feeding and hands the bottle to Dan. As she releases her grasp on the baby's head, it flops backward. She lifts Adele in a jerky, awkward manner up over her shoulder by grabbing her with both hands under the armpits and swinging her around before seating her, as before, on her right forearm. Again Monica's right hand remains extended and unsupporting as she pats Adele's back with her left hand. After a short time, she grabs the baby awkwardly around the chest with both hands, lowering her first to a sitting position and then face down across her knees before patting her some more. Adele's head is not supported during this maneuver, and it is not supported when Monica picks the baby up to place her supine along her thighs with Adele's head toward her knees. She brings Adele closer by taking hold of her feet and pulling her toward her. The baby lies unsupported along her mother's thighs, except for Monica's right hand behind the head, which rolls somewhat as nursing is resumed. Monica is holding the bottle with her left hand as she leans forward and watches Adele suck vigorously. After several minutes, Monica leans back and crosses her left leg over the right so that the baby comes to lie with her head elevated along the incline of the left thigh.

During another over-the-shoulder burping session, Monica begins to cough. She briefly holds the baby's thigh with her right hand to steady her. Otherwise, that hand is held extended as before. When nursing is resumed, Adele is placed lengthwise along Monica's left thigh, unsupported except for Monica's grasping of Adele's head from behind with her left hand. The baby seems quite relaxed, not moving except for some jerky, flailing movements of her arms. This time she rejects the nipple and Monica soon gives up and hands the almost empty bottle to Dan, while resting her right hand on the arm of the chair. Now, Adele's only physical contact with her mother is her back resting on her mother's thigh while her mother holds her head from behind with her left hand. Hence, when Monica shifts her position ever so slightly, Adele's arms extend sharply in a typical Moro reflex response. Monica responds by bringing her right hand to the baby's side, but only for an instant, returning it to the arm of her chair almost at once.

One more feeding scene just before the session ends differs only in that this time Adele is placed diagonally across Monica's thighs, her head resting on, but not fully supported by, Monica's left hand as before.

Monica's manner of feeding her baby struck us as so unusual and in such contrast to her husband's that it came up for discussion several times during the visit.

V.H.: Is this the way you always hold her?
  M.: Yeah. It's easier for me. My arms ache if I hold her up. . . .
V.H.: Your arms ache if you hold her like this? (She demonstrates.)
  M.: This way [as she is doing it at the moment] is more comfortable for me . . . and it's just as comfortable for her. (Monica feeds Adele silently for two minutes.)
V.H.: When she gets a little bigger, there won't be as much room for her across your lap.
  M.: When she gets a little bigger, she's going in that little nip-nap when she gets fed (said with emphasis and a laugh).
V.H.: I see. (V.H. laughs with surprise.)
  M.: Every now and then I'll put her in the nip-nap if I. . . . Like last night, she wanted to eat when we wanted to eat . . . so I was feeding her while I was eating, so I put her in the nip-nap and fed her while I was eating too. Can be a bother when you can't cut your meat with one hand.
V.H.: Does she seem to register a preference as to which way she is fed?
  M.: She doesn't care either way.

Monica gives exactly the same response to Franz Reichsman's (F.R.) inquiry. He also tries to find out how Joanne feeds her new little grand-daughter.

F.R.: How does she [Joanne] feed the baby?
  M.: I don't know. I never paid that much attention. I think she does it the same way I do, doesn't she, just about? (She turns to Dan for confirmation, but he does not respond.) Anyway, it's comfortable this way for me 'cuz my arm tires with her head on my arm too long, the way Dan was holding her. [Actually she is never seen holding the baby as Dan does.]

COMMENT. During this and all subsequent feeding sessions, Dan's discomfort and disapproval of Monica's manner of feeding were unmistakable in his facial expressions and body movements as he sat beside her watching. However, he said nothing.

12 Weeks Old (December 8, 1972)
In this videotape taken in the laboratory, the baby is in the nip-nap and Monica is standing up feeding her cereal with a spoon. She brings the spoon to Adele's mouth and puts it in her mouth quite skillfully, wiping away the excess cereal with the edge of the spoon. All the while she is talking encouragingly to the baby as she continues to spoon-feed at a rapid and regular rate, which Adele has no difficulty keeping up with. At home, she says, she puts the nip-nap on the couch so that she can sit down while spoon-feeding the baby.

When the cereal is all finished, Monica wipes Adele's mouth and, leaning close, asks whether she wants her bottle. She picks her up by grasping her with both hands under the arms and placing her over her shoulder, supporting her with her arm under Adele's buttocks. She does not use her hand to hold her. As Monica sits down in a chair, she swings Adele around so that she reclines in the crook of her mother's left arm. At the same time she is grasping the baby's left thigh with her left hand. Dan hands her the nursing bottle and Adele eagerly grasps the nipple as soon as Monica brings it to her lips. Almost as quickly as the baby begins to nurse, Monica first releases her grasp of the thigh and then a few seconds later removes her arm from under Adele's head and places her flat across her lap (Fig. 1-4). Monica's left arm now rests loosely on the arm of the chair and is used from time to time to gesture and point as she talks animatedly with her husband and V.H. Her right arm also extends along the arm of the chair, with the hand resting on the baby's chest as she props the bottle by extending her wrist.

The feeding continues in this fashion for only a few minutes when she decides to put the baby in the crib and prop the bottle. Adele is placed on her right side in the corner of the crib and Dan helps Monica roll up blankets as props for the bottle until they finally succeed in getting it in a position so that the baby can grasp the nipple.

Later the baby is fed once more. Monica begins the feeding with Adele lying across her lap. The baby's head and shoulders are resting in the fold of her elbow, but as usual Monica's hand hangs loose and gives no support. Within less than a minute, she removes her arm from under the baby's head, which comes to rest on her mother's left thigh. The baby's buttocks are on her mother's right thigh and her legs hang down over the other thigh. Again Monica props the bottle with her hand on the baby's chest. She is leaning forward looking into Adele's face while with her free hand she occasionally fingers the baby's hand or cheek. The baby is sucking actively but does not seem altogether relaxed. Whenever Mon-

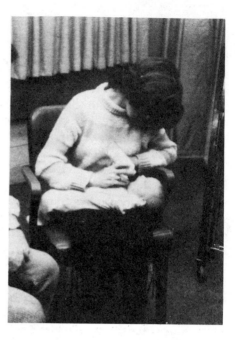

Fig. 1-4. *Monica feeding Adele (12 wk): lap, unsupported.*

ica shifts position ever so slightly, Adele sharply extends her arms and legs and arches her trunk forward. As the baby grows more restless, Monica interrupts the feeding to burp her over her shoulder.

Resuming nursing, she rests the baby's head on the fold of her elbow, letting her legs hang down limply over her thigh. Now Adele seems quite relaxed. Monica rests her left hand on her own knee rather than using the hand to help support the baby. She looks in Adele's face as she feeds her.

After a few minutes, the decision is again made to complete the feeding with Adele in the crib and the bottle propped. Monica comments, "I prop her on her side at home. I don't hold her. She seems to eat better when she's laying [sic] down by herself." For the first time she acknowledges that she has been doing this since Adele was 2 weeks old.

Again Monica emphasizes how her arms tire out if she holds the baby for more than a few minutes. "When you hold her for a while, she feels like a ton of bricks." If she just lays the baby across her lap, she can smoke a cigarette or have a cup of coffee. She says she gets bored "sitting still and feeding her, unless I'm watching TV."

According to Monica, her sisters hold their babies in their arms when feeding, at least until they get "too big," and then they also prop them. Joanne has yet to comment on how Monica feeds her baby, but to Monica she seems vaguely disapproving, as does Dan. Monica comments, "I don't care. It's *easier* to feed her [Adele] that way . . . really . . . and she doesn't mind it, so I don't see where's there any difference in which way you feed her as long as she is fed. She likes it. If she fussed, I wouldn't feed her that way. . . . I used to put my hand underneath her head when I fed her her bottle, but now she likes it better just laying *[sic]* down on my lap. I think my hand is a little boney for her head."

On this visit Monica acknowledges that "like every new mother," she worried a little whether "I was feeding her right, you know, giving her the right amount, burping her the right times." But with the doctor's good report on the first monthly checkup she decided "I must'a been doing something right." It turned out that she was not referring to how she fed her baby but to what she fed her.

COMMENT. Monica's explanations and rationalizations for her manner of feeding Adele make it clear that at some level she is aware that it deviates from the expected. For Monica not to conform with the expected was decidedly out of character. Over the many years that we had worked with her, Monica typically presented as a person low in initiative and innovativeness. She was more prone to imitate and follow the model of those on whom she was most dependent [6, 7, 10, 14]. Her insistence that her approach was more comfortable for her and more natural for the baby, so to speak, suggests a degree of inner conviction and certitude (i.e., autonomy) that we had not so far observed in any other sphere of her behavior; that it should involve this particular aspect of behavior will be discussed later.

14 Weeks Old (December 12, 1972)
In this super-8 mm film taken at home, Monica is seated on the edge of the bed with Adele lying across her lap completely unsupported. Her legs hang over Monica's thigh. Monica holds the nipple to the baby's mouth with her right hand, which rests on the baby's abdomen, and she is supporting herself with her left arm extended stiffly to the mattress beside her. When Monica changes her position, the baby suddenly extends her legs, which for a moment remain outstretched higher than her head before she lowers them once again over her mother's thigh.

COMMENT. From this time on Monica reports that she no longer holds her baby when giving her the bottle. "I don't hold her . . . she's getting too big to hold," she explains. Films at home and videotapes in the laboratory reveal that once Adele could hold the bottle herself, there was virtually no further physical contact between Monica and her baby during feedings. At home she goes about her housework; in the laboratory she sits chatting with the investigators, from time to time glancing in the direction of the baby lying by herself with the bottle. Once again Monica rationalized her behavior with: "It's easier for her and for me to do it that way."

4 Months Old (January 18, 1973)
On a home visit by the technician, Adele is photographed on the living room couch lying on her left side against the back of the couch. The bottle is propped with a pillow and a diaper (Fig. 1-5).

4½ Months Old (February 8, 1973)
A technician who visited Monica at home recorded the following note: "She played with the baby often, picked her up, cuddled her, squeezed, nuzzled her, and talked baby talk with her. When it was time for a bottle, she put the baby into the playpen, propped her into a feeding position

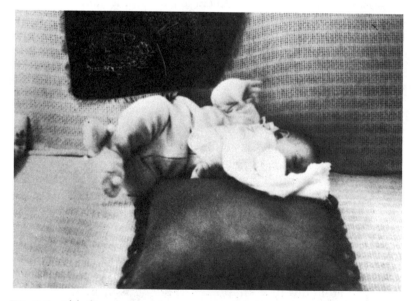

Fig. 1-5. *Adele (4 mo): propped.*

with an elaborate arrangement of blankets and pillows. This seemed awkward, since the baby was at floor level, the bottle kept falling out of the mouth, and much bending and reaching was required. Nevertheless, no mention was made of holding the baby for the feeding."

Joanne Feeding Adele

Although Joanne rarely had occasion to feed her granddaughter, we nonetheless thought it would be informative to see how her handling of Adele compared with Monica's. Hence we asked her to join the little family on the next visit (May 25, 1973) when Adele was 8 months old. Although Adele was now husky and active and quite capable of bottle-feeding herself, Joanne nonetheless enfolded her snugly in her arms on her lap as she held the bottle for herself, all the while fondling, patting, kissing, stroking, and murmuring to her little granddaughter. Adele, in turn, lay back contentedly in her grandmother's arms. When asked, Joanne commented that this is how she always holds babies when feeding them. Her attention was fully devoted to the baby with only occasional glances at the interviewer (Fig. 1-6).

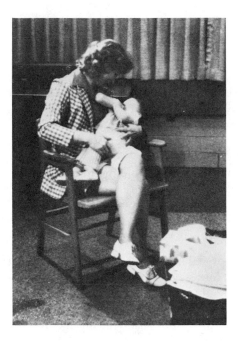

Fig. 1-6. *Joanne feeding Adele (8 mo).*

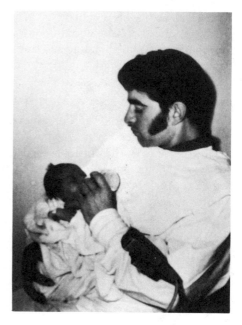

Fig. 1-7. *Dan feeding Beth (1 day): en face.*

BETH (BORN MARCH 15, 1974)

1 Day Old (March 16, 1974)

A Polaroid photo taken in the hospital nursery of Monica sitting upright in a hospital bed feeding Beth shows the baby to be resting on her lap with her head and upper torso resting on Monica's left arm and hand. Monica's head is tilted forward and she is looking into Beth's face. The baby's eyes are closed, perhaps in response to the flash. We do not know for how long she sustained this position.

The photo of Dan shows him sitting in a chair holding the baby snugly against his chest with his right arm and hand in the en face position (Fig. 1-7).

2 Days Old (March 17, 1974)

A super-8 mm film taken in the hospital nursery shows Monica feeding Beth in the hospital bed (Fig. 1-8). She is resting comfortably against the back of the bed, which is elevated only to an angle of about 50 degrees. Her left knee is drawn up and her right leg is outstretched. Beth lies diagonally and almost at arm's length with her back resting against her

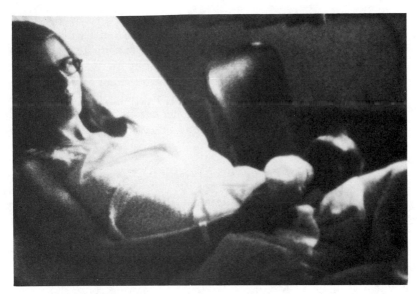

Fig. 1-8. *Monica feeding Beth (2 days): lap, unsupported.*

mother's upraised left thigh, her head above the level of the thigh and her legs extending toward Monica's right elbow. Monica is grasping the baby's neck from behind with her left hand, while with her right hand she is holding the formula bottle tilted into the baby's mouth by resting her forearm on the baby's legs. She then elevates her knee so that the baby's head comes to rest against it, enabling her to withdraw her left hand from behind the baby's neck and let it lie freely beside her. The baby is now almost in a seated position. From time to time we see Monica moving her free left hand. When she wants to readjust the position of the baby's head, she does so by shifting her leg. At the beginning of the feeding, she is leaning her head slightly forward, but soon rests it back on the pillow so that her face is a full arm's length away from the baby's face. After a few minutes, she interrupts the feeding to burp the baby, whose head she rests on her right shoulder with their faces close together. During the burping Monica turns her head and murmurs to Beth, patting her gently on the back. She then returns her to the position just described and resumes the feeding.

Next, Dan, in a hospital gown, is seen feeding Beth. He holds her so closely in his right arm that little of her body is not in contact with his. Their faces are less than a foot apart.

7 Days Old (March 22, 1974)
The super-8 mm film taken at home shows Monica in a white quilted bathrobe sitting on the edge of her bed at home feeding her baby, who lies across her mother's lap with her head resting on her mother's left forearm. Monica's left hand lies alongside the baby, not supporting her, while she is holding the bottle with her right hand, which rests on the baby. On this occasion, Monica is tilting her head forward and has good eye contact with the baby. From time to time, she looks up, evidently conversing with someone.

3 Weeks Old (March 4, 1974)
In this super-8 mm film taken at home, Dan gives Beth her bottle holding her closely and tenderly in his arms as he rocks slowly back and forth in a rocking chair.

4 Weeks Old (April 12, 1974)
A Polaroid photo of Monica in the hospital waiting room shows her feeding Beth in the partially supported position (Fig. 1-9).

Fig. 1-9. Monica feeding Beth (4 wk): lap, partially supported.

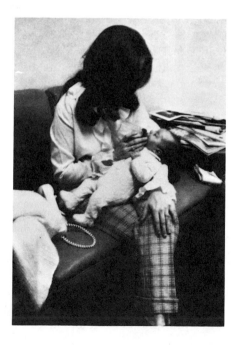

In a 16 mm film taken in the laboratory, Monica enters carrying the baby in a carryall, which she puts down on the crib. Dan and Adele follow. Beth is crying, evidently hungry. Monica at once lifts the baby up with both hands around her chest and shifts her onto her left arm, grasping her left thigh with her hand as she leans over to take the bottle of milk from the bag on the chair. The baby's right leg dangles loosely Straightening up, she offers the baby the bottle with her right hand. Because Monica's supporting arm is extended rather than flexed at the elbow, the baby is held almost erect against her, her head near her mother's left breast and her feet toward her mother's right hip. Discomforted by this, V.H. suggests to Monica that she sit down. As she does so, Monica relinquishes her grasp of Beth's left thigh, letting both legs fall limply.

Once seated, Monica crosses her left knee over the right. She seats the baby on her right thigh with her back against her elevated left thigh and resting against her left forearm. Monica's left hand simply extends along the baby's thigh and provides no support. Beth is thus in a semiupright position with her feet resting on the chair seat. She literally has to hold her head up by herself in order to grasp the nipple because her head and shoulders are not supported by Monica's left forearm. Even so, Monica soon shifts her left hand away from the baby's side to rest it on her own knee. When at one point she raises her hand sharply in a warning gesture to Adele who is playing nearby, she jostles Beth's head. Beth, however, appears unperturbed, remaining motionless and quite relaxed in her peculiar sloping position, from which there is little change during the 20 minutes of feeding.

At the beginning of the feeding, Monica is leaning forward to bring her face close to the baby's. But after a few minutes, she thereafter only glances to the baby from time to time while talking with V.H. or watching Adele play. When the bottle is empty, Monica grasps Beth under her arms, picks her up, and turns her so that they face each other. Then, smiling and cooing, she brings her face very close to Beth's before placing her over her shoulder for burping.

When it is Dan's turn to feed Beth, he holds her snugly with his face close to hers, as on earlier occasions.

On this visit, Monica tells us that she was already propping the bottle for Beth by the time she was 2 weeks old. "If I'm busy doing my housework, I'll prop a bottle and just keep an eye on it." She also puts her in the nip-nap to give her the bottle.

Responding to F.R.'s inquiry about what she knows about how she was fed as a baby, she says, "I know I'm having a lot easier time than Mom did with me . . . cuz I don't have to feed 'em through tubes. . . . I feed 'em *through* a bottle." That she should repeat "through" when speaking of bottle-feeding suggests an unconscious link in her mind between the two procedures.

14 Weeks Old (June 24, 1974)
In this 16 mm film taken in the laboratory, Monica reports that she rarely holds Beth during feeding. Either the bottle is propped or she is fed in the nip-nap. But they forget to bring the nip-nap with them on this visit, so we get one last look at Monica feeding Beth on her lap. Monica's ankles are crossed and her lap is flat. As before, the baby lies across her lap with her neck resting on Monica's left thigh and her head extending slightly beyond and not otherwise supported. Monica's right hand, with which she is holding the bottle, rests on the baby; her left hand mostly hangs loosely from the arm of the chair on which she is leaning her forearm, or she rests her left arm across her lap between herself and the baby. Monica's left hand is also used from time to time to smooth her hair and adjust her glasses, as well as one time to pick up a block that Adele had dropped from the baby-tender.

At the outset of the feeding, Monica gazes intently, but briefly, at Beth's face and thereafter, as usual, engages more with the others in the room than with the baby she is feeding. When she interrupts for a burping, Monica first brings Beth very close to her, smiling, cooing, and kissing her and then hugs her briefly before resuming the feeding.

Dan did not give the baby the bottle on this visit.

COMMENT. Monica's feeding of Beth followed the same pattern as with Adele, even to the extent of propping her by the end of the second week. Dan, too, remained consistent. Again, Monica engaged more actively with the baby when not feeding her than when feeding her.

CAROL (BORN OCTOBER 29, 1976)
Although the home movies had clearly demonstrated that Monica fed her first two babies in essentially the same way at home as in the laboratory, we nonetheless thought it would be of interest to visit Monica with her third baby in her own home setting.

1 Month Old (November 29, 1976)
This 16 mm film taken at home showed that throughout most of the four-hour visit, Monica sat on the living room couch from which she

directed her children, and later her husband when he got home from work, and played hostess to her guests. (We were reminded of her lying in her crib during her many months of crib-bound existence in the hospital, watching and influencing those around her on the busy hospital unit.)

Monica fed Carol basically the same as she had fed Adele and Beth. What was different in the home setting was the extent to which she arranged things conveniently to keep herself busy while nursing the baby. Thus, next to her on the couch were cigarettes, an ashtray, and a coffeepot and mug. In front of her was the TV. When ready to give the baby her bottle, Carol, not otherwise supported, was stretched out cross-wise over Monica's knees with her head to Monica's left (Fig. 1-10). To

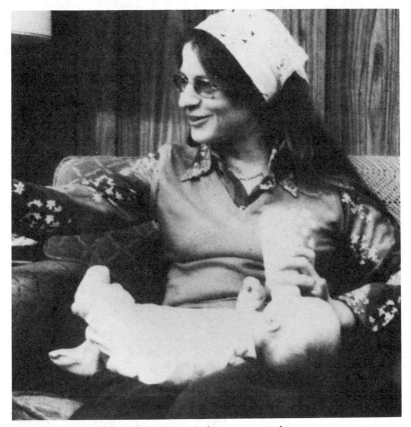

Fig. 1-10. *Monica feeding Carol (1 mo): lap, unsupported.*

hold the bottle to her lips, Monica rested her right hand on the baby's torso. During the feeding she talked animatedly and with many hand gestures to her visitors and gave directions to the children while pointing, beckoning, and admonishing them. With her free hand, she adjusted her eye glasses, straightened her hair, scratched her cheek, sipped from her mug of coffee, and finally smoked a cigarette, careful to get the ashes in the ashtray. For her coffee and cigarette she used her right hand, requiring her to shift the bottle to her left hand, which she held in an awkward back-handed position (Fig. 1-10). Throughout all this activity, the baby nursed contentedly. There was no period during which Monica fixed her gaze for any length of time on her baby as she sucked.

Again Monica's relative lack of attention during the feeding contrasted with her more active engagement with the baby when not feeding her. Before and after the feeding, we saw her bring her face close to Carol's, smile and talk to her, gently touch and stroke her around the lips and cheeks, and rub and pat her on the back.

Monica was feeding Carol when Dan got home and he readily took over at our request. Again, he held her closely en face with his attention entirely fixed on her, ignoring the goings-on around him (Fig. 1-11).

While in the neighborhood, we decided to visit with Joanne. She commented on how Monica fed her babies. Spontaneously Joanne (J)

Fig. 1-11. Dan feeding Carol (1 mo): en face.

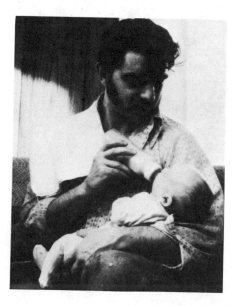

associated Monica's method of feeding her babies with the way she herself had had to feed Monica.

J.: Last Wednesday I was up and she was just feeding the baby. . . . She put her in that little plastic thing facing her on the couch. . . . Even with the other children, I noticed she lay [them] facing her on her lap and fed them that way, you know, with her hand kinda beside the head and. . . . Well, course, I'm different, I guess. I always liked to hold them the other way (chuckles). I always liked to kinda hold 'em like this . . . cuddle 'em. But, of course, with Monica you couldn't do that. When I had to feed her through the tube, I had to lay her on the bed . . . or lay her on my lap. . . . You couldn't cuddle her . . . not while you were feeding her. . . . You just didn't have enough hands.

COMMENT. Joanne's descriptions of how she had fistula-fed Monica and of how Monica was bottle-feeding her babies were remarkably similar.

DONNA (BORN JULY 19, 1980)

3½ Months Old (October 31, 1980)

In this videotape filmed in the laboratory, Monica reported that Donna takes her bottle so fast that she does not get as fatigued feeding her as she did with the others. Hence she has not propped the bottle as often with her. Also, Donna was precocious in how actively she went after the bottle, first with her mouth and then with her hands. In the laboratory, Donna reached for the bottle and directed the nipple to her mouth as soon as Monica produced it. In her usual fashion, Monica stretched Donna out across her lap (Fig. 1-12). For only a matter of seconds until Donna had the nipple firmly between her lips, did she let the baby's head rest on her arm. Monica then crossed her left ankle over her right knee so that the baby came to rest with her head elevated on the inner side of Monica's left knee while her feet dangled over the other thigh. With her left hand free, Monica either rested it on the arm of her chair or used it to gesticulate as she talked with Dr. Harway. At no time was it used to support or fondle the baby. When Dr. Harway commented on how well Donna was keeping control of the bottle, Monica gazed at her baby admiringly. But only once during the feeding did she lean forward smiling and murmuring to capture Donna's attention.

Dan's manner of feeding Donna was the same as with the other babies (Fig. 1-13).

Fig. 1-12. Monica feeding Donna (3½ mo): lap, unsupported.

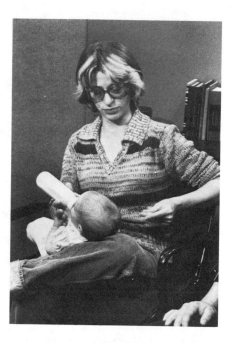

Fig. 1-13. Dan feeding Donna (3½ mo): en face.

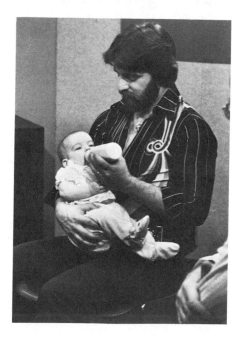

COMMENT. After Donna's birth, Monica had her tubes tied, bringing her reproductive career to an end. The consistency of her mode of feeding all four babies leaves no question that no learning of new behavior or modification of old behavior took place over the eight-year span.

How Monica Play-fed Dolls and Baby-sat

Once we had seen how Monica fed her first baby, we realized that we had already encountered similar observations in her doll-feeding and baby-sitting techniques. However, until all such data had been reviewed, we could not know how representative those examples were. Between ages 4 and 13 years, two films and eight descriptions by observers of Monica play-feeding dolls revealed that only twice — once on film at age 4 years, 3 months but only for a few seconds, and once at age 7 years, 10 months as noted by an observer — did Monica ever hold the doll in her arms while feeding it. More characteristically, the doll was fed lying across her lap, its head supported only fleetingly or not at all; or it was placed on a flat surface with Monica either holding or propping the bottle. Monica's account of bottle-feeding as a baby-sitter yielded the same picture.

Doll play and Rorschach responses also document unconscious memories of Monica's oral-feeding deprivation and of the presence of the gastric and esophageal fistulas. These include references to the presence or absence of the mouth, "open tum" (tummy), and leakage from the doll's neck.

These data strengthen the evidence indicating a developmental continuity between Monica's fistula-feeding experience as an infant and her feeding practices with her own infants as a mother.

OBSERVATIONS

The two films of doll-feeding taken at the ages of 4 years, 3 months and 5 years, 2 months were reviewed and descriptions were written in 1982. All other accounts are taken from notes or transcripts of recordings made on the dates specified.

4 Years, 3 Months (October 12, 1956)

A 16 mm film, audiotape, and observer's notes revealed Monica (M.) with mother (J.) in the laboratory seated on a couch. Monica's baby brother Alvin is just 8 days old. At home Monica has spent a lot of time watching Joanne take care of the new baby. Monica refers to the doll as "baby" or "baby dolly." It is about 10 inches in length.

M.: Can I play with the baby? Oh, there's a bottle! (Squeals with pleasure)

J.: Now you can feed the baby, can't you?

M.: Yeah.

Monica sits with her legs apart and her right knee elevated. With her right hand she is holding the doll by its head and resting it against her inner thigh at an inclination of about 70 degrees. With her left hand she inserts the nipple into the doll's mouth. Then she lowers her knee so that the doll is lying flat across her knees (Fig. 1-14). After but a moment she puts the nursing bottle down and "burps" the doll by holding it upright against her abdomen.

J.: Can you put the baby over your shoulder and pat it on the back like Mommie does?

M.: Like you do?

Monica does so briefly, looking to her mother for approval. Then she lowers the doll so that it is more or less standing on her right thigh with

Fig. 1-14. Monica (4 yr, 3 mo) feeding doll.

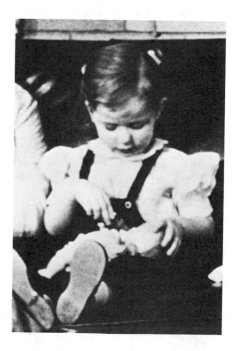

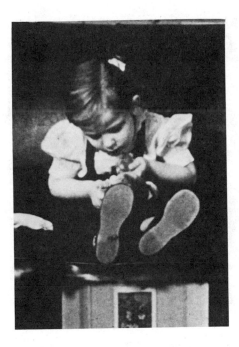

Fig. 1-15. *Monica (4 yr, 3 mo) feeding doll.*

its back resting against her elevated left knee while she inspects the nipple. To resume the feeding she lowers her left leg, which again brings the doll to a flat position across her knees, and inserts the nipple into the doll's mouth. Her left hand is along the side of the doll's head, slightly holding but not supporting it. Periodically she removes the bottle to see how much "milk" is left.

Other feeding positions were noted on this film, as follows:

The doll rests lengthwise along Monica's thighs with the head toward her feet. The bottle is sometimes held with both hands (Fig. 1-15).

Monica supports the doll at an angle of 40 degrees with one hand under the buttocks and lower back. The doll's head extends unsupported beyond her arm.

The doll lies unsupported across one or both thighs with its head extending beyond the thigh. She holds the bottle to its mouth with one or both hands. The hand holding the bottle rests on the doll's abdomen.

The doll lies across one thigh with the head extending beyond the thigh while Monica's hand holding the bottle rests on the doll's abdomen.

The doll is held by the head in an upright or semiupright position, sometimes facing Monica and sometimes facing away from her.

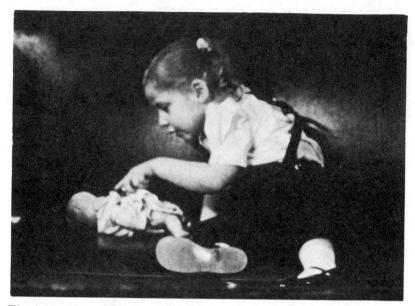

Fig. 1-16. *Monica (4 yr, 3 mo) feeding doll.*

The doll is placed flat or slightly propped up on the couch next to Monica (Fig. 1-16).

In one scene F.R. criticizes Monica's handling of the doll and tries to show her the proper way.

F.R.: That's the right way to feed the baby. The way I am doing it. (He demonstrates the en face position.)

M.: What? I want to do it.

F.R.: You want to do it?

M.: Yeah. (He gives her the doll.) Like this? (She rests the doll against her thigh at a slight angle and inserts the nipple.) See, I can.

F.R.: Oh, Monica, that's not the way to feed the baby. Uh-uh! [no].

M.: Uh-uh?

F.R.: Uh-uh. That's not the way to feed the baby.

M.: I do that. I do that (showing how she holds it).

F.R.: But that is not the right way.

M.: (Monica takes the nipple from the doll's mouth and invites F.R. to have a drink.) "Here, do you want a drink?"

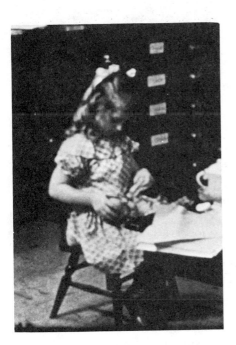

Fig. 1-17. *Monica (5 yr, 2 mo) feeding doll.*

COMMENT. This particular exchange was not intended as a lesson on feeding for Monica. On the preceding visit (June 6, 1956), we had filmed some remarkable withdrawal behavior when her father criticized her. What we actually wanted to find out was whether she would react the same way to F.R.'s verbal disapproval; she did not. Nor did she modify how she held the doll while feeding it.

5 Years, 2 Months (September 18, 1957)
This is a film of Monica and her mother with Dane Prugh[3] in the laboratory. Alvin, her baby brother, died of pneumonia in December 1956, so there was no baby at home being fed. Monica sits down on a chair and places the doll across her lap, holding it with her left hand under its neck as she brings the nursing bottle to the doll's mouth (Fig. 1-17). She has difficulty getting the nipple into the mouth, so she briefly

---

[3] Dane Prugh, M.D., currently Professor of Psychiatry and Pediatrics at the University of Colorado Medical Center, Denver, was a member of the research team from 1956 to 1963. At that time, he was Associate Professor of Psychiatry and Pediatrics and head of the Division of Child Psychiatry at the University of Rochester.

leans forward and brings the doll closer so that she can see better. Once the nipple is inserted, she returns the doll to its original position across her lap, supporting its head with her left hand. After about 30 seconds, she removes the nipple, reaches for a tissue, and vigorously wipes the doll's mouth. With the doll lying on her lap unsupported, she again brings the nipple to its mouth, but only for about 15 seconds before wiping the mouth with a paper towel. Next, with her left hand she lifts the doll up by its head until it is at an angle of about 45 degrees and reinserts the nipple into its mouth with her right hand. The doll is then lowered to her lap and her left hand comes to rest on the doll's forehead as the bottle is held with her right hand. The doll thus lies completely unsupported for the brief time the "feeding" continues.

6 Years, 8 Months (March 25, 1959)

An observer's notes on a play session with Monica and Dane Prugh (D.P.) reveal that: "She finds a nursing bottle and goes at once to the sink to fill it with water. . . . She then instructs D.P. to put the nipple on it, while she turns to cut out a piece of paper with scissors. She puts the paper aside, picks up the bottle, and moves over to nurse the doll that she holds awkwardly in her left hand, not supporting it. After a few minutes of giving water, she squeezes the doll vigorously to see if it would wet. Then she lays the doll down on a table and gives it the bottle from that position."

7 Years (July 17, 1959)

Below are an observer's notes on a play session with Monica and D.P. when Monica's mother is five-months pregnant.

"Monica has filled the nursing bottle and is feeding the doll intermittently while telling D.P. about the new baby (Randy) due soon at their house. (There is no description of how she is handling the doll during the feeding.) Monica gets up and puts the doll in the crib saying to it, 'Go to sleep.' She turns to D.P. and says, 'Wanna cup of tea?' While they are having their 'tea,' she turns back to the doll in the crib and says, 'I guess she's thirsty. I better give her her bottle.' With that she goes over to the crib and props the bottle against the doll's mouth. She herself remains standing next to the crib drinking from her own toy cup and talking with D.P.

"Later in the same session she again goes with the nursing bottle to the doll lying in the crib. This time she kneels down and holds the bottle to the mouth of the doll.

"The same is repeated a little later in the session."

7 Years, 2 Months (September 2, 1959)
Monica's mother is seven-months pregnant. An observer's notes during a play session with Monica and D.P. reveal that: "She picks up the bottle, lays the doll across her lap, and begins to feed it. Then, concerned that her dress will get wet, she holds the doll in the palm of her hand away from her body."

7 Years, 10 Months (May 5, 1960)
Below are an observer's notes during a play session with Monica and D.P. Randy, her half-brother, is 6 months old.

"Monica fills the baby bottle with water, picks up the doll from the table, and starts feeding it cradled on her arm. She spills water on her apron and gets up to wipe it off. The feeding is not resumed."

COMMENT. This is the only observer note where "cradled on the arm" is used. There was no elaboration of exactly what that meant or how long the position was held.

8 Years, 3 Months (October 7, 1960)
Randy is 11 months old. An observer's notes on a play session with Monica and D.P. reveal that: "Monica has filled the baby bottle with water. . . . She sits down and picks up the large baby doll and starts nursing it, laying the doll across her lap. She then holds it in her hand well away from her lap, explaining that she does not want to get wet."

8 Years, 11 Months (June 21, 1961)
Below are an observer's notes on a play session with Monica and D.P.

"Standing up, she holds the bottle to the doll's mouth as it lies on the cart. She undresses the doll and still standing, holds it on her arm and nurses it. Her attention is not on the doll but directed to D.P. with whom she is conversing. A few minutes later she sits down and continues to nurse the baby, holding it close to her chest. Again she stands up and holds the doll in her hand away from her body so that she will not get wet as she gives the bottle. The doll is leaking from the neck."

COMMENT. During this phase Monica was preoccupied with getting wet while giving the doll the bottle. This suggests that the observer's notes on how close to herself Monica was holding the doll had more to do with the wetting issue than with how she was supporting the doll for feeding.

9 Years, 1 Month (August 18, 1961)
An observer's notes on a play session with Monica and D.P. reveal that: "Monica picks up the doll and places it on the table to nurse it. She just supports the bottle with her hand."

11 Years, 4 Months (November 15, 1963)
Below are an observer's notes on a play session with Monica and Dr. D. Wilson Hess (W.H.).

"Monica is standing in front of W.H. holding a baby doll in her left hand and a bottle filled with 'milk' in her right. She now starts feeding the baby, which she is holding by its head and away from her body. She makes the baby doll squeak and then puts it and the bottle on the table.

"After a minute she picks the doll up again, sits down, and begins feeding it. This time she holds it on her lap rather carelessly and awkwardly. She is concentrating more on the bottle than on the doll. After a minute or so she puts the doll on the table and gets up."

That such childhood doll play did indeed anticipate how Monica (M.) would feed her own babies as a mother is suggested by her associations to a comment by V.H. when she was seven months into her first pregnancy (July 28, 1972).

V.H.: When we first got to know you, you were just a little baby and now you are going to have a baby.

M.: (Recalling the doll she used to play with in the laboratory) I remember this one little doll. I was gonna take all her clothes home and wash 'em and bring 'em back, remember? I never did take 'em home, did I? But that doll was so cute. It really reminded me of a real baby, you know. Now it would be too tiny, it wouldn't remind me of a baby at all (laughs). I couldn't have been only 5 or 6 years old. I loved (with emphasis) dolls. I always used to pretend they were my babies, that I took care of the baby.

Her description of feeding an infant as a baby-sitter also anticipated how she would feed her own babies years later.

13 Years, 3 Months (October 2, 1965)
Monica is telling V.H. about feeding and changing the 1-month-old baby for whom she is the baby-sitter.

V.H.: Well, now, when you feed her, how do you hold her?
  M.: Oh, I just put her across there (indicating her lap), put her head right here on my leg (indicates left thigh). Just lay her at an angle like this; she'll be all right. You have to tilt the bottle up so far (demonstrates).

13 Years, 3 Months (October 2, 1965)
W.H.: What's it like to feed the baby?
  M.: O-o-oh. I love it. I don't know what it's like, but I love it. But, boy, when I burp her, she burps all over!
W.H.: How do you feed her?
  M.: I just lay her on your *[sic]* lap, put the bottle in her mouth, then let her suck on that. After she drinks it down, you burp her.

Unconscious Residues of Gastric Fistula-feeding and Oral-feeding Deprivation

Random items recorded during Monica's childhood document the persistence of unconscious residues of her not being fed by mouth during the two-year fistula period.

2 Years, 9 Months (May 13, 1955)
Monica has been eating by mouth since she went home early in July 1954. The unused gastric fistula, contrary to expectation, did not heal spontaneously. She is admitted to the hospital for its surgical closure. We have her in the laboratory with F.R. for a final examination of gastric juice before the fistula is permanently closed. Monica is lying on her back with a small doll in her hand. As F.R. is trying to insert the tube into the fistula, she pulls it from his hand and puts it to the doll's mouth. When he takes another tube and inserts it into the fistula, she cries out irritably, "What you do?"

3 Years, 10 Months (June 6, 1956)
Monica is undressing a doll in a play session with V.H.

M.: I'm gonna take my baby's pants off.
V.H.: Who is that baby?
   M.: That baby's mine. It got pants. It's [got] baby's *mouth* (with emphasis).

4 Years, 3 Months (October 12, 1956)
Monica is seated on the couch by herself feeding the doll. F.R. walks in.

F.R.: Hi!
   M.: (looking up at him with a broad smile) I'm feeding the baby by her *mouth* ("mouth" uttered with pleasure and emphasis).

4 Years, 3 Months (October 12, 1956)
Later in the same session Monica is holding the doll and talking with F.R.

   M.: See her hands?
F.R.: I see her hands.
   M.: And her mouth?
F.R.: And her mouth.
   M.: I feed her like this. (She brings the nipple to the doll's mouth.)

4 Years, 3 Months (October 12, 1956)
D.P. is meeting Monica for the first time. She is trying to get the nipple into the doll's mouth.

D.P.: Gonna get that little thing in her mouth?
   M.: Huh?
D.P.: Can you get that little thing in her mouth so she can drink?
   M.: Huh? What'd you say?
D.P.: Can you get that little thing in her mouth there?
   M.: (laughs) I'm trying.
D.P.: You're trying. I'll say. Kinda hard though, isn't it?
   M.: Now she gets it! (Said with satisfaction)
D.P.: Does the baby like it?
   M.: No.
D.P.: She doesn't?
   M.: She likes it a little bit.

4 Years, 8 Months (March 13, 1957)
Monica is trying to get the nipple into the doll's mouth in a play session
with D.P.

M.: Poor baby (said softly and sympathetically) . . . you ain't got a
mouth.
D.P.: You haven't got a what?
M.: Hasn't got a mouth, does he?
D.P.: Doesn't have any mouth?

Monica starts to undress the doll.

M.: Can you take this off?
D.P.: Well, I'll help you if you want me to. Why do you suppose he
hasn't got any mouth?
M.: He got a little teeny mouth right there.
D.P.: Do you think something happened to his mouth?
M.: (Unintelligible)

5 Years, 11 Months (July 1, 1958)
Monica's first Rorschach responses are confirmatory. Heads and mouths
are missing.

CARD I. Monica says, "Looks like a man . . . has no head."

CARD IV. Monica comments, "That looks like a bird. . . . It don't have
any mouth . . . because they cut it off."

CARD V. Monica responds, "Like a girl, a half a girl. She has no head."

7 Years (July 17, 1959)
Rorschach response indicates awareness of the fistula.

CARD VI. Monica says: "That looks like a cat. Whiskers, head, feet, and
here's his open tum (tummy). I had one too, only mine was more than
that."
    The abdominal scars are a constant reminder of which she is quite
aware, even proud. When she was 9 years old, her mother reported, "She
gets a big kick out of showing her scars."

11 Years, 4 Months (November 15, 1963)
Monica is standing up holding the doll by its head and is trying to get the nipple into its mouth. Monica exclaims, "Watch! This baby will drink fast. Hey! Where's your mouth?"

On two occasions Monica made remarks while doll-feeding that suggested unconscious memory of the esophageal fistula draining from her neck.

8 Years, 11 Months (June 21, 1961)
Monica is feeding the doll but is holding it away from her body. She comments, "No wonder. It's coming out of her neck."

10 Years, 4 Months (November 14, 1962)
Monica is giving water to the doll when she exclaims: "Hey! I think some of it is coming through her neck! Sometimes it does with dolls. Unless it's coming from the back of her, unless she's wetting her pants. I think I'll see if she wet them. [She looks] She didn't *wet* on me; she *drooled* on me."

How Monica's Daughters Play-feed Dolls

Once we appreciated how closely Monica's doll-feeding play replicated how she herself had been handled during fistula-feeding, it became of great interest to note the evolution of her children's doll-feeding behavior. They, after all, were subjected to two contrasting styles of feeding, relatively unsupported or propped by Monica and well enfolded, en face, by Dan.

There were nine occasions when Monica's three older daughters were filmed or videotaped play-feeding a doll. On two visits, when 19 months and again when 26 months, Adele, the oldest, fed her doll exactly as she saw her mother doing, either unsupported across her lap or placed flat on the floor or on a low table. In the remaining seven examples when the girls were older, from 4 to almost 10 years old, all play-fed the doll well enfolded in their arms, sometimes closely, and en face, even in the presence of Monica feeding a baby in her usual way. When one of the girls brought Monica her doll to feed, Monica did so across her lap, unsupported, just as she had been feeding the baby a short time earlier. Detailed observations follow.

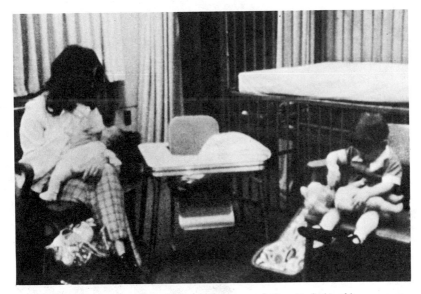

Fig. 1-18. *Adele (1 yr, 7 mo) feeding doll; Monica feeding Beth (4 wk).*

April 12, 1974
This film taken in the laboratory shows Adele, 19 months old, sitting on the floor in front of Monica who is feeding 1-month-old Beth unsupported across her lap. Adele is leaning over a doll (circa 14 in.) lying on its back on the floor and alternates between briefly giving it the nipple and then taking a drink herself, glancing toward her mother as she does so. In another scene Adele is sitting in a chair with the doll lying across her lap unsupported. She is holding the nipple to its mouth with her right hand while her left hand rests on the doll's tummy. From time to time she looks toward her mother seated in the chair next to her, still feeding Beth. Her imitation of her mother is quite exact, except that she has the doll's head to her right while Monica has the baby's head to the left (Fig. 1-18).

November 22, 1974
This laboratory film shows Adele (2 years, 2 months) who has just been watching 8-month-old Beth take her bottle by herself lying on her back on the floor. Adele is seen sitting on a low table leaning over a small doll lying on its back, alternately giving it the nipple and wiping its face with a paper towel (Fig. 1-19).

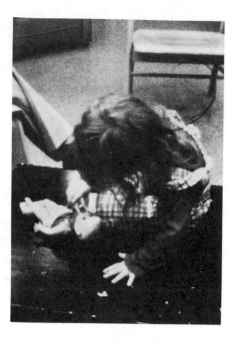

Fig. 1-19. Adele (2 yr, 2 mo) feeding doll.

November 29, 1976
This film, made on a home visit, shows 4-year-old Adele sitting on the couch next to her mother, who is feeding 1-month-old Carol, who is lying flat and unsupported across her lap. Adele has a rather large doll (circa 14 in.) on her lap, its feet toward her and its head extending beyond her knees. She leans forward trying to bring the nipple to the doll's mouth, but then rotates the doll so that it is on her lap enfolded in her arm with its head elevated (Fig. 1-20). As she puts the nipple to its mouth, she brings her face close to the doll's. After a few minutes, she puts the bottle down beside her and hugs the doll closely with both arms, patting gently with one hand. She resumes feeding the doll enfolded in her left arm, interrupting to shake the bottle playfully in the doll's face. After a bit, she leans the doll semiupright against her chest with her arm around it and her face close and feeds in that position. Adele periodically glances at Monica still feeding Carol who is stretched out unsupported across Monica's lap.

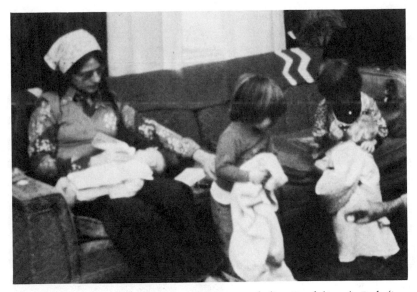

Fig. 1-20. *Adele (4 yr, 2 mo) feeding doll; Monica feeding Carol (1 mo); Beth (in middle) watching.*

May 8, 1981
In this videotape, Monica, Dan, and the children are in the laboratory with V.H. From time to time, one of the children picks up a large (18 in.) nursing doll to feed.

Adele, 8½ years old, is seated feeding the doll (Fig. 1-21). She is holding it close to her well enfolded in her right arm, her hand is under the doll's buttocks, and the bottle is in her left hand. She is rocking the doll slowly back and forth. Even when distracted by the activity around her, she continues to hold the doll well supported. From time to time with her right hand she gently fingers the doll's hand or strokes its thigh, even while her attention is briefly elsewhere.

Beth, age 7, is standing up leaning her back against the desk observing all the activity. She is holding the doll in a semiupright position enfolded in her left arm with her left hand either grasping the thigh or under the buttocks (Fig. 1-22). She brings her face close to the doll's as she tilts the bottle to the doll's mouth (the en face position). She continues to hold the doll well supported in her arms, even while watching, listening, and responding to the others.

Fig. 1-21. Adele (8½ yr) feeding doll.

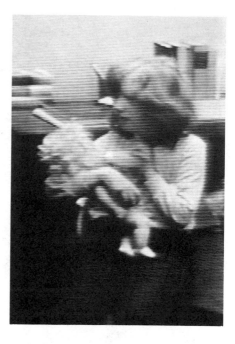

Fig. 1-22. Beth (7 yr) feeding doll.

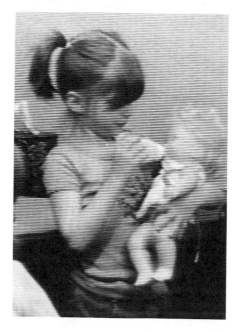

Carol, 4½ years old, picks up the doll as soon as Beth relinquishes it. She enfolds it in her left arm with the bottle in her right hand, just as Beth had done. The doll seems big and awkward for her and its legs keep slipping out of her grasp. She puts it down and tries again, this time with her right arm encircling the head, holding the bottle to the lips with her right hand. Her left arm encircles the doll's buttocks.

Later we see Carol seated with the doll lying flat on her lap, its head resting on her right arm at the elbow, her right hand on its shoulder. Her left hand is under the doll's buttocks. The bottle is protruding from the doll's mouth by itself, apparently not requiring to be held.

Carol then brings the doll over to her mother and asks her to feed it. Monica does so exactly as we have seen her feed her babies, unsupported across her lap (Fig. 1-23).

May 8, 1982
In this videotape of a home visit, each of the three older girls was in turn given a doll and a nursing bottle by V.H., who suggested that the doll is hungry. V.H. and the child sit next to each other on the couch and talk while the doll is being fed.

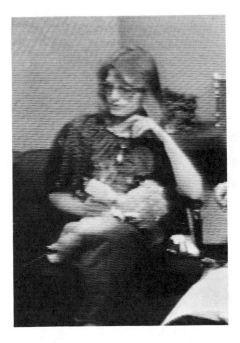

Fig. 1-23. *Monica given doll to "feed" by Carol.*

Adele, 9½ years old, never does get involved in feeding the doll; she is mainly engaged talking with V.H. The doll is partly on her lap and partly resting against the arm of the couch so that its head is somewhat elevated. Three times she brings the nipple to the doll's mouth, but each time for only 10 seconds or less. The first time she has her hand behind the doll's head; the other times the doll lies unsupported. Yet while preparing the doll for the feeding, she commented to V.H., "You have to hold the head because you'll break the neck if you don't."

Beth, 8 years old, is immediately and totally absorbed in feeding and taking care of the doll. As she inserts the nipple, she holds the doll snugly in her left arm, her face close to the doll's face (Fig. 1-24). She smiles and says, "She's cute." This en face nursing position is maintained steadily for several minutes at a time, interrupted only to gently wipe the doll's mouth and to burp the doll over her shoulder. After burping, she hugs the doll closely and tenderly kisses it. When she resumes feeding, she holds the doll high in her arm so that her face is within inches of the doll's, her head cocked so that she can gaze in its eyes. All the while she remains attentive to V.H., with whom she carries on a conversation, looking at her only for a few seconds at a time before turning back to the doll. She tells how much she likes baby dolls because she likes real babies and how

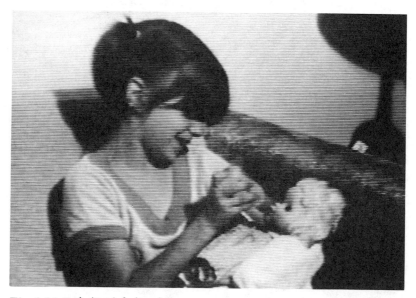

Fig. 1-24. *Beth (8 yr) feeding doll.*

she fed Donna when she was a newborn. The overriding quality of Beth's doll-feeding in this scene is tenderness.

Carol, age 5½ years, has the doll lying across her lap and is holding the nursing bottle in her hand looking at V.H. expectantly. As soon as feeding the doll is suggested, she places her hand behind the doll's head, brings the doll closer to her and leans forward to insert the nipple (Fig. 1-25). As V.H. continues to talk to her, she removes her hand from behind the doll's head and briefly uses both hands to hold the bottle, the left hand actually resting briefly on the doll's face. After but a minute, she burps the doll over her shoulder. When she resumes, she is responding to Dr. Harway's questions and is only partly attentive to the doll that lies across her lap unsupported or with her hand behind its head. But when asked whether she would like to care for a baby of her own, Carol nods, smiles, and immediately brings the doll close to her by enfolding it in her left arm, grasping its hand with hers. Thereafter, she holds the doll enfolded in her left arm with her hand sometimes on its hand or thigh and sometimes grasping its head, alternately gazing in its face and turning to respond to V.H.

Donna, 22 months old, was asleep, so we did not have an opportunity to see how she might play-feed a doll.

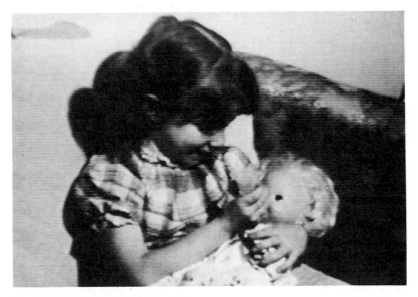

Fig. 1-25. *Carol (5½ yr) feeding doll.*

January 9, 1985
An unexpected visit of the family to the Rochester area enabled us to reassess the children's doll-feeding behavior after a lapse of 2½ years. Adele (now a 12-year-old), Beth (approaching 11 years), and Carol (a few months past 8 years) all now fed the doll held snugly and well supported on the left arm (en face). Both Adele and Beth, on request, accurately demonstrated Monica's mode of feeding, lengthwise along the thigh or across the lap. They reported that while feeding a month-old baby under Monica's supervision, their mother cautioned them not to hold the baby's head "too high"; she also advised putting a pillow under the arm "just in case [your arm] gets tired" (Beth). Both girls prefer their own method; "more comfortable," says Beth.

Donna is now 4½ years old, but this was our first view of her feeding a doll. Easily distracted in the unfamiliar setting, she moved the doll quickly from one position to another, unsupported across the lap, standing up, partially supported on either arm, all the while chattering and only casually attending to the feeding. However, when asked how she held the real baby she had once fed, she brought her right arm up and her head forward in the en face position; she then repeated this with the doll, though awkwardly and only fleetingly.

COMMENT. Earliest doll-feeding closely imitated Monica's style. By age 5 all the girls were beginning to hold their dolls in their arms during feeding, at least briefly. Thereafter the en face position became the preferred ("comfortable") one and was clearly differentiated, at least by the two older girls, from Monica's preferred, unsupported position.

Discussion

This study began in 1953 when Monica was 15 months old. It was intended to be only a time-limited psychophysiologic research study. There was no anticipation that it would evolve into a developmental study, certainly not one that would extend into Monica's motherhood. Indeed, we did not even know whether Monica would survive the surgical correction of the esophageal defect. And while immediate and long-term developmental consequences of gastric fistula-feeding and oral-feeding deprivation soon enough became major foci of attention, we hardly expected in those early years to be able to trace such influences into Monica's own maternal feeding behavior. Our first view of Monica feeding Adele at 3½ weeks in 1972 was stunning (see Fig. 1-3). It immediately evoked a picture of Monica herself being fistula-fed as an infant, along with recollections of how we had seen her play-feed her dolls. Fortunately we had more than our individual memories on which to rely. Numerous tape recordings and films, some never before studied in detail, were on file and available for review. The documentation thereby provided in this report is thus based on observations recorded at the time, uninfluenced either by anticipation of some particular outcome or by memory biased by knowledge of outcome.

Accordingly, we believe we have reliably documented a close correspondence between how Monica was fistula-fed during her first two years of life and how later she handled feeding, first with dolls as a little girl, then with babies as an adolescent baby-sitter, and finally with her own four babies as a mother. In all these regards her feeding behaviors differed significantly from those of family members, including her own children, at least with respect to doll-feeding. Further deserving of our attention is that the distancing and lack of engagement with the babies that Monica manifested during their feeding stood in contrast with her more active involvement with the babies at other times, such as when burping, diapering, or bathing. While the latter observations remain to be fully analyzed, it would appear that behavior displayed during feeding cannot be generalized to other situations.

That Monica virtually never holds her dolls or babies in her arms while feeding them is notable considering the innumerable opportunities she had to see babies so handled, all the more so since an unusual proclivity to imitate had early been identified as a conspicuous aspect of her cognitive development [14]. During her nine-month hospital stay in her second year, Monica watched daily, often attentively, as infants were fed cradled in arms. By the time she was 8 years old, she already had frequently been present, indeed had even helped, as each of her four younger siblings was held snugly in mother's arms while being bottle-fed. When her own babies came, Monica regularly saw her husband thoroughly enfolding the baby in his arms during feedings. Both he and her mother were surprised at how Monica fed Adele, and they remarked about it to her, though how often or how forcefully we do not know. Her two younger sisters, each of whom also has four daughters, both are reported to bottle-feed their babies cradled in their arms. Despite her well-established susceptibility to the influences of others, Monica's pattern of maternal behavior persisted unmodified with four babies [6, 7, 10].

The demonstrated continuity between Monica's fistula-feeding experience in infancy and her subsequent doll- and baby-feeding behavior supports the notion that feeding experiences in infancy can have enduring consequences for maternal behavior in humans, as has already been demonstrated in lower mammals [2, 13]. Involved are biological processes fundamental for the survival not only of the infant, but, in the long run, of the species as well — namely, the establishment of the symbiotic, feeding (alimentary) relationship between infant and mother. Studies in rats and infrahuman primates have convincingly demonstrated that the development of maternal behavior already begins with the newborn's experience of being manipulated by its mother through the period of dependence. Birch has shown that mother animals repeat actively the mothering behavior they experience passively as infants [2]. Harlow's experiments demonstrate that female rhesus monkeys raised from birth onward without recourse to real monkey mothers ("motherless mothers") have major defects in their subsequent ability to care for their own young [13]. Maternal incompetence has long been known to occur among mammals in zoos when lone specimens acquired as infants or born in captivity are not raised by their own kind.

For the human infant, gastric fistula-feeding imposes a major distortion on the development of the mother-infant alimentary symbiosis. If the animal experiments are any guide, this would be expected to have consequences for the subsequent maternal behavior of the woman so fed as an infant, as indeed we have found with Monica. Dowling has shown that some of the adverse effects of fistula-feeding on the development of these children can be prevented by contriving an arrangement whereby the fistula-fed baby be held in his or her mother's arms and allowed to nurse from a bottle (the contents of which will drain from the esophageal fistula) synchronously with the fistula feeding [4, 5, 10]. Such experiments offer an opportunity to study eventual infant-feeding behavior of adults who, as fistula-fed infants, were handled in different ways during their fistula-feeding periods. Even more importantly, they suggest practical models for animal experiments to elaborate further the significance of the findings on Monica and her children.

Monica's children, in doll play, are tending toward feeding in arms, despite the fact that their own infant-feeding experiences were more often unsupported than supported. But in two important respects, their feeding experiences differed significantly from Monica's. First, they were fed cradled in father's arms from time to time, whereas Monica never was fed cradled in anyone's arms. Second, the act of feeding was an integrated experience for Monica's children — from lips to stomach and from hunger to satiety; whereas for Monica, the act of feeding was a disjointed experience. She was disconnected anatomically (stomach disconnected from esophagus) and psychologically (disconnected from her mother's arms during the life-sustaining, hunger-satisfying, comforting process of being fed). The basic conditions for the alimentary emotional symbiosis as defined by Benedek existed neither for Monica, nor for that matter, for Joanne, her mother [1].

To the extent that doll-feeding behavior predicts eventual baby-feeding behavior, Monica's children's form of doll-feeding suggests that to bring about the distortion in infant-feeding exhibited by Monica, a prolonged and consistent deviation from the norm may be required. For Monica, this type of deviation lasted two years. This hypothesis makes sense from an evolutionary perspective. Survival of the species would favor the newborn's being biologically biased toward the "being held and holding" mode, without which breast-feeding would be difficult, if possible at all. Monica never had a "fed-in-arms" experience. Her children did, perhaps enough to activate development of the biological organizations required for eventual competence to breast-feed their young.

We have referred to Monica's infant-feeding behaviors as "enduring." That is not to say they were totally unmodifiable, although she did successfully resist such pressures as were brought on her, chiefly by her family. But for Monica to have to conform with the expectations of others would have involved changing a body behavior that felt "natural" to her. We speculate that such body feelings of naturalness reflect processes embedded deeply in one's very being, the earliest body learning with which psychological development begins. Perhaps the deviant experiences in infancy most likely to have truly enduring consequences are ones that implicate biological processes essential for the infant's development, if not for its very survival. Their very essentiality would enhance the probability that the behavior altered thereby would be felt by the affected individual as "natural" regardless of how deviant it may appear to others. If Monica's maternal-feeding behavior truly was shaped in the matrix of her peculiar feeding experiences as an infant, such would constitute deep biological roots and would explain why her behavior feels "natural" to her. Even if she had altered her behavior to satisfy another (e.g., the nurse who instructed her how to feed Adele), it probably never would have felt "right." In this sense, Monica's infant-feeding behavior reflects her "natural" self, a genuinely enduring effect.

Finally, what still remains to be established is the incidence in the general population of the infant-feeding behavior displayed by Monica, along with more information about the kinds of experiences in infancy that might predispose to such behavior. Along with fistula-feeding, being propped during feeding may be one.

Dedication

Therese Benedek (1892–1977) became involved in the Monica case from its very beginnings and maintained an abiding interest right up to her death. At the time she was developing her ideas about the psychobiological aspects of the development of mothering and parenting. At the first presentation in 1955 when Monica was not yet 3 years old, Benedek, commenting on the gross distortions consequent to oral-feeding deprivation and passive fistula-feeding confidently predicted: "We might be prepared to find traces of this unusual maturational process in her future psychology" [8]. The same year she put forth her key formulation about the development of maternal behavior [1]. *"The psychodynamic tendencies which motivate maternal behavior—the wish to feed, to succor the infant—originate in the alimentary (symbiotic) relationship with the mother which she as an infant has experienced with her own mother."* Benedek lived to see support for her thesis in Monica's manner of feeding her own infants. Her predictions have been fulfilled.

Acknowledgments

This research has been supported by grants from the Foundations Fund for Research in Psychiatry (1952–1957), The Commonwealth Fund (1953–1957), National Institute of Mental Health (1954–1978), Ford Foundation (1957–1964), Fund for Psychoanalytic Research (1978–1981), and The William T. Grant Foundation (1980–1983).

The number of individuals who have contributed to the effort over the 30 years certainly must be well over a hundred. We acknowledge here only technicians involved two or more years: Deanna Anderson, Royce Solomon, Claire Hubbell, Patricia Horton, and Jean Vincent.

References

1. Benedek, T. Psychological aspects of mothering. *Am. J. Orthopsychiatry* 26:272, 1956.
2. Birch, H. G. Sources of order in the maternal behavior of animals. *Am. J. Orthopsychiatry* 26:279, 1956.
3. Dale, W. A., and Sherman, C. D. Late reconstruction of congenital esophageal atresia by intrathoracic colon transplantation. *J. Thorac. Surg.* 29:344, 1955.
4. Dowling, S. Seven infants with esophageal atresia: A developmental study. *Psychoanal. Study Child* 32:215, 1977.
5. Dowling, S. Going forth to meet the environment: A developmental study of seven infants with esophageal atresia. *Psychosom. Med.* 42 [Suppl.]:153, 1980.

6. Engel, G. L. Ego development following severe trauma in infancy: A 14-year study of a girl with gastric fistula and depression in infancy. *Bull. Assoc. Psychoanal. Med.* 6:57, 1967.

7. Engel, G. L. Ego development following severe trauma in infancy. *Bull. Philadelphia Assoc. Psychoanal.* 19:234, 1969.

8. Engel, G. L., and Reichsman, F. Affects, object relations and gastric secretion. Panel, American Psychoanalytic Assoc., May 1955. (Reported by G. E. Gardner.) *J. Am. Psychoanal. Assoc.* 4:138, 1956.

9. Engel, G. L., and Reichsman, F. Spontaneous and experimentally induced depressions in an infant with a gastric fistula: A contribution to the problems of depression. *J. Am. Psychoanal. Assoc.* 4:428, 1956.

10. Engel, G. L., Reichsman, F., Harway, V., et al. Monica: A 25-year longitudinal study of the consequences of trauma in infancy. *J. Am. Psychoanal. Assoc.* 27:107, 1979.

11. Engel, G. L., Reichsman, F., and Segal, H. L. A study of an infant with gastric fistula. I. Behavior and the rate of total hydrochloric acid secretion. *Psychosom. Med.* 18:374, 1956.

12. Engel, G. L., and Schmale, A. H. Conservation-withdrawal: A primary regulatory process for organismic homeostasis. In R. Porter and J. Knight (Eds.), *Physiology, Emotion and Psychosomatic Illness,* Ciba Foundation Symposium 8 (new series). Amsterdam, Holland: Elsevier-Excerpta Medica, 1972. Pp. 57–85.

13. Harlow, H. F., Harlow, M. K., Dodsworth, R. O., and Carling, G. L. Maternal behavior of rhesus monkeys deprived of mothering and peer association in infancy. *Proc. Am. Philos. Soc.* 110:58, 1966.

14. Reichsman, F., Engel, G. L., Harway, V., and Escalona, S. Monica, an infant with gastric fistula and depression: An interim report on her development to the age of four years. American Psychiatric Association, *Psychiatric Research Report,* 8:12, 1958.

2

From psychological birth to motherhood: the treatment of an autistic child with follow-up into her adult life as a mother

Anni Bergman

Ellie, an autistic little girl, began treatment at the age of 3. She was profoundly withdrawn, was mute, and avoided all eye contact. She was pretty and clearly intelligent. Her outstanding musical talents later developed into creativity that extended into several fields. Her treatment lasted for sixteen years. In reflecting about this long period of her life that covered her early childhood, her latency years, and finally her adolescence, I am struck by the feeling of pain that permeated her life. The autistic withdrawal and, later on, her psychotic preoccupations were ways in which she defended her vulnerability against the onslaughts of her untamed drives, the painful relationship with her mother, and, eventually, her own feelings of being damaged and inferior. She feared that she would never have a normal life, never be lovable or loving, and never find the world around her enticing.

In this chapter, I shall concentrate on the following aspects of Ellie's life history and treatment.

1. Her early history, which was colored by her mother's difficulties in her own life to attain the capacity for empathy with the child's needs for separation and individuation.
2. The period in her treatment that I consider her psychological birth, culminating in the ability to use language and symbolic communications.
3. The period of her psychotic obsessions.
4. Her young adulthood, and, in particular, her motherhood.

As I consider Ellie's separation-individuation process as it emerged in treatment, I will focus on the transition points or shifts from one subphase to the next. Each of these shifts can be looked at as a miniature or potential crisis entailing a measure of object loss, which is built into each successive step toward separateness and individuation. Yet with increasing differentiation and separation, there is a concomitant development toward autonomy and attachment to the love object. The points of miniature crisis in normal development become major crises in the psychological birth of a psychotic child. There are two major shifts I will consider: the shift from symbiosis to differentiation and practicing and the shift from rapprochement toward the attainment of a measure of object- and self-constancy.

The separation-individuation phase begins at the height of symbiosis, around 4 to 5 months of age, with the first subphase, differentiation. This subphase results in the hatched state at about 7 months in which can be seen a definite turning to the outside world and a more permanent state of alertness [2]. The brightening of this period has been described by Resch [3].

After smiling, hatching becomes observable as a microcosm; it is the next of the crucial organizers. The baby's first social smile lights up everyone around. The infant's world is warmed emotionally by that smile, and ordinary adults respond powerfully to it. As Spitz has shown, this smile reorganizes the infant's symbiotic world.

In hatching, I think that we see a similar affective warming, this time for the infant—an infusion of pleasure into the link between the infant's new sense of instrumental functioning and the world about him. The infant for the first time actually gets hold of the world and goes after it—and that not only produces "interesting new sights" (to borrow Piaget's phrase), but is joyously satisfying to the infant (pp. 429–430).

This coincides with the beginning of the practicing period, which one might think of as a love affair with the world. In contrast, the symbiotic phase might be thought of as a love affair with the mother. At 9 months, stranger anxiety develops and, according to Emde [1], is the time when fearfulness in general becomes possible. An important change occurs at this time in the mother-child relationship: only the mother is able to comfort the infant who is distressed.

The other critical period, the period of the rapprochement crisis that occurs around 18 months, centers around the conflicts of separation and autonomy. The toddler has to come to terms with his now much more clearly perceived separateness and vulnerability and the fact that he experiences a state of distress that the mother cannot always allay. Furthermore, a period of conflict between the powerful wish for autonomy and the equally powerful wish to maintain the earlier state of oneness with the mother comes into play. I believe that Winnicott [5] describes the same process in his paper, *The Use of an Object.*

. . . first there is object-relating, then in the end there is object-use; in between, however, is the most difficult thing, perhaps, in human development; or the most irksome of all the early failures that come for mending. This thing that there is in between relating and use is the subject's placing of the object outside the area of the subject's omnipotent control; that is, the subject's perception of the object as an external phenomenon, not as a projective entity, in fact recognition of it as an entity in its own right. (P. 89)

The resolution of the rapprochement crisis takes place by way of internalizations and identifications that result in intrapsychic structure and self-other differentiation. This is the point at which language and symbolic play become possible, and from then on remain important tools for mastering intrapsychic conflict as well as traumatic situations that are incurred in further development.

These ideas about early mental life serve as a backdrop to the description of the treatment of a psychotic child and her mother. The pivotal points in the development toward psychological birth, self- and object constancy, and the capacity to love and bear ambivalence are important to keep in mind when trying to understand the long, arduous road of a treatment for a child whose early stages in the development of object relations did not unfold naturally.

Early History

Ellie was almost 3 years old when she began treatment. She was the only child of two young artists. Her mother (Mrs. E) had been an only child who had lost her parents when she was 3 years old. She had grown up on a farm with her grandparents. She hated her grandmother and had no happy memories of her childhood. Her only refuge and consolation was roaming the wide-open spaces of the countryside. There were no children to play with; she was a frightened, subdued, and lonely child. But she loved to go to school, was a good student, and eventually learned from the other children that she could fight back. In college she met her husband, who also was an only child and rather lonely, withdrawn, and shy. Both were devoted to their studies. They married and soon planned to have a child. Mrs. E married because she wanted to have the life of a normal woman. She thought that by becoming a mother she would be able to undo some of the deprivations of her own childhood.

The conscious and unconscious fantasies of Mrs. E about the functions that a child was to perform for her seemed to have played a great role in the pathology of the mother-daughter relationship. Because of her own deprived childhood, Mrs. E had a rather small repertoire of possible actions and feelings that she could allow her child to have. Also, the need for her child to confirm her own femininity was so great that the pathology in the child, which would have been a blow to any mother, was quite intolerable to her and often kindled murderous rages. From the beginning, she was enraged when the child tried to assert her own will.

Mrs. E could understand the child's responses only in terms of her own childhood. Thus, the child either represented Mrs. E's grandmother, thereby becoming the dreaded persecutor; or Mrs. E would identify with the child and see the child's responses as complete repetitions of her own, which in turn would make her into the bad grandmother. Thus, no matter how things went, the tragedy of the mother's own childhood would be repeated over and over again.

Ellie was a full-term baby, the birth was normal, and her condition at birth was described as good, although she cried steadily for an hour. She was active at birth and cried frequently throughout infancy. She cried when hungry, wet, sleepy, and sometimes for no apparent reason. She was breast-fed for seven months, and weaning from the breast was accomplished without difficulty. Mrs. E was very happy with her infant. Ellie started to crawl and walk at an average age, but she did not develop speech beyond a few words. Sleeping difficulties were present from the very beginning, and her mother remembered the child's bouts of waking up in distress that started at an early age.

During Ellie's first year of life, her mother suffered several losses of close relatives, which depressed her greatly. She recalled that there were periods during that time when she ignored almost everything around her and tended only to the physical needs of her baby.

Mrs. E remembered three incidents of rage toward her infant daughter. The first of these occurred when Ellie was about 3 months old and kicked off her covers and laughed. After putting the covers back on several times, the mother finally got furious, pinned the covers down, and said, "Now you can laugh all you want." Mother said that she remembered the child's laughing hysterically for a long time after she left the room. Thus, she already attributed defiance to Ellie at the age of 3 months. The second attack of rage in the mother's memory happened when Ellie was about 8 months old, at the time when mother and child were visiting the grandmother's home together. One night the baby cried and the mother could not stop her by feeding her. She did not know what to do and remembered wanting to hit her and then being horrified at her own rage. At 9 months, there was a further rageful incident between mother and child. The baby was alone in the crib; she had a bowel movement in her diaper, which she smeared all over herself and the crib. Mother, on seeing this, was overcome by rage. The child from then on would not touch her bowel movement or look at it, and would not have a bowel movement except when she was wearing a diaper. Later on she was extremely difficult to toilet train. What we see here is typical for a psychotic child — namely, the fact that she could not forget or overcome traumatic incidents between her mother and herself.

Two further significant incidents occurred around 18 months of age. One was that Mrs. E decided to put a sudden halt to the night-feeding that was still taking place. Ellie cried for two nights, then no more. Also, at that time, Ellie had insisted on climbing on a dresser that had a lamp on it that fascinated her. One day, when her mother was in another room, she heard a crash and found the child under the dresser. Mother removed the dresser but did not pick up the child or make any move to comfort her. Immediately after this incident, Ellie crawled into a corner and seemed terrified of the lamp that had previously fascinated her. This terror appeared to spread to other things.

In looking back over this history, it is interesting to note that the traumatic incidents that were reported occurred at the critical points in development: at 3 months, which is the beginning of symbiosis; at 9 months, which is the height of differentiation with fearfulness of strangers; and finally at 18 months, during the rapprochement crisis.

According to Mrs. E's reports, Ellie was a wild and destructive child at an early age. She needed constant supervision. Therefore, her mother, when she needed to be by herself to play the piano or do work around the house, often put Ellie into her room, where she then had terrible temper tantrums.

Ellie was a child who possessed unusual musical ability. By the time she came to treatment at the age of 3, she was already able to play the piano, imitating pieces that she had heard her parents play. When in front of the piano, she was completely entranced and could not be interrupted. The piano was understood as Ellie's psychotic fetish. The fact that it both tied her to her parents and was a rival for their attention was an important fact throughout her whole life.

Treatment

OVERVIEW
1. From autism to symbiosis (ages 3 – 6)
   a. Changing the autistic balance by working with mother and child
   b. The piano as a psychotic fetish
   c. The piano's destruction

2. The emergence of symbiosis and words (ages 6–9)
   a. Giving up the piano
   b. Beginning of drawing and symbolic play as communication
   c. Separation from mother and therapist
   d. Emergence of affect of sadness
   e. Exploration of her own and mother's body
   f. Doll play
   g. The first words
3. The emergence of communicative language (ages 9–12)
   a. Reconstruction of old traumas in tripartite treatment sessions with the help of mother
   b. Preoccupation with sexual difference
   c. Further elaboration of play and drawings
   d. Emergence of oedipal themes in play
4. Therapeutic alliance and observing ego (ages 12–14)
   a. Mother no longer present in therapy sessions
   b. Analysis of dreams and psychotic preoccupations
5. Early and late adolescence
   a. Looking back and facing her illness
   b. Writing of stories and diaries
   c. Interest in sexual activity
   d. Continuing analysis of psychotic preoccupations
   e. Suicidal depression, paranoid attacks, and acting out
6. Termination — the search for normality
   a. Reconciliation
   b. Leave-taking
   c. The first heterosexual relationship
7. Follow-up study
   a. Marriage and motherhood in a foreign country

For the purposes of this chapter, I have restricted my description of the treatment to the first four phases and the follow-up study.

PHASE 1

During the beginning phase of treatment, the therapeutic task consisted in altering the autistic balance between mother and child. First, I, as the therapist, slowly lured the child out of her autistic shell and then attempted to make a bridge between her and her mother. In the case of Ellie, this phase lasted for about four years, during which she was completely mute. Although she did not speak, she understood what was said to her and also communicated thoughts and feelings by way of piano playing. Many sessions took place at the piano. When not at the piano, the child tended to be destructive — writing with crayons on walls and furniture, gouging plaster out of the walls, and attacking the therapist physically. An important early communication to Ellie was that her rage would not be responded to with anger in her therapeutic sessions. Slowly, a close relationship developed between her and me, as well as between her and her mother. There were times when the attachment to the mother was very specific, and she would be taken care of or comforted only by Mrs. E.

Ellie reacted to anxiety by becoming hyperactive and dashing about the room, the playground, and the building with the speed of lightning. As one would expect, during the symbiotic phase of her development she became more and more difficult to take care of. She was destructive and intractable, though there began to be moments of tenderness between her and both mother and myself. Music and piano playing were her only sources of pleasure, but, on the other hand, she also treated the piano with great destructiveness. She explored the insides of the piano as a normal child might explore the body of his or her mother. She jumped on the piano and banged on it aggressively. It seemed important to allow these explorations and yet also to preserve the piano from her aggressions. Therefore, a second piano that Ellie was not allowed to attack aggressively was put into the playroom. Communications by way of piano playing were often exquisitely specific and poignant. Often, Ellie was ecstatic while at the piano.

Unfortunately, in the midst of this partly tender but often rageful symbiotic period, Ellie's mother became ill and had to be hospitalized for a week. Ellie reacted strongly to what she experienced as abandonment by her mother. Her reaction took the form of instantly destroying the piano that she had been allowed to explore freely. This symbolic destruction of the love object was difficult and painful to live through with her. It was the beginning of a pattern that continued through much of her treatment. I feel that this pattern can best be understood using Winnicott's [5] conceptualization about the use of an object, which suggests that the object must be destroyed *and* survive before it can be used as something real and separate.

Ellie was not toilet trained, which became more and more unbearable for her mother. She began, however, to signal her need for a bowel movement at the piano and preferred to have her bowel movements at the piano.

Separations from me during the summer became more and more painful and intolerable to Ellie's mother in the end. Dealing with the child without therapeutic support became too difficult for the family. In order to safeguard the treatment, it became clear that Ellie would have to be away from home during the summer months to provide a respite for her parents.

PHASE 2

When Ellie returned from her summer camp experience, she had become toilet-trained, which apparently had been easily accomplished as she followed along with the other children. Once more, she seemed, on the surface, more serene, but it soon became evident that this serenity was a kind of repetition of her former autistic withdrawal. She seemed more self-sufficient and had acquired some self-help skills in addition to toilet training, but seemed to have lost her emotional connection. But, even more dramatically, Ellie no longer played the piano. Although a piano had been available to her during the summer, she never touched it; from then on, Ellie never went back to piano playing, and she lost the ability to use the piano as a vehicle for both pleasurable contact and communication. In the therapy sessions, a kind of hopeless mood prevailed for a while.

During one session that took place in the late afternoon when her mother was not present, Ellie went to the window as it became dark outside. She seemed suddenly very anxious. Both she and I were exhausted from a long session during which she had been completely unwilling to make contact with me. This had even taken the form of not touching any object or toy once I had touched it. Ellie found a scissors and started to cut things; she tried to cut her own hair. She was completely out of contact with me. It was only the next day that I understood her anxiety and realized that the darkness must have reminded her of being away at camp — of being away overnight for many nights. Seeing it get dark made her feel that her parents would never come back to her.

The next day Ellie was able to play for the first time since the summer. She first played with little cars in the sandbox and then built a rather elaborate highway with blocks. Then she found a piece of black paper and put it on top of the highway; she looked to the window. I thought that she was thinking of the darkness, and I reminded her how it had been dark last time, how she had been worried because her mother had not come back to pick her up, and how it must have reminded her of the summer when it used to get dark and mommy did not come. At this point, I felt that Ellie was resuming her connection with me. For the first time since the summer, she was reluctant to leave a session.

Two days later in an interview, Mrs. E reported that Ellie had experienced a terrible night. Ellie had woken up during the night and had not been satisfied with having her mother comfort her and lie down next to her. Instead, she had insisted on getting up. Mother was furious, finally turned on the light, and said, "Do what you want. If you've decided that it is daytime, we'll make it daytime." Mother, at this point, was filled with murderous, sadistic fantasies and eventually withdrew and went back to bed, leaving Ellie to her own devices. Quietly, to herself, she decided that she would send Ellie away the next day.

As mother and I discussed this event, she could only slowly and reluctantly realize that Ellie might have missed her during the summer. She much preferred to think that Ellie was now missing summer camp with all the freedom that it had afforded her. Mrs. E believed that it must have been a great relief to Ellie not to be around her, the angry mother. This in turn reminded Mrs. E of the only way in which she could get freedom for herself as a child — roaming the countryside to get away from her grandmother.

Following these events and my understanding and interpretation of Ellie's feelings of sadness over the separation during the summer and the fear that this would never end, there was a very marked change in Ellie. She was able to look at me, smile at me, and allow me to enter into her games. She continued to build highways, built a tunnel, and enjoyed our hands meeting inside the tunnel. Then she found some scissors and again wanted to cut her own hair and the doll's, but she accepted cutting paper as a substitute. She finally cut out a tall house with many windows. This was her way of saying that in the summer she had missed her house in New York City. Then she played in the sandbox. She put a babydoll into the bathtub and buried the bathtub and the babydoll in the sand. She was determined that the babydoll had to stay there. In burying the babydoll in the sand, she conveyed the desperate feelings she experienced at summer camp, which had been at the seashore, when she had feared that she would be forgotten and buried in the sand. She had experienced this separation as a kind of death.

At this point, Ellie's play became more symbolic and her communications were less frantic and more organized. In one session when her mother was present, Ellie pretended that a doll had a temper tantrum and kicked the door, as she herself had done many times during her severe temper tantrums. Then she went outside with the doll — mimicking those times when her mother had asked her to go outside after she had had a tantrum — and threw the doll down the stairs. When her mother suggested a reconciliation, she was willing to have a reconciliation with the doll. This seemed symbolic of the reconciliation that she was willing to make with her mother and with me.

In Ellie's more organized communications, she was able to use drawing. For example, when she wanted to go outside to the playground, she drew a swing, a slide, and a jungle gym, rather than just pointing and screaming. With the doll, she continued to enact the fights that were so characteristic of the relationship between her and her mother. She fed a big babydoll with a bottle but then threw it down the stairs. She would retrieve it or want me to retrieve it, only to throw it down again. In this way, Ellie enacted with the doll aspects of the ambivalence that she felt toward her mother and that she experienced from her mother. In her current life, battles with her mother were particularly concentrated on Ellie's insistence on raiding the refrigerator whenever she felt that her mother was not paying attention to her. This was especially hard for Mrs. E to tolerate, since she herself used to get severely punished as a child for taking food without permission.

In spite of the seemingly irrational and driven aspects of Ellie's behavior, she was clearly emerging slowly and becoming a more coherent and cohesive individual in her own right. She began to be interested in her own body as well as mine and her mother's. The way in which she showed this was very much reminiscent of a baby's method during the subphase of differentiation, from 5 to 8 months of age. She touched different parts of her own and her mother's body and began to say the words for different body parts. In particular, she was interested in ears, and she would affectionately approach her mother, touching mother's ears and saying "little ears." Her interest in ears, clearly overdetermined, eventually reached obsessional proportions, with tenderness and aggression in close proximity. She also touched and played with my beads—always a favorite preoccupation of normal babies during differentiation. The process of differentiation went hand in hand with oral, incorporative fantasies; these emerged in various kinds of play.

Ellie played with a number of small dolls and clearly indicated the one that represented herself, which was the prettiest one that had a ponytail. She created scenes in which all the dolls would sit around the table to eat. The plate of the Ellie-doll was heaped high with food. Ellie took candy and put all of it into her mouth at once. She played out various school scenes in which the Ellie-doll was always clearly at the center of attention. Her mother reported that in bed at night, Ellie masturbated in an affectionate, gentle way. Thus, she was clearly beginning to cathect her own body as well as the body of her mother in a more libidinal way. Mrs. E recognized the growing attachment between them but at the same time remarked on Ellie's basic mistrust. Ellie always expected the worst and never believed that her mother would fulfill her wishes until this actually occurred.

As Ellie cathected and took cognizance of her own body, she also became cognizant of sexual differences. She started to draw boys with penises and girls with holes. She became preoccupied with wounds and asked interminably for Band-Aids (Fig. 2-1). She played at filling the pants of dolls with sand, making sure that there was sand both in front and back. Then she would feed the doll and put the doll to bed, thus making sure that the doll had everything (i.e., food, penis, bowel movement). At home, a rather dramatic scene was reported in which she put clay into her own pants, then put on several pairs of pants, wrapped herself in blankets, and went to bed. This was understood as a regressive enactment of her wish to merge with her mother, possibly a womb fantasy establishing closeness.

At a different time, when the mother was angry with her, Ellie put the lights out, went to bed, and pulled the mother to lie close to her. Around the same time, more and more words emerged. She said, "hi," "bye-bye," and, finally "mommy." She said "mommy" both directly to her mother and in doll play. More and more, Ellie was struggling with her ambivalent feelings, and this emerged in her doll play as well as in the transference.

I will quote briefly from a therapy session around the time she first started to say "mommy."

Ellie plays with the small dolls at the beginning of the session, again using much detail. When I brought in tea, she spontaneously said "hot." She talked mostly during the beginning of the session while the mother was present. Mother, however, did not involve herself. She then asked if she could leave and do her grocery shopping. Ellie settled down to play in the sandbox. I sat very quietly and during that period she was close to me, leaning against me, and at moments being quite affectionate. There were other moments during this play when she became aggressive. She would hit me, scratch and bite, but not hard. Her anger at me started as it was getting dark outside, and I therefore connected again the darkness with her longing for mother during the summer, with her anger at me because she had been sent away during the summer, reminding her how she may be responsible for the bad things that happen, namely when mommy left her. I reassured her that she could be angry with me and still love me. She took a baby doll, treated it very roughly, throwing it, biting it, but then putting a Band-Aid on it. She dashed away from me very quickly, and then laughed when I went to catch her.

One could describe this period in Ellie's treatment and development as a period of hatching, characterized by increasing body narcissism, incor-

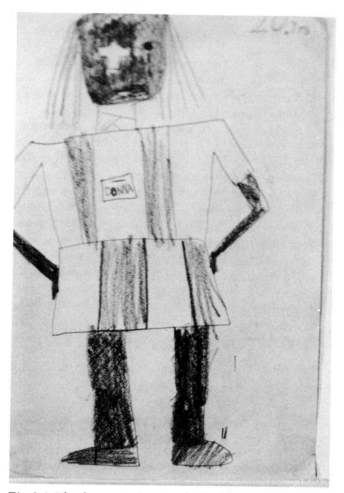

Fig. 2-1. *This drawing is characteristic of Ellie's art work during the period of her preoccupation with the anatomical difference.*

porative fantasies, and some sense of differentiation, which for her also included sexual differentiation. Both introjective and projective mechanisms could clearly be observed as Ellie was struggling to somehow differentiate between herself and the object. Mood swings, battles, and reconciliations were the order of the day, and as Ellie's therapist — or rather as the therapist of the mother-child pair — it was my function to endure their continuously shifting moods and destructiveness directed at each other, at me, and at the treatment process.

Ellie made important progress in ego development, especially in communication and symbolization. Phenomena related to a delayed practicing period also appeared: Ellie became more curious and explorative (Fig. 2-2). For example, in the large apartment building in which she lived, she wanted to go to each apartment and ring the door bell. She loved to go on walks to the park and on bus rides, and a therapeutic companion accompanied her on many of these excursions. An important aspect of these excursions was to put herself in danger so that she would have to be rescued. This represented a transition to her own version of a rapproche-

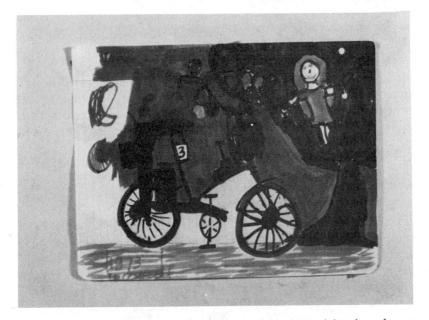

Fig. 2-2. *Ellie went through a period of intense preoccupation with bicycles and motorcycles and drew them endlessly. They symbolized her growing wish to explore, as well as phallic excitement.*

ment struggle that was colored by intense fears of abandonment and the mutual destructiveness between her and her mother.

As would be expected, the rapprochement struggle was intense and had an all-or-nothing quality. In her therapy sessions, it often took the form of violent escapes (e.g., rushing up four flights of a fire escape with lightning speed — her psychotic version of the darting-away behaviors of the normal toddler during rapprochement). Negativism took the form of refusing to stay in the playroom because closeness at this time was too dangerous; violent temper tantrums continued over the course of a year, and during that year, if often felt as if the therapeutic process had inexorably ground to a halt. The situation in her outside life was also difficult, since she had to change schools, and a teacher whom she liked very much left suddenly. With her mother, the struggles had a more cautious quality in which she seemed much more ready for compromise and reconciliation. But her insatiable demand for food and toys remained rampant. Sometimes she was able to use drawings for wish fulfillment and be satisfied, at least at times, with drawing the thing tht she wanted. On the whole, though, the year of rapprochement was extremely trying and at times gave me the feeling that I was engaged in a hopeless struggle. Yet Ellie was also making progress, especially in her cognitive development and her ability to draw, write, say more and more words, and distinguish among past, present, and future.

The exhaustion of the struggle eventually came to a dramatic climax. Mother had an accident in which she hurt her foot and had to walk with crutches, which enraged the child who tortured her by taking her crutches away. Shortly afterward, Ellie herself had a serious accident that happened while her mother was out of the house. While she was with a babysitter, she pulled a heavy filing cabinet down onto herself. This, in part, was certainly a reaction to her mother's accident but also a repetition of an accident in her earliest childhood (when she had pulled a dresser with a lamp on top of herself while her mother was in the next room practicing the piano). This self-inflicted accident caused a large wound in Ellie's leg. Her mother was able to respond to her with tenderness and care. The working through of this accident lasted for many months because Ellie demanded that all the details of the accident be gone over and over again in drawing and writing. The causes of this accident were clearly overdetermined: identification with the damaged mother; guilt and punishment; feeling herself to be the cause of mother's suffering; rage against the mother and myself for leaving her and not taking care of her; memory of earlier hopeless times; and ultimately, possibly some suicidal intent that had already emerged earlier in her play of burying the little doll in the bathtub in the sand.

Following this accident, Ellie's treatment seemed once again to proceed. It took the form of reenacting and reconstructing events from the past, mostly through doll play. Ellie's vocabulary slowly increased, and the most important words that were added were "yes" and "why."

Ellie's treatment described so far covers the period of development that, in normality, would be negotiated approximately during the first two years of life. From the psychosexual point of view, this would be the oral and anal phases; and from the object relations and ego development point of view, this would be the phases of symbiosis and separation-individuation. For Ellie, who was now 9 years old, it involved six years of intensive treatment. Even after this time, one could by no means feel that Ellie's development was a healthy resolution of the delayed early developmental processes. But, given both her constitutional endowment and maternal environment, it was probably the best solution she could come to at this time. It was a triumph for Ellie that she had been able to emerge as a coherent person who was capable of experiencing affects of sadness and longing, tolerating delay, being able to anticipate, and using play and imagination. Although splitting was still present as a defense mechanism, it was not constant, and she was able to tolerate ambivalence and experience love and hate for the same object. She was also beginning to be able to perceive the object as objective, rather than just subjective. In her self-development, sound secondary narcissism was beginning to emerge; though she experienced a great deal of self-hatred, she also experienced self-love. Most importantly, Ellie had definitely emerged from an autistic situation and had established meaningful emotional experiences and relationships.

PHASE 3

During this period (ages 9 to 12), there was a marked change in Ellie. Language now developed rapidly, and though it was not always easy to understand her, she would express herself well with words. Her drawing improved enormously and was another very important avenue of expressiveness for her (Fig. 2-3). Fantasies became more and more elaborate and reached an oedipal level. Many of them were acted out in puppet shows. Ellie now became jealous of my other patient at the center and asked questions about her. She developed fears of thunderstorms and of death (Fig. 2-4); she developed counterphobic mechanisms for dealing with

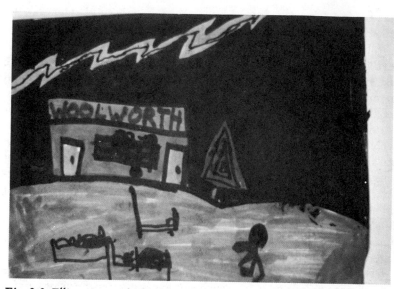

Fig. 2-3. *Ellie, now on a higher level of development, developed conflicts. Here we see the temptation of her greedy acquisitiveness (symbolized by the Woolworth store), as well as the imagined punishments, symbolized in hospital beds and thunderstorms.*

these fears, e.g., jumping off diving boards. She began to think about a future: What would she be like? Would she find a husband? Would she have babies? She began to ask her mother questions about her childhood, and did the same with me. She developed conflicts about masturbation and asked me if I had ever masturbated. Destructive rages and splitting diminished markedly. She moved from the stage of oral narcissism to a capacity for object love, developing the ability to show and give love to others. She became more feminine and wanted to know about childbirth and menstruation.

While Ellie functioned on a much higher level in many ways, she developed an intense psychotic preoccupation with crowded highways. In part, this preoccupation was used defensively whenever anything was discussed that made her anxious. She would begin to concentrate all her attention on thinking and talking about the crowded highway. At the same time, fantasies about the highway were condensations about present and past concerns. She now occasionally went away on weekend trips with a therapeutic companion and her husband, both of whom she loved intensely. She had a good time on these weekends but then seemed

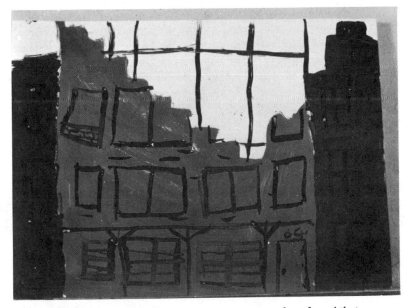

Fig. 2-4. *Fear of punishment gave rise to the ever-present fear of annihilation.*

to worry that her mother would retaliate and leave her. Thus, the highway fantasies contained memories of her badness for which earlier on she had been threatened with abandonment. Ellie also had a fantasy of getting stuck in a traffic jam, not being able to go to the bathroom, and defecating in her pants. She talked about her early memories of being away at camp and thinking about highways while in bed at night. Cars and motorcycles had become very important phallic symbols; she demanded that her parents buy the biggest, most flashy car and was very dissatisfied with the actual car that the parents had.

PHASE 4

Ellie had now reached the stage of full verbal communication. She was no longer interested in playing. She also had developed an observing ego and a desire to work on her problems. She said: "You must help me with these hang-ups. I cannot stand them any more." Thus, there was a conscious decision to attempt to free herself from her psychotic preoccupations. She brought rich dream and fantasy material into her sessions.

Now that Ellie had clearly emerged as a person — as a separate individual with an observing eye — she began to be tortured by two aspects of her life. She realized that she had not had a normal childhood, and she did not know whether it would be possible for her to have a future. Her problems were now no longer directly concerned with the immediate interactions between her and her family; conflict had become internalized as she was trying to deal with her place in the world.

The realization that she had not had a normal childhood was so painful to her that for a while she could not bear to see little children; it was especially intolerable for her to see a little child happy with his or her mother. She attempted to deal with the problem by externalization and projection, blaming her mother for not having forced her to talk, be normal, and have friends. She also blamed her mother for having sent her away to the dreadful summer camp, which she now saw as the cause of all her problems. She told elaborate stories of having been beaten in the camp, of having been locked up in a room by herself, of having been forced to do things she did not want to do, and of having been punished for bowel accidents. By blaming the summer camp, she could at least partially protect her parents and myself from being the sole culprits of her suffering.

As Ellie started to travel to different places in the city on her own, including my office, she had to face herself in relation to the world around her. She was deeply ashamed of herself and felt awkward and unable to initiate or sustain social contacts. She noticed other children talking and laughing together on the bus or subway. Not knowing how to participate and having no friends of her own, she became absorbed in staring at and trying to read the backs of newspapers that were hiding some of the people on the buses. She developed a psychotic preoccupation with The New York Times and "all that was fit to print." Subsequently and simultaneously, she also developed a psychotic preoccupation with the Attica Prison revolt. In thinking about this, she identified with both the victims and the victimizers. She felt sorry for the poor prisoners and at the same time was clearly sexually excited by the stories and drawings that she did about tortures (Fig. 2-5). These were quite wild and out of control. Contained in them, of course, was the fear that she would have to end up in an institution. She became more and more impressed with what she considered to have been her own insanity and attempted to understand where it came from or what it was about. In that connection, she became very interested in people who had had to fight

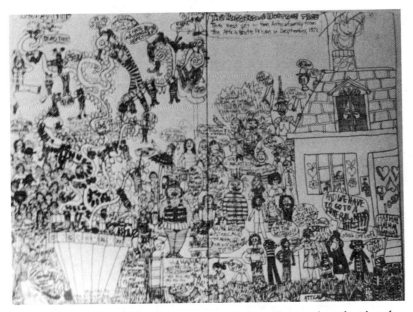

Fig. 2-5. *This is a drawing typical of the period when Ellie was obsessed with and fascinated by the Attica prison revolt. The earlier fear of crowds and crowded highways took on a new form in the fantasies about crowded prisons.*

physical handicaps; in particular she became interested in studying the life of Helen Keller. I will quote from a session of that period.

Ellie came in and complained that she did not know what to talk about. She was thinking about Attica again but she did not want to talk about it because she knew I must be bored with it and she was bored too, that she did not talk about it any more except with me and sometimes at home but her mother did not like it. She was silent for a while and then said that she was nervous or restless. I said that we knew that she often thought about Attica when something had happened that was worrying or upsetting her. She thought for a while and said that last night her mother could not sit with her in the evening when she was in bed because her mother was feeling sick and her father did not have time either, and that she thought that she must have felt lonesome last night and maybe that made her think of prison. And then she said: "And I think I'm still jealous of the little kids in school who never had the kind of trouble that I had, who were able to talk, and who did not have to go to camp." I agreed that it was hard to get over the jealous feelings. I knew that she was still worried about herself and that the other day she had asked me about state hospitals which also reminded her of prison. She then told me that once her father had said that crazy people go there. For example, if somebody would walk in the street without their clothes on. She said that she would never do that. I pointed out that there was a big difference between thinking and doing, and she then said that she still likes to touch herself and that she thought that that could be a crime or make her crazy. She said that when she thought about it, it made her think of all the terrible things — prisons, jails, tombs, churchyards. She wondered if other people did it too, and then said it was even worse to think that I or her friends or her parents would do such a thing. She said it was disgusting. She said it was sticky between the legs, like the stuff that comes out of the nose. She had seen her mother dry herself with a towel and that was disgusting. She has good feelings at night when she does it, but the bad feelings come the next day when she thinks about it and then she thinks of all the terrible things and the punishments. I asked her what she thinks about when she touches herself and she said that then she thinks about being a little child. She knows that you cannot go to a state hospital until you are 18. And I said that that could help us understand why she was so worried about growing up. She said that she was afraid that if she went to a state hospital there might be a riot there, like there was in Attica, and she would get caught in it.

Ellie retained her old insatiability, but now it switched from food to clothes. She hoped that by finding the right clothes she would become the right person. She insisted that her mother and others take her on endless shopping trips to Macy's, and she did endless drawings of children in all kinds of different clothes.

During this period Ellie spent one summer with both her parents at a beautiful beach with her father's family. This made her very happy, and she then drew many pictures about this experience, which was serene and beautiful (Fig. 2-6). She made a book about happiness and in it she said such things as: "Happiness is the sun early in the morning on the beach; happiness is gathering egg shells; happiness is gazing at the moon at night, near the ocean, in the window of the attic." She made a particularly beautiful drawing of a little girl (representing herself) looking out of the window at the moon. This drawing was especially meaningful because this had been the first summer in many, many years she had spent with her parents.

Ellie tried valiantly to overcome her obsessions, but it was only at rare moments that she could get away from them. The narcissistic injury of her illness was too profound. There were two aspects of her personality that seemed to have saved her. One was her natural beauty and appeal, along with her now deeply felt desire for human relationships. The other, her artistic ability, helped the process of sublimation (Fig. 2-7). She spent hours and hours drawing and writing and eventually wrote a very interesting autobiography, weaving together reality and fantasy. It was the story of her life and of her treatment.

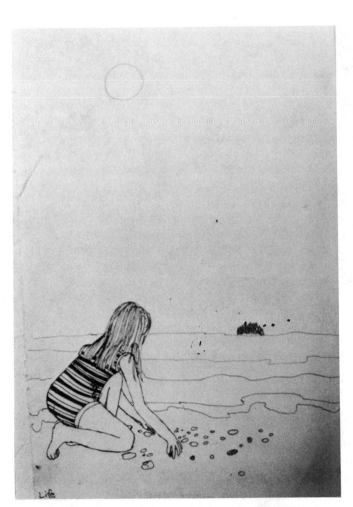

Fig. 2-6. One of a series of idyllic beach drawings which followed a summer vacation spent with both parents.

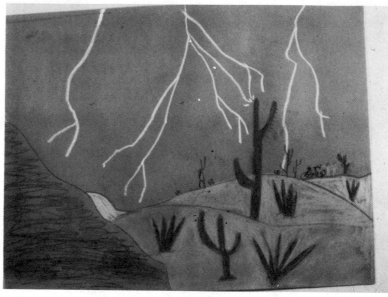

A

Fig. 2-7. *Ellie continued to be haunted by feelings of loneliness and isolation. She deeply wished to find relationships but had great difficulty doing so. These feelings are represented by the small lonely figures in the desert and among the skyscrapers.*

Discussion of Treatment

As I have told of Ellie's development during her childhood treatment, I have described the first four phases, concentrating on two: namely, the emergence from symbiosis and the time when she had truly become a separate person, suffering acutely from her obsessions, which, by then, had become true symptoms. We might ask: How did Ellie manage to change? How did she make the transition from one phase to the next? It is striking that each change was preceded by a crisis. The change from autism and symbiosis to hatching, the first words, and the beginning of symbolization, which happened between the ages of 6 and 8, was preceded by her separation from her family in the summer camp. The change from a violent rapprochement crisis to beginning object constancy and the emergence of communicative language, which happened at the age of 8, was preceded by first her mother's and then her own accident. And, finally, the change toward a therapeutic alliance, an ob-

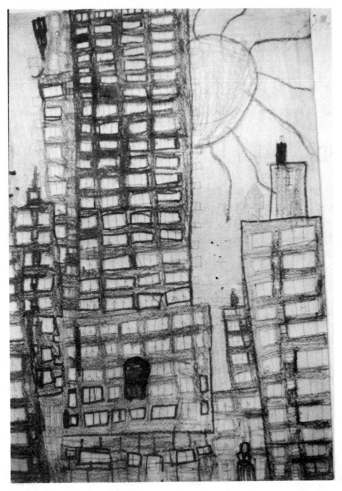

B

serving ego, and the initial working through of her obsessions happened at the age of 11 when our treatment center closed and she began to come to therapy sessions on her own in my office.

Each of these important steps, then, was preceded by a challenge and crisis that her treatment could help her weather and use in a way that produced further growth. The mutative point in the first transition seemed to be the recognition of her feelings of despair when she was left at camp, saw it get dark, and had the feeling that her parents would never come back. The loss she experienced was dramatically expressed by her giving up her psychotic fetish and love object — the piano. The recognition of and working through of her despair produced the real affect of sadness and brought her closer to both me and her mother. The most important event of the following period was the emergence of words (most importantly, "mommy") and symbols.

In normal development, the rapprochement crisis is resolved by way of identification and internalization. It is dramatic that in Ellie's case, the identification was with her mother as the victim of a painful accident for which undoubtedly she felt guilty. Through her own accident and identification with her mother, she could then bring about a reconciliation which, during the next period of treatment, resulted in relationships on a much higher level with me and both parents — her oedipal phase.[1] During that time, many of Ellie's fantasies and preoccupations had to do with narcissistic aggrandizement and exhibitionism (e.g., she saw herself as a famous cello player commanding a large audience).

Finally, the change toward a true therapeutic alliance occurred when Ellie's mother no longer came to treatment sessions. However plaguing her obsessions were and however hopeless the struggle against them often seemed, Ellie struggled valiantly to become a more independent person and create a life of her own.

From a clinical point of view, one could say that the therapeutic task in the first two changes was to bring her closer to her love object; whereas the therapeutic task in the next stage was to help her achieve greater autonomy and separateness.

Marriage and Motherhood

After a long, difficult adolescence during which therapy proceeded, treatment was terminated when Ellie graduated from high school. Ellie

---

[1] I have not discussed Ellie's oedipal phase in this chapter inasmuch as I am concentrating on her separation-individuation process and its influence on her experience of motherhood.

married a man whom she had met during her last year of high school. She went with him to a faraway country to live in a foreign culture where she had to learn a new language. Once more she was a stranger in the world in which she lived. But this time, she could feel herself to be a legitimate stranger because she was a foreigner. She could repeat actively and by choice her childhood experiences of not being able to talk, of understanding more than anyone knew she did, of being different, and of being dependent on her caretakers. Ellie soon became pregnant.

The material that follows is taken in part from her long, extensive, and informative letters. It is also taken from a follow-up study.[2]

Ellie's first letter to me was written during her first pregnancy and was entitled "To an old friend." In this letter she expressed fears about whether or not she was well enough to have a normal life, a loving husband, and a child. She worried about whether or not she would make it as a mother, and she worried about whether or not her husband would ever become disenchanted with her and reject her. She said: "I feel awful if I have displeased him in any way, even worse than I had with my two parents in the past."

Ellie attributed the sickness that she felt during pregnancy to the baby's rejection of the food she was eating. Here is the first sign of one of the themes that has been important in the mothering of her first child, a boy, namely the fear that he might reject her and her need for him to love her. She believed that the baby in the womb already had a great deal of control over her by rejecting or accepting the food that she ate.

The birth of Ellie's first baby, Jamie, was a difficult one. There were some complications that necessitated his staying in the hospital for a few days after she had gone home. Breast-feeding was not encouraged, and thus she soon gave it up. Ellie's mother-in-law was ready and waiting to take care of the new infant. Ellie felt inferior and incompetent next to her and relinquished much of the baby's early care to her mother-in-law. She looked on enviously and sadly when her mother-in-law was feeding her infant. All of these circumstances, as well as the difficulties and insecurities emanating from within her, probably interfered with the full expression of her primary maternal preoccupation [4] and, even more, interfered with a full establishment of mutuality and reciprocity during the baby's symbiotic phase.

After the birth of this first child, Ellie suffered quite a bit from homesickness. She contemplated taking a trip home with her husband and

---

[2] The follow-up study was supported by the Margaret S. Mahler Psychiatric Research Foundation and was undertaken by Anna-Marie Sacramone.

leaving the baby behind with his grandmother. Her reason for contemplating this was that she worried that she and her husband would be unable to take care of him. She was afraid that the baby would be noisy and difficult. It was as if at that point she felt that she had to leave behind not only her baby, but the noisy, demanding, and needy part of herself if she were going to go back home to her parents. After some contemplation and encouragement from her parents not to leave her baby behind, she decided against the trip home.

Ellie then became deeply involved with her child. She made great efforts to please him and win him back from her mother-in-law. But she had great fears about not being competent as a mother, and therefore allowed her mother-in-law to do much of the caretaking, which consisted mostly of feeding the baby and putting him to sleep. She wrote: "Well, my baby gets more beautiful every day and he seems happier now than before (I hope I'm right). He even laughs out loud once in a while when I play with his hands. When I'm not busy with him, I make toys for him like stuffed animals and blocks."

Thus, Ellie began to take great pleasure in her child during the symbiotic phase, but did not fully feel herself to be his mother. As he began to grow up and move about, she became his faithful companion in his explorations. Contrary to the culture in which she lived, she encouraged his freedom from restraint, locomotor behavior, exploring, and playing with toys. She read to him and talked to him a lot, but she continued to leave some of the basic caretaking functions to her mother-in-law. Jamie's primary attachment seemed to be to his grandmother, whose bed he shared. Ellie often felt herself to be more like an older sister than a mother. She repeated some of her own mother's feelings about her when she was a baby — namely, the feeling of not being competent as a mother and a primary caretaker.

Recalling the isolation of her own childhood, Ellie felt very reassured and happy when Jamie started to relate to other children. Ellie was fearful of Jamie's aggressiveness, as well as of her own. She feared that the culture in which they lived allowed children to express their aggressive feelings too openly. She felt that her husband and mother-in-law tended to indulge all of Jamie's whims and desires.

Ellie took great pleasure in Jamie's developing language capacity, his musicality, his sensitivity, his brightness, and his warmheartedness.

Some of the more pathological aspects of Ellie's developing relationship to her child were her intense need for love and approval from him, and also her intense overprotectiveness because of her anxiety that harm could come to him. Although she was very involved with him and needy of his love and approval, there were times when she was not sensitive to his demands because she was too preoccupied with her own. During the period of Jamie's rapprochement struggles, Ellie became unhappy because there were times when she felt herself to be too impatient with him. She would lose her temper and then beg his forgiveness. When she had to be briefly hospitalized for a physical illness, she was delighted that Jamie cried for her. She believed that this was proof that he loved and missed her.

When Jamie was 2 years old, Ellie became pregnant again. It was a planned pregnancy because she wanted Jamie to have a sibling to play with; she did not want him to have a lonely childhood like her own. She said that she wanted a daughter. "Maybe it's because I feel I could identify with her, and she'd be living or reliving my dream childhood, a normal, happy and easy childhood I wish I could have had myself. As for me, I try to identify with Jamie, but in vain because in spite of myself I can't help but think things are different for a boy, and that boys are somehow tougher." Ellie said that she felt perfectly comfortable discussing male genitals with her son, but imagining that she might have a daughter and need to discuss female genitals with a girl child made her blush. She enjoyed her pregnancy. She made romantic-looking maternity clothes and seemed to be able to enjoy her femininity more than ever before. At the same time, she said that Jamie needed her more than ever now that she was pregnant. She was very sensitive to Jamie's feelings about her pregnancy and the fact that he might feel left out once she had the baby. She planned to include him in baby care as much as possible.

Ellie's second child was a healthy baby girl named Mimi. She wrote: "She's the sweetest little baby in the world. In spite of difficult labor, I was really happy when I saw Mimi for the first time."

Ellie's mother came to help her at the time of the birth of her second child. She wanted to help Ellie have the opportunity to be the primary caretaker. She supported breast-feeding and supported Ellie in asserting herself as a mother to her mother-in-law and husband. Ellie truly appreciated her mother's help at that point and was sad when she left to go back to the United States. She wished her mother could have stayed longer, and she said: "At twenty-three I'm still a baby in many ways."

Ellie worried that she was more of a mother to Mimi than she had ever been to Jamie, and she said: "Because I breast-feed her and take almost complete responsibility for her care. Also, she's a girl, which in itself forms a unique bond between us. We are both females." She felt guilty about her older child, and she said that she tried not to look back but to see him as he is now and help him to become a secure person, "at least more secure than I was when I was a kid. I try to spend time with him, I try to be understanding, since I think that that's what Jamie needs."

Jamie was very attached to his father and Ellie tried to encourage him to be patient with Jamie as well. Ellie compared Jamie's sensitivity to her own as a child. She thought that he was very much the way she had been. Although she thought that she identified more easily with her daughter, she, in fact, strongly identified with her older child. She could not bear to take him to the doctor's office because, she said, "I get upset when I hear little kids crying. In fact, I get so caught up in the crying child's emotion that I often find myself on the verge of crying myself." She was acutely aware of reliving aspects of her own childhood memories of unhappiness and she was constantly concerned about providing a happier childhood for her children.

It seemed that Ellie saw herself in Jamie, and saw some of her own difficulties, sensitivities, and disagreeable qualities (e.g., her quick temper) repeated in him. Mimi, on the other hand, seems to have been experienced as the ideal child—the good child that she could not be herself. Through Mimi, Ellie seems to have found, at least for the moment, her lost, good baby- and childhood.

Ellie spoke lovingly of her husband, and felt that he was patient and kind. However, she was also aware of the fact that sometimes he treated her more as a child than as an adult partner, and that he tended at times to confide more in his mother than in her. Although she could not yet speak the language perfectly, she understood everything they said and realized that her husband often discussed serious matters with his mother rather than with her; this hurt her. Her reaction was to become more acutely aware of her own internal struggle, which she named the struggle between the child and the woman in her — the child was demanding, had a quick temper, and tended to be resentful; the woman was appreciative, patient, giving, and kind. She had high standards for herself and blamed herself for not being able to meet them.

When Ellie was an adolescent, she had seen her childhood illness as an angry turning away and escape from the realization that she could not be perfect. Now, as a mother, Ellie once again tried very hard to be perfect and suffered from the imperfections, vulnerabilities, and weaknesses she perceived in herself. It is impressive that at this time she no longer has to deal with these imperfections with denial, projection, and avoidance. She seems capable of genuine love and concern for her children. Her need for their love for her is very great, and so is her need to love them. As a

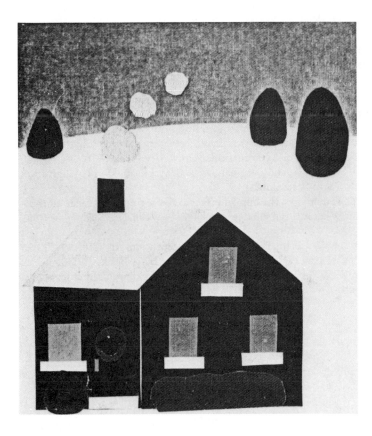

Fig. 2-8. *This recent handmade Christmas card from Ellie, although it does not contain people, seems nonetheless very much alive. The home does not look empty; it is well lit and warm, and the memory of the snow shows that Ellie still misses and thinks about home. This picture clearly reflects Ellie's sense of being a part of a family.*

mother, Ellie seems to relive and repair her own childhood. The pain of her childhood is forever vivid in her mind. Through the birth of her daughter, Ellie seems to have been able to experience a kind of rebirth; in nursing and caring for her baby girl, she experienced complete happiness and bliss, probably for the first time in her life. As her daughter has entered the separation-individuation phase, Ellie herself seems to be emerging stronger and a bit more rebellious, as well as eager to become more fully adult. She talks about wishing to take over more of the household chores, to be more of a companion to her husband, and, in general, to be more in charge of her life (Fig. 2-8).

Acknowledgment

The author wishes to thank David Pollens for his assistance in the preparation of this chapter.

References

1. Emde, R., Gaensbauer, T., and Harmon, R. Emotional expression in infancy: A biobehavioral study. *Psychological Issues, Monograph Series,* Vol. 10, Monograph No. 37. New York: International University Press, 1976.
2. Mahler, M. S., Pine, F., and Bergman, A. *The Psychological Birth of the Human Infant.* New York: Basic Books, 1975.
3. Resch, R. C. Hatching in the human infant as the beginning of separation-individuation: What it is and what it looks like. *Psychoanalytic Study of the Child* 34:421, 1979.
4. Winnicott, D. W. Primary Maternal Preoccupation. In *Collected Papers: Through Paediatrics to Psycho-analysis.* New York: Basic Books, 1958.
5. Winnicott, D. W. The Use of an Object and Relating through Identifications. In *Playing and Creativity.* London: Tavistock, 1971. Pp. 86–94.

3

Generational repetition of the maltreatment of children

Brandt F. Steele

Several of Therese Benedek's classic papers concerning the early mother-infant interaction and the dynamics of parenting provide much of the framework for our understanding of the disturbed patterns of care observed in cases of child abuse [1, 2, 3, 4]. Our studies through the years have amply illustrated and validated the concepts she developed in her pioneering work; this chapter will indicate the continuing pertinence of her ideas in the exploration and understanding of an intriguing aspect of the child maltreatment syndrome, namely, the recurrence of maltreatment in successive generations.

Parents and other caretakers who have neglected or abused the infants or children in their charge commonly give a history of having been significantly deprived or neglected with or without accompanying physical abuse in their own early years [15, 33, 34, 35]. In our own experience it has been rare in any thoroughly studied case not to obtain such a history. The same phenomenon has been noted by other investigators, although some observers have not been so impressed by its frequency [6, 23, 25, 30, 31]. Undoubtedly there are some child abusers who were not maltreated in their early lives, but lack of such a history is most often due to other factors. Occasionally there is a true amnesia for early life events that is alleviated only after considerable therapy, at which time specific details of abuse are clearly recalled. More common is a simple denial of abuse, but on further questioning about family discipline, the explanation is brought forward that frequent, severe beating with belts or whips could not be called "abuse" because it was deserved punishment for bad behavior. More attention has been drawn to the history of physical abuse than emotional abuse because it can be more clearly pictured. It is easy to describe beatings, bruises, lacerations, burns, and fractures. On the other hand, the history of neglect and emotional deprivation is more difficult to elicit. It tends to be more vague, often more difficult to put in clear words, and it is related to a pervasive, negative atmosphere as well as to specific events.

Early deprivation is described in many ways: feelings of never having

121

been really loved or cared about; the sense of never really being listened to or heard; rarely feeling close to anyone; an inability to recall much real pleasure; feeling unwanted, empty, and lonely since the beginning. Although such feelings may be expressed by many unhappy people, they are significantly more intense, more pervasive, more persistent, and of an earlier origin in child abusers. In addition to the picture of a generally bleak emotional environment, their histories may reveal more concrete factors such as grinding poverty, parental alcoholism, drug taking and depression, multiple foster-care placements, frequent change of residence, and lack of loving relatives or friends. We consider neglect more important than the physical abuse that overshadows it.

Physical abuse would not occur if the caretaker did not lack adequate empathy for the state and needs of the child and neglect his or her welfare. Deficient empathy is a common denominator in the background of all types of maltreatment. The relative significance of abuse and neglect was clearly stated to me by a man who had seriously injured his two baby sons. He said, "I could understand and forgive my father in a way for beating me with boards because he thought he was doing the right thing, but I can never get over the idea that my mother wouldn't protect me." For this man, as for many others, it was much easier to describe the attack than to tell how much love was not there.

The phenomenon of generational repetition in matters of child care is not in itself unusual. It seems that most patterns of caretaking, either good or bad, tend to be similar in each succeeding generation. Parents bring up their own children in much the same way they, themselves, were reared. Two main streams of influence enter into this repetition of child care patterns. One is the general influence of the beliefs and behaviors of the society and culture into which the child is born. The other is the more specific influence of the child's individual caretakers during the dyadic relationships of the first months of life.

Cultural Influences
Culturally determined patterns of infant and child care are fairly obvious and are largely directed toward the "craft" of parenting (i.e., the more mechanical behaviors of feeding and clothing; carrying in arms, shawls, or baby carrier; types of food; types of toilet training). The knowledge of these patterns is gained by direct observation of child care of growing children, and often by experiences of direct involvement in child care during such activities as baby-sitting. New parents are also molded into

cultural patterns by knowledge of child care and advice given them by older authorities including their own parents (especially mothers), in-laws, midwives, nurses, doctors, and baby books. These influences on baby care may change in detail from time to time according to fads, technology, or "scientific" theories. Common patterns of dressing babies have changed from frocks and gowns for babies of either sex to pants, T-shirts, and overalls for both boys and girls. Feeding patterns may change from breast to bottle and back to breast; cloth diapers often are replaced by disposable diapers. None of these factors seems to have a real bearing on the abuse of children, but there are other cultural factors that do.

The belief in the value of punishment as an essential tool of proper child rearing has been pervasive since our earliest history, especially in Western culture. It provides the rationale for physical punishment of children and also the means of rationalizing and excusing the injuries of children by maltreating parents. Certain religiously based beliefs in the innate sinfulness of children are used as a justification for severe physical punishment. Parents have frequently quoted to us passages in the Bible that support the concept of "Spare the rod and spoil the child" [26]. There are still occasional reports in the press of children dying as the result of beatings administered with excessive zeal during cultist exorcism of evil spirits that have possessed the children. There are also laws that provide parents with not only the right but also the duty to properly discipline their children as a means of ensuring good behavior.

Although maltreatment of children may occur in successive generations of people exposed to these cultural patterns, the influence of culture does not seem to be crucial or very significant considering that only a minority of people so exposed show the maltreatment behavior. While it is statistically true that abuse and neglect of children are reported more commonly among families of lower socioeconomic levels living with the problems of poverty, unemployment, poor housing, and core city decay [36], these adverse living conditions do not seem to be necessary and sufficient causes for the abusive patterns; only a minority of such unfortunate people significantly abuse their offspring. It is also well known that abuse and neglect occur in all socioeconomic levels with all varieties of religious beliefs or ideology and from all kinds of cultures and subcultures. In short, while cultural patterns, subcultural patterns, and social factors may have a significant effect on many patterns of general child care and parenting behaviors, they are not able to account for the occurrence of maltreatment patterns in specific family constellations.

Individual Caretakers

The origin of the maltreatment syndrome seems to reside in the very early idiosyncratic caretaking interactions during the earliest months and years of life. The kind of care given by the individual caretakers has an earlier, more profound effect on the child's development than do elements that appear later when the child leaves the confines of the family and is exposed to the larger world of neighborhood, school, and society.

The basic patterns of "mothering" or "mothercrafting" can be learned and carried out by almost any adult or older child of either sex. It is not a gender-linked, biological function, nor is it an expression of a "maternal instinct." Fathers, other males, and unrelated females can all provide good "mothering" to natural, adopted, or unrelated babies and children. The more subtle aspects of parenting — the empathic awareness of an infant's state and needs and the corresponding ability to respond appropriately — are not transmitted intergenerationally through cultural or social channels. These qualities that we call "motherliness" and that Winnicott [39] described as "good enough mothering" are acquired during the ongoing interactions of individual baby and caretaker, beginning with the first contacts after birth and continuing through ensuing months for years. Benedek has emphasized the intense ongoing, repetitive interactions in the mother-infant dyad during the baby's early postnatal life in what she called the "symbiotic" phase [2]. It is out of the matrix of this early stage when the infant has not yet separated from the caretaker that the early primitive identifications begin to develop; they will be enhanced and consolidated by later experiences in the dyad. Benedek [4] ascribes the origins of parenting behavior back to this early period.

Becoming a parent arouses two kinds of memories, largely unconscious. One is of what it was like to be a child; the other is of how one was cared for. These two identifications determine the caretaking behavior of the new parent. This phenomenon described so clearly by Benedek provides the central core of the generational transmission of child abuse patterns. If the experiences of early life were good, the parent repeats good caretaking with the new baby; if the early life was fraught with neglect and abuse, neglect and abuse will be repeated in the pattern of child care in later life.

The early "incorporative" identifications with the libidinal object of the oral phase are not the same as those identifications that occur in later phases of the child's life (e.g., during the resolution of the oedipal conflict). Sigmund Freud [8] described them as being different from the identifications occurring in mourning in which "an object cathexis has been replaced by identification." He wrote:

We must also take into consideration cases of simultaneous object cathexis and identification cases, that is in which the alteration of character occurred before the object has been given up.

In the individual's primitive oral phase object cathexis and identification are, no doubt, indistinguishable from each other.

This same process in terms more relevant to the problems of child maltreatment was described by Anna Freud [7] as it occurs in the earliest mother-infant interaction.

Due to their inability to care for themselves, infants and children have to put up with whatever care is given them. Where child management is not extremely sensitive, this causes a number of disturbances, the earliest of which are usually centered around sleep, feeding, elimination, and the wish for company. Inconsiderate handling of the infant's early needs has some further repercussions for pathological development.

In his growth toward independence and self reliance, a child accepts the mother's initial gratifying or frustrating attitude as a model which he imitates and recreates in his own ego. Where she understands, respects, and satisfies his wishes as far as possible, there are good chances that his ego will show equal tolerance. Where she unnecessarily delays, denies, and disregards wish fulfillment, his ego is likely to develop more of the so-called "hostility toward the id," that is, a readiness for internal conflict, which is one of the prerequisites of neurotic development.

The poorly cared for infant is provided with ample opportunity to recreate in his own developing ego hostile caretaking attitudes as well as a hostile attitude toward him- or herself.

Although aggression is obviously involved in all maltreatment, there is no good evidence of an unduly strong aggressive drive present in child abusers, nor any other evidence of common genetic, hormonal, or organic reasons for aggressive discharge. Rather, maltreatment is related to two types of identification with the early-life caretakers. The more obvious one, of course, is that of identification with the aggressor. The other is a more subtle and earlier identification with aggression itself. As noted above, Anna Freud described how the caretaker's attitude is taken in and made part of the infant's developing ego; it is a common observation that an infant tends to resonate with the mood of the caretaking mother, be it positive or negative. Spitz [32] discussed the relationship of affective states in the child to those of the mother.

The mother's depressive mood generates in the child an inclination toward depressive tendencies. The depressed mother retreats from the child and the child, in Anna Freud's words, "follows her into the depressive mood."

Anna Freud [7] made it clear that she considers this phenomenon to be in the nature of

. . . infection and that it is not an imitation of the mother's gestures that produced this mood in the child. The child simply responds to the affective climate, not to the cause of the affect. He is thus infected by the affective climate.

Just as infants respond to maternal depressive affect, it seems likely that infants exposed to repeated aggressive behavior on the part of their caretakers develop a proneness to the expression of anger and aggression that can be released under appropriate stimulation at any time later in life. This fundamental "identification with aggression" is established in the ego before the infant's object relations have developed to the point in the second year of life when he can identify with the aggressor. The latter is considered to be one of the early elements entering into the formation of the superego and it is not surprising that maltreating parents, identifying with the aggressive behavior of their own parents, often show a very righteous attitude about their punitive behavior. A beautiful example of this is a letter written by Henry IV of France to Madame de Montglat who was in charge of the nursery where the infant dauphin (Louis XIII) was being cared for [12].

I have a complaint to make: you do not send word that you whipped my son. I wish and command you to whip him every time he is obstinate or misbehaves, knowing well for myself that there is nothing in the world which will better him than that. I know it from experience, having myself profited, for when I was his age I was often whipped. That is why I want you to whip him and to make him understand why.

Another aspect of the internalization of the affect expressed by parents during caretaking activities is the infant's basic acquisition of the quality of empathy. The empathic talent that we call "motherliness" is acquired by the experience of being empathically cared for in the first few months of life, as has been described by Kohut [16] and Olden [21, 22]. Deficiency in the empathic mothering experience during infancy results in the lack of empathic ability to care for an infant in later life. Inability to be empathic is probably more basic in all forms of child maltreatment than is the release of aggression. It is in the background of all forms of maltreatment, whether they be aggressive physical abuse or the simple inability to care for infants manifested by neglect and failure to thrive. It is also lack of empathy that accounts for the fact that both male and female caretakers can be equally abusive and neglectful; both boy and girl babies can be equally exposed to unempathic caretaking in infancy and identify with it. Josselyn [14] wrote that the ability to show tenderness, gentleness, and empathy "is not a prerogative of women alone; it is a human characteristic."

Diminished capacity for empathy as a consequence of the lack of an empathic caretaker with whom to identify seems to remain unchanged unless in subsequent years a new, responsive, loving caretaker appears and remains for some time in the child's life. The original identifications with aggression and the aggressor may undergo some developmental changes. The element of retaliation or revenge against the parent as well as the suppression of such anger can be seen in toddlers.

Dicky, age 2 years, 8 months, was observed as his mother yanked him out from under the kitchen table and spanked him with a very hard swing. When she turned her back to pull a younger brother, Carl, from under the table, Dicky raised his arm in anger as if to strike her. Then he stopped, brought his arm down slowly and barely touched her. Later he went outdoors without permission and she chased after him. He dropped a plastic pail, causing her to trip and fall; it appeared to be deliberate. Dicky also hits Carl and bites him.

In somewhat older children we can see evidence of the aggression being directed toward a baby in a fashion quite like the adult abuser.

Johnny was born while his mother was feeling lonely and abandoned by her husband and mother. She had a cesarean section for pre-eclampsia, was sick, did not attach well to her baby, was depressed, and had trouble caring for him. During his first year he did not thrive well, and she often shook, choked, or bruised him in her frustration over his poor responses. Two years later after psychotherapy she delivered a girl under much better circumstances and was a very good mother. When Johnny was 4½ and his sister was 2, he became angry at her, choked her, and shook her. Mother asked him why he did it and he answered quite simply, "Mommy, that's what you used to do to me."

In older children and adults the residual aggressive drive for revenge is usually displaced onto other adults or offspring and is manifested as delinquent behavior, rebellion against authority, or child abuse and neglect. Crying babies are often seen as frustrating the parents' need for love and sense of competence or as embodying their own critical scolding parent, and aggression is released against them in retaliation. We have also seen abusive parents who as teenagers exploded on a few occasions with violent physical attacks on their own maltreating parents; in a few instances, this has gone as far as parricide. In all such cases, there is the common denominator of lack of empathy for the human being who is attacked.

The time of birth and the ensuing weeks and months of dyadic caretaker interaction seem to be the pivotal periods in which the psychological influences essential for maltreatment are transmitted to the next generation [10, 20, 24]. It is then that the crucial ability or inability to be empathic will be established. Maltreatment syndromes can in one sense be considered a disorder of attachment. An unempathic mother cannot attach well to her baby; the baby grows up to be an unempathic parent who does not attach well to his or her children, and the cycle is repeated. The process begins, however, much earlier — certainly as soon as pregnancy is confirmed and parenthood will be a reality. The parents' hopes and fears for the future child will be highly colored by their memories of childhood and of being parented, as Benedek described. A kind of tripartite "identity" state occurs with elements of three generations that are not completely integrated. While present in the father, it is more clear in the mother whose baby in utero is both a part of her and a separate being. This "fluid identification" can be astoundingly apparent in its distorted form in maltreatment situations. Penny, the mother of Johnny previously described, suddenly developed acute anxiety during her second pregnancy and told me, "If it's a boy, I know now how to take care of him. But if it's a girl, I'm likely to treat it the way mother treated me, and she'll be angry at me as much as I'm angry at mother. It will be a mess." These interlocking identifications as herself, her mother, and her baby occur in all mothers, but fortunately are healthy in most families and only cause trouble if the original objects of identification are unempathic and abusive or neglectful. The misperception of the baby as a reincarnation of the bad childhood is a common feature in maltreatment. Common expressions are, "He's as bad as I was when I was a kid" and "She looks like me, poor kid."

During a woman's pregnancy, her longing and need for her own mother is heightened, and the relationship between them, both past and present, has a deep influence on the mother's attitude toward her unborn child. Benedek [5] elaborates on this point.

The prospective grandmother remembers not only her pregnancies but she recalls what her own mother told her about childbearing. It is not unusual that the "expectant" grandmother in her wish to protect her daughter, conveys her anxieties to the pregnant woman. (P. 406)

In the same vein, Jessner and associates [13] call attention to the strong revival during pregnancy of the mother's relationship to her own mother. She is flooded with memories that may be either pleasant or horrifying and result in either enhancement of positive identifications or a struggle against negative ones. Bertie provides an example of this [35].

Bertie had often been told by her mother how she had "ruined" her mother's marriage because father began drinking and being unfaithful during the pregnancy, and how she had ruined mother's body during a difficult delivery. The labor had been long and painful and dismemberment of the baby had been considered. Mother often showed Bertie the scar of an operation allegedly done to repair the damage. Mother had rarely been warm or close to Bertie and had routinely physically abused her by whipping with a razor strop and coat hangers. During Bertie's pregnancy her mother repeated these stories to her and she dreamed of having a girl who would take her husband away from her, ruin her pelvis, and make her unattractive. She occasionally expressed a wish that the baby would die, wondered how soon she could start spanking it and thought of giving it away. Her labor and delivery were difficult, painful, and deeply resented. At age one month, her baby girl's femur was broken, and at age 3 months there was a fractured skull with subdural hematomas. Bertie was particularly vulnerable because of the wish and need for maternal closeness which is a normal aspect of pregnancy, but which led her back into the early identifications with a punitive, unempathic mother and into the identification of her baby in utero and after birth as a reincarnation of her own "bad self." She clearly depicts the two "memories" and identifications described by Benedek. During her pregnancy and in the period after delivery she regressed and revived the residues of early life experience and reenacted the behavior of her mother. (P. 110)

The early primitive identification with the caretaking parent can be repressed and intellectually denied or counteracted, only to surface later as a response to becoming a parent and experiencing the stresses of infant care. This is exemplified in the not unusual statement we hear from young people, "I will never treat my children the way I was treated as a child." However, after a brief period of trying to be more kindly parents, they regress under the frustrations of baby care and revert to the abusive, neglectful patterns of their own parents. Credence in the importance of the early identifications is illustrated by the following example of an opposite form of the process.

A wealthy young woman described a totally socially conforming life of going by the rules since early childhood, and could recall only aloof formality in relationship to both parents. She went to proper schools, met the proper people, went to the proper functions, and married a proper young man. All of her relationships including that with her husband were quite correct, but were superficial, cool, and devoid of any deep sense of pleasure, commitment, or true interest. She became pregnant and was somewhat puzzled and anxious over feelings of being rather deeply involved with her unborn child. After delivery she was astounded and overwhelmed by feelings of love and closeness to her baby. These were feelings that she was not aware she was capable of having. She then began to recall memories of how as a little girl she had been extremely happy and closely involved with a beloved nurse-governess who had cared for her from birth on and of happy, warm relationships with maids, the cook, and the chauffeur. She further recalled that her father and particularly her mother had told her before she started in kindergarten that she must never again feel close to these servants — that she, herself, was of an upper class and should never have anything more to do with these other lower grade people. When her own baby was born, in a regressive identification with her good, earliest caretakers and love objects, she became an excellent, empathic mother.

Sexual Abuse

Clinically, sexual abuse is a much more complex problem than neglect or physical abuse, although the three may coexist in various combinations or occur quite separately. The sexual abuse may be either heterosexual or homosexual with children of any age from infancy through adolescence, and the type of activity may be anything from simple touching and fondling to genital intercourse, all kinds of perversions, incest, and rape. Despite this broad spectrum of behaviors, the sexual abuser shows basic characteristics similar to those who neglect or physically abuse, which is not surprising considering there is often an overlapping of the different kinds of maltreatment.

Most obvious is the sexual abuser's lack of empathic concern for the age, state, needs, and appropriate interests of the child; the sexual activity is in the service of satisfying the adult's need while exploiting the vulnerable child's obedience, helplessness, and malleability. Like other maltreaters, sexual abusers commonly give histories of unempathic care with neglect or physical abuse in their early lives [11, 19, 29, 37, 38]. More specifically, a majority of perpetrators have themselves been sexually abused as children or have witnessed a great deal of sexual exploitation or chaotic sexual activity in their childhood homes [9, 17, 18, 27, 28, 40].

The generational repetition of sexual abuse may be largely that of a rationalized imitative behavior, exemplified by variations of the often heard statement, "My father had sex with all my sisters, so why should I not do the same with my daughters?" Sometimes there is an almost uncanny repetition of the early life experience as when a father seduces his son or stepson at exactly the same age and in the same way as he, himself, was seduced by his father in childhood. Frequent, but more complex and less well understood, is the more or less unconscious, and often denied, complicity in subtly allowing, condoning, or instigating incest or other abuse by a spouse, other relative, or persons outside the family. Fathers may surreptitiously encourage sons in such behaviors through covert interest or amusement while overtly condemning sexual activity. Some mothers, despite dismay and anger at their own experience of incest with their fathers, seem unable to protect a daughter and behave in such a way as to permit or promote the sexual exploitation of the daughter by the husband or others. For instance, a woman who was furious at her father and her unprotective mother because of being subjected to incest in her early teens, nevertheless sent her 14-year-old daughter to spend summer vacations with the grandfather, who had "promised to be good." The daughter was sexually exploited and the mother was again outraged.

The overt behavior of the sexual abuser seems to be determined to a large extent by knowledge gained in later childhood and adolescence through cognitive learning from observation, social learning, and role models. There is always, however, the inevitable underlying matrix of lack of empathy and of aggressive tendencies, residual from the inadequate care of earliest life and the identification with the caretakers of that time. Present also are the complex psychodynamics of the various perversions and paraphilias related to individual distortions and conflicts during psychosexual development, which are described in the standard psychiatric and psychoanalytic literature. Particularly prominent is the sexualization of aggressive drives, which channels the aggression that is released because of lack of empathy into the sexual sphere and reaches the extreme form of rape. Throughout the tragedies of sexual maltreatment run the threads of various levels of identification with the caretakers of the previous generation in their unempathic and aggressive attitudes.

Summary

In understanding the generational repetition of patterns of child maltreatment, the individual's identification with caretakers during the earliest months of life is crucial and most basic. It is more important in determining subsequent parenting patterns than are the later enhancing and channeling influences of social and cultural factors and cognitively learned behaviors. The most significant core identification is with the unempathic, depriving, insensitive attitude of the parent, to which identifications with aggression and with the aggressor are added. From this foundation, established during earliest experiences in the infant-caretaker dyad, arise the later maladaptive parenting behaviors of neglect, physical abuse, and sexual exploitation of infants and children.

References

1. Benedek, T. Adaptation to reality in early infancy. *Psychoanal. Q.* 7:200, 1938.
2. Benedek, T. The psychosomatic implications of the primary unit: Mother-child. *Am. J. Orthopsychiatry* 19:642, 1949.
3. Benedek, T. Psychobiological aspects of mothering. *Am. J. Orthopsychiatry* 26:272, 1956.
4. Benedek, T. Parenthood as a developmental phase: A contribution to the libido theory. *J. Am. Psychoanal. Assoc.* 7:389, 1959.
5. Benedek, T. *Psychoanalytic Investigations.* New York: Quadrangle, 1973. P. 406.
6. Curtis, G. Violence breeds violence—perhaps? *Am. J. Psychiatry* 120:386, 1963.
7. Freud, A. *Normality and Pathology in Childhood.* New York: International Universities Press, 1965. Pp. 155–157.
8. Freud, S. The Ego and the Id. In J. Strachey (Ed.), *The Standard Edition of the Complete Works of Sigmund Freud.* London: Hogarth, 1961. Vol. 19, pp. 28–30.
9. Gebhard, P. H., Gagnon, G. H., and Pomeroy, W. B. *Sex Offenders: An Analysis of Types.* New York: Harper and Row, 1965.
10. Gray, J., Cutler, C., Dean, J., and Kempe, C. H. Perinatal Assessment of Mother-Baby Interaction. In R. E. Helfer and C. H. Kempe (Eds.), *Child Abuse and Neglect. The Family and the Community.* Cambridge, Mass: Ballinger, 1976.
11. Hartogs, R. Discipline in the early life of sex-delinquents and sex-criminals. *The Nervous Child* 9:167, 1951.
12. Hunt, D. *Parents and Children in History.* New York: Basic Books, 1970. P. 135.
13. Jessner, L., Weigert, E., and Foy, J. The Development of Parental Attitudes during Pregnancy. In E. J. Anthony and T. Benedek (Eds.), *Parenthood: Its Psychology and Psychopathology.* Boston: Little, Brown, 1970.
14. Josselyn, I. Cultural forces, motherliness and fatherliness. *Am. J. Orthopsychiatry* 26:264, 1956.
15. Kempe, C. H., Silverman, F. N., Steele, B. F., et al. The battered-child syndrome. *J.A.M.A.* 181:17, 1962.
16. Kohut, H. Forms and transformations of narcissism. *J. Am. Psychoanal. Assoc.* 14:243, 1966.
17. Langsley, D. G., Schwartz, M. N., and Fairbairn, R. H. Father-son incest. *Compr. Psychiatry* 9:218, 1968.
18. Lukianowicz, N. Incest. *Br. J. Psychiatry* 120:301, 1972.
19. Lustig, N., Dresser, J. W., and Spellman, S. W. Incest: A family group survival pattern. *Arch. Gen. Psychiatry* 14:31, 1966.
20. Lynch, M., and Roberts, J. Predicting child abuse: Signs of bonding failure in the maternity hospital. *Br. Med. J.* [Clin. Res.] 1:624, 1977.

21. Olden, C. On adult empathy with children. *Psychoanal. Study Child* 8:111, 1953.

22. Olden, C. Notes on the development of empathy. *Psychoanal. Study Child* 13:505, 1958.

23. Oliver, J. E., and Taylor, A. Five generations of ill-treated children in one family pedigree. *Br. J. Psychiatry* 119:552, 1971.

24. Ounsted, C., Oppenheimer, R., and Lindsay, J. Aspects of bonding failure: The psychopathology and psychotherapeutic treatment of families of battered children. *Dev. Med. Child Neurol.* 16:447, 1974.

25. Parke, R. D., and Collmer, C. W. *Child Abuse: An Interdisciplinary Analysis.* Chicago: University of Chicago Press, 1975.

26. Proverbs XIII:24, XXIII:13-14.

27. Raphling, D. L., Carpenter, B. L., and Davis, A. Incest: A genealogical study. *Arch. Gen. Psychiatry* 16:505, 1967.

28. Raybin, J. B. Homosexual incest. *J. Nerv. Ment. Dis.* 148:105, 1969.

29. Reimer, S. A research note on incest. *Am. J. Sociology* 45:566, 1940.

30. Silver, L. B., Dublin, C. C., and Lourie, R. S. Does violence breed violence? Contributions from a study of the child abuse syndrome. *Am. J. Psychiatry* 126:404, 1969.

31. Spinetta, J. J., and Rigler, D. The child-abusing parent: A psychological review. *Psychol. Bull.* 77:296, 1972.

32. Spitz, R. *The First Year of Life.* New York: International Universities Press, 1965. P. 259.

33. Steele, B. F. Parental Abuse of Infants and Small Children. In E. J. Anthony and T. Benedek (Eds.), *Parenthood: Its Psychology and Psychopathology.* Boston: Little, Brown, 1970.

34. Steele, B. F. Psychodynamic Factors in Child Abuse. In C. H. Kempe and R. E. Helfer (Eds.), *The Battered Child* (3rd ed.). Chicago: University of Chicago Press, 1980.

35. Steele, B. F., and Pollock, C. B. A Psychiatric Study of Parents Who Abuse Infants and Small Children. In R. E. Helfer and C. H. Kempe (Eds.), *The Battered Child.* Chicago: University of Chicago Press, 1968.

36. Straus, M. A. Family patterns and child abuse in a nationally representative sample. *Child Abuse and Neglect* 3:213, 1979.

37. Weiner, I. B. Father-daughter incest: A clinical report. *Psychiatr. Q.* 36:607, 1962.

38. Weiner, I. B. On incest: A survey. *Excerpt. Criminol.* 4:137, 1964.

39. Winnicott, D. W. Ego Integration in Child Development. In D. W. Winnicott (Ed.), *The Maturational Processes and the Facilitating Environment.* New York: International Universities Press, 1965.

40. Yorokoglu, A., and Kemph, J. P. Children not severely damaged by incest with parent. *J. Am. Acad. Child Psychiatry* 51:111, 1966.

II
The parental experience

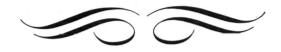

4

The flow of empathy and trust between mother and child

Judith S. Kestenberg

Modern infant research has discovered many differentiated cognitive apparatuses in the newborn and young infant. However, it has not disproved that symbiotic dual unity [22] is the precursor of love. Within the dual unit, mother and child resonate, attune to one another, and regulate the child's input and output. The resonance initiates maternal [21] and infantile empathy, while the regulation of input and output creates the basis for mutual trust [5]. No doubt, these mechanisms develop even before the symbiotic phase, but they blossom forth when an intrinsic unity between mother and child is established. Empathy and trust develop further, coming to a new peak in the rapprochement subphase when emotional and cognitive aspects of togetherness and separateness converge [7, 17, 22]. Within the first two years, the early affective contagion [11] and communing [16, 17] become transformed into a higher form of empathy, and the early mutuality develops further into a confident expectation that maternal presence will bring comfort. Without going into details regarding the later phases of empathy and trust, suffice it to say that later identifications are based on empathy, and constant relationships are based on trust.

Kohut [21] speaks of a primary empathy with the mother that prepares us for the recognition that the basic inner experiences of our children remain similar to our own. Buie [3] is convinced that the event necessary for the initiation of the empathic process is perception through ordinary sensory input. Insofar as the organs through which we perceive are functional before birth, we can assume that a sensorimotor apparatus is available from the start that permits the transmission of movement qualities and underlying feelings such as changes in the degree and type of tension. Tension-flow rhythms are comparable to the rhythmic vibration of musical tones that initiate a resonant response. The dual unity of

This is the fourth in the series of papers "Prevention, Infant Therapy, and the Treatment of Adults." For "Prevention, Infant Therapy, and the Treatment of Adults" Parts I and II, see reference [18]. For Part III, see Call, J., and Galenson, E. (Eds.). *Frontiers in Infant Psychiatry.* New York: Basic Books, 1982.

mother and child is comparable to the dual unity of musical instruments with their two distinct components: vibrator and resonator.

Buie distinguishes several factors in empathy; among them are resonance and imaginative imitation [3]. Sigmund Freud [9] spoke of a path that ". . . leads from identification by way of imitation to empathy . . ." (p. 110). Fenichel [6] defined empathy as "narcissistic identification" in which the subject takes over the object's expressive movement, and Shapiro [26] referred to empathy as based on the child's reading of the mother's face. Although tension changes are perceived visually, it is hardly possible to imitate them; they can be reproduced from visual perception by way of remembering the resonant response to touching another person whose tension flow made our own body vibrate. The principal apparatus for the conveying of moods via mirroring and imitation is the flow of shape; it is the basis of our expressiveness.

The knowledge we gain from perceiving the tension changes of another person pertains to such feelings as tension, calmness, or impulsiveness. These and other basic feeling states represent the gamut of the organism's responses to safety and danger, but they do not convey the processes involved in relatedness to others. The impressions we have from assessing tension changes are akin to intuition. The simultaneous changes in the shape of the body, especially the face (e.g., its broadening to smile and its narrowing to frown), are the formal elements from which we infer whether a person is happy or angry. Empathy utilizes tension-flow changes to feel what the other person feels. Our innate understanding of changes in the configuration of the face and body makes it possible for us to infer the meaning of these feelings.

Buie [3] describes patients who strain the limits of our empathy. Some become rigid and do not allow their flow of empathy to be mobilized; others are distrustful and fail to give the right cues for our understanding of them. Longitudinal observation of mothers and babies led Kestenberg and Buelte [18] to believe that empathy thrives on tension-flow attunement, and trust is transmitted via mirroring of shape flow. However, these processes cannot develop without the conditions of mutual holding and support that Winnicott [32] refers to as the "holding environment." Empathy and trust in the therapeutic holding environment differ from their precursors in the mother-child milieu. Although they originate in this milieu, they are sustained by higher ego functions such as judgment and reasoning.

In this chapter, I describe the apparatuses of tension and shape flow, which underlie empathy and trust respectively, and give examples of failure in empathy and trust to illustrate the distinction.[1] Excerpts are given from the psychoanalysis of a mother whose difficulty in understanding her young children was explored in depth and who was enriched by insights derived from the observation of her tension and shape changes. The dependence of these rhythms on the feeling of being held and supported are briefly elucidated. A glossary of movement terms is provided at the end of the chapter.

Tension Flow and Empathy

When we speak of tension, we do not mean the tension of psychoanalytic usage, which refers to the discrepancy between the intensity of the drive and its fulfillment. To us, tension pertains to the elasticity of our tissues, and its qualities reflect the changes and sequences in neuronal innervation. Free flow of tension reflects the facilitation of neuronal transmission, and bound flow reflects its inhibition. Free flow initiates movement and promotes continuity of motion; bound flow effects cessation of movement and thus promotes discontinuity. Free flow in muscle action results from a lack of restraint by antagonistic muscles; bound flow results from the simultaneous action of agonists and antagonists. Changes in tension are mediated by the gamma system. Spindle stimulations are relayed via the reticular zone to the hypothalamus. The connection to the centers of breathing and to those regulating emotions appears to be established after birth.[2]

The simplest form of a tension-flow rhythm is sucking, in which free and bound flow alternate. An attunement between the infant's sucking rhythm and the mother's rhythm of milk excretion results in the free-flow pumping of the breast and simultaneous milk secretion, which is followed by bound flow during swallowing and a simultaneous stoppage of milk flow. If this attunement is out of kilter, the child may gulp, cough, or be unsuccessful while pumping. Such a failure often forebodes a failure in mutual empathy, at least during the early oral phase of development.

---

[1] In the following sections only the basic apparatus of tension flow and shape flow as the core of empathy and trust are discussed. For the ego-controlled motor apparatuses that mature later and are operative in the cognitive aspects of these processes, see Kestenberg and Buelte [18].

[2] The reticular zone is also responsible for changes in alertness, which manifest themselves in tension changes and in related alterations in the autonomous nervous system. High tension in the contractile tissues of blood vessels has an adverse effect on circulation. Binding of tension in the contractile excretory ducts, such as the mammary ducts, can stop the flow of the secretion.

The affects that emerge from experiencing free and bound flow are characterized by the alternation of a feeling of freedom or safety and a feeling of impending danger. Bound flow inhibits us, giving a signal that mobility is to be curtailed. In addition to these two basic tension elements, there are six attributes, called intensity factors. Three of these signal safety for leisure.

1. Adjustment of tension levels, as can be seen in a cat's response to rubbing and in all activities that give subtlety to changes in feelings.
2. Decreasing tension to a low level, as in abatement of excitement or relief.
3. Gradual increase or decrease of tension, as seen in deliberate actions and leisurely walks.

The other three intensity factors signal that preparedness for action is needed.

1. Keeping tension on an even level, as a cat does before pouncing.
2. Increasing tension to a high level, as seen in rapidly mounting excitement.
3. Abrupt increase or decrease of tension, as in startles, surprise attacks, and quickness of reflexes.

There are countless combinations of tension-flow attributes, and there are countless sequences and intervals between changes. Certain combinations of attributes prevail in specific rhythms (e.g., even flow in high intensity that is seen in straining). Intrinsic to all rhythms are qualities that evoke certain affective tones and are evoked by these affects. For instance, even flow suggests indifference or poise; feeling unruffled will express itself in keeping the level of tension on an even keel. Flow adjustment is associated with shyness and flirtatiousness; high intensity with anger or anxiety; low intensity with calm or soothing; abruptness with impatience; and graduality with patience and leisureliness.

The popular view of the empathic mother is that she knows almost telepathically how the child feels; she provides relief without excitement or impatience with the irritable or "colicky" infant. This view is not accurate. To know how the child feels, the mother must attune to him or her and resonate his or her high tension and abruptness, not only his or her low tension and graduality. Although the empathic mother becomes excited with her excited child, this alone would only constitute a state of contagion. Once she feels how high the child's tension has risen, she can begin to lower it. The baby feels her resonance, and it is only then that he or she can accept a change in lead and allow the mother's lowered tension to resonate with his or hers.

When two people attune, one is usually the leader and the other the follower, but they can change positions in midstream. When the attunement proceeds, we do not expect a complete synchronicity or exactly the same degree of tension. Synchrony and sameness occur with regard to certain elements, but not all. Vennard, a voice teacher [28], speaking of instruments says: "The resonator takes the product of the vibrator and increases (or decreases) its intensity or improves its timbre or both. Sometimes the line between these two elements of an instrument is hard to draw. This will not worry you if you remember that the resonator is really a secondary vibrator. One vibrator must dominate the other. If they are equally strong . . . more often than not they cancel each other out" (p. 15). At times, the resonator and the vibrator are out of phase, working against each other. A resonator may refuse to be the slave of the vibrator and may produce interference. In the language of mother-child interaction, we speak of clashes between them [19]. However, clashing is part and parcel of the interaction in which a mother calms the baby or vice versa. A clash occurs, for instance, when the mother lowers her tension while the infant's remains high. If the mother lowers her tension gradually, there comes a point at which the baby follows suit, and a harmony between their tension qualities can be reestablished. A feeling of sameness is recreated that is an intrinsic aspect of empathy.

Clashing that is not followed by a reattunement creates battles between mother and infant. One can teach them to find a common denominator by "tuning" them to each other. This attunement is difficult to accomplish, however, when there is an interference within the transmission of flow through the body. This happens when certain parts of the body remain in a state of high tension (i.e., tension spots) or lose elasticity and remain in what we call "neutral" flow that gives the feeling of inanimateness (i.e., dead spots). Generally speaking, dead spots are reminders of injuries, scars, or localized illness, and tension spots may build around them or in their vicinity as leftovers of emergency measures that continue to signal that inhibition is in order. Sometimes, such spots are located in the neck or shoulders, and they make mothers uncomfortable when they hold the baby. Under conditions of what could be called an empathic alliance, babies can help relax their mothers' tension spots or animate the dead spots by rubbing and fingering them. Babies who are premature or suffer from birth injuries present difficulties in transmission of flow from the start. Frequent massage helps them to a better distribution of tension flow and circulation [25]. However, even under the best conditions the empathic alliance is not a perfect instrument. Normal maternal failure [30] is based on a breakdown in empathic communication.

Most people are not aware of the tension changes in themselves and others, but they do recognize their own affects and those of others without knowing that they have accomplished the recognition through attunement in tension flow. Certain conditions enhance attunement, and others diminish it. Pregnancy makes women more sensitive to the baby inside of them, and they are more likely to learn tension-flow notation in a shorter time than others [16].[3] Anger, defensiveness, fatigue, and illness all reduce one's ability to react to tension-flow changes in others [2].

The perception of tension changes is best achieved through touch and pressure, but one can also attune by responding to another person's intonation and the characteristic rhythms of his or her singing and speech [27]. It is also possible to attune visually, but this has to be learned via intersensory connections from touch to vision. This distance attunement becomes the basis of distance empathy [15], familiar to us from our therapeutic knowing of the patient's feelings. However, tension changes in the face observed at a distance are not, as we shall see, easily recognized unless they are mediated by changes in the shape of the face.

Winnicott's [30] idea that a mother will recognize and feel her baby's rhythms in a proper holding environment is derived from his observations of mothers actually holding babies. Holding is an act of taking possession, of being there and being available. When the holder allows the baby to use his reflexes to hold him or her, the baby, too, takes possession, is there, and becomes available. Using the metaphor of an instrument once more, we can point out that the vibrator and the resonator are contained in the instrument. They are held together by a framework that is the instrument's holding environment. When a mother has a problem holding the baby or allowing the baby to hold her and when a baby is unable to hold the mother, the conditions for attunement are not favorable [18]. Through the transitional loss of boundaries when free flow blurs them and through the reinstatement of boundaries through bound flow, the mother-child couple can transmit their feelings without running the danger of losing their individuality. The bliss of the early nursing situation comes from getting to know one another via the unob-

---

[3] Because people judge other people's feelings by their tension-flow rhythms, it is not surprising that quite a few researchers assign feeling tones to the fetus [29]. The less attuned a professional is, the more he or she is inclined to use mechanical, inanimate remedies to help a woman deliver.

structed transmission of the proper doses of safety and caution, facilitation, and inhibition. By holding one another, the partners discover where there is free passage of vibration and where there is an obstacle, such as tension spots or dead spots. Defensive people who keep their bodies largely rigid present an insurmountable obstacle to the sending and receiving of feelings.

Shape Flow

Buie [3] described two types of patients whose nonverbal communications do not reach us. One type blocks the cues so they cannot be transmitted, and the other miscues so that the therapist cannot make proper inferences from what he or she perceives. Patients who block the flow of tension underlying their feelings allow us to recognize the blockage but not the feelings that are defended against. The miscuer transmits his feelings, but does not allow us to make proper inferences from them. He or she may smile when unhappy or frown when cheerful. We cannot trust what the miscuer's body tells us. There is still another type who keeps a poker face while speaking; this noncuer's tension changes may be coming through, but we do not know what significance to attach to them because there is no change in the shape of body and face. Both the miscueing and noncueing patients are untrustworthy. They may be dependent on others, but nevertheless they do not trust them. The miscuer may be "deceitful"; the noncuer does not know how to trust or evoke trust in others.

The apparatus of shape flow is the conveyor of trust in the environment. It is the foremost vehicle of relatedness to others. The trustworthy parent is one who provides the nutrients for the child's body; the trustworthy child is one who takes them in and eliminates the waste. While the tension-flow apparatus is a kinesic reflection of the intensity and sequence of nervous impulses, shape flow is the visible reflection of our intake and output. The neuromuscular system is not directly dependent on the caretaker's actions. In fetal life all nutrients are provided by the mother; at birth the baby begins to control his or her own intake and output, but he or she continues to be dependent on nutrients from the environment. The shape-flow apparatus has many functions that all are programmed for interaction. It is most useful in the functions of respiration, alimentation, and expressiveness.

With the first intake of breath, the body grows in inhalation and shrinks in exhalation. These are the primary elements of the flow of shape. There is reason to believe that maternal respiration produces a very small rocking action in utero. This and the small inspiratory movements of the fetus provide a preparation for extrauterine life, when the mother's own respiration has a regulatory effect on that of the newborn. Leaning on the maternal chest, the baby feels the beating of the mother's heart and her breathing rhythm. Inhaling, they grow closer to one another; exhaling they separate, leaving a minute intermediate space between them [14, 31].

A coordination between tension flow and shape flow reflects the interaction of the reticular zones and the breathing centers. Inhalation is initiated by free flow; if the limit of expansion is reached, bound flow sets in to discontinue the motion, and reversal into free flow initiates shrinking and exhalation.[4] Bound flow and shrinking are maintained when noxious substances threaten to invade the respiratory system. The transmission of tension flow helps us to experience the feeling tones that go with respiration; the transmission of shape flow allows us to interpret these feelings and develop trust in ourselves and others.[5]

What we ordinarily call trust is composed of alternations between our anticipating something good to come to us from the environment and expecting relief when noxious substances leave our body or fail to reach us. Growing and taking in allows the salutary environmental substances to enter our body in comfort, whereas shrinking emerges from the discomfort of being exposed inside or outside to noxious substances or stimuli. The psychological attitude "trust" is born from the expectation that discomfort will be followed by relief or comfort. However, without the discomfort that precedes relief, the experience of comfort would not impinge on our consciousness. When a child is uncomfortable for too long, he or she loses trust in his environment and may assume a habitual shrunken body attitude [2].

Breath, especially inhalation, gives us support. Every action we take and every sentence we speak (and perhaps every thought we think) rides on the waves of breath. The proper regulation of breath intake and output regulates our behavior. This regulation is more complex than is the mere alternation between growing and shrinking. The following shape-flow attributes, which we call the dimensional factors, modulate our intake, output, and expressiveness: widening, as in smiling; narrowing, as in frowning; lengthening, as in beginning of laughter; shortening, as in the clenching of teeth; bulging, as in the ballooning out of a

---

[4] This version of coordination between tension flow and shape flow is more accurate than the one given in Kestenberg [14].
[5] The word "transpires" is derived from this experience.

satiated baby's belly; hollowing, as in doubling up or compressing the abdomen in pain.

We turn to salutary stimuli and shrink from noxious stimuli. These experiences help us focus on the principal parts of our body: the sides and the middle in the horizontal dimension, the top and the bottom in the vertical dimension, and the front and the back in the sagittal dimension. These dimensions are projected into space, forming the vectors for our relationships to objects in space. When we grow toward someone "nice," we inhale, widen, lengthen, or bulge in response. When we shrink from someone or something "bad," we exhale, narrow, shorten, or hollow. The former shape dimensions serve attraction and approach, the latter serve repulsion and withdrawal. A balance between these shape changes constitutes the mainstay of the mental attitude of trusting the trustworthy and mistrusting the suspect. An imbalance may result in an unrealistic appraisal of the environment and in undue optimism or pessimism. A balanced response to environmental objects [1] is at the core of our capacity to infer the meaning of what we perceive and relate to as good or bad.

Glaser [12] speaks of the inborn transsensus, a primary outgoingness on which trust is based and relationships develop. He gives many examples of how we relate to people trustingly and in a trustworthy manner when we incorporate their images into our own. Conversely, a mechanical approach becomes a tedious task rather than a joyous interaction. The deeper the inhalation in growing toward the environment, the more relatedness is experienced. The less conspicuous inhalations and exhalations that are coordinated with the changes in the shape of the face, called facial expressions, are not easily perceived. Their excursions become larger and breathing becomes labored when emotions are strong and facial changes are exaggerated.

In the following quotations from Darwin [4] we must keep in mind that he is describing shape-flow changes. To make this clear I shall put the appropriate shape-flow terms in parentheses.

"While thus screaming their eyes are firmly closed (shortening) . . . and the forehead contracted in a frown (narrowing) . . ." (p. 147). Darwin further says that in violent or unrestrained crying, there is forceful expiration and the eyes are closed (shrinking). In violent retching the glottis is closed and the expiratory muscles contract strongly (shrink) to expel the stomach content, and the eyes are shut tightly (shortening).

Darwin observed that frowning occurs regularly when one encounters obstacles in the train of one's thought. People frown instantly when they perceive a bad taste in their food. Darwin described deep exhalations in violent desires to get rid of the unpleasant, but did not pay attention to the more subtle narrowing of the chest that accompanies narrowing of the brow when people want to eject something bad or want to prevent the entrance of a noxious stimulus into their bodies. Darwin noticed that when the infant is uncomfortable or unwell a series of frowns "may be seen incessantly passing like shadows over his face" (p. 223). To prevent the entrance of too much sunlight into the eyes, people contract their brows.

Darwin further states: "During rage, the chest heaves. . . . hence the expressions as 'breathing vengeance' and 'fuming with anger'" (p. 239). Rage seen in the face reveals a contraction of nasal muscles, pulling the corners of the nose upward while the eyes are shut and pulled down, and the mouth is generally closed firmly, with teeth clenched or ground together (all shortening).

Darwin cites Bell, who spoke of the ". . . sympathy (i.e., habitual coaction) of all respiratory muscles . . ." (p. 239). Bell implied that facial muscles act in sympathy with such respiratory muscles as the intercostals and the diaphragm. According to Bell, "In all exhilarating emotions the eyebrows, eyelids, nostrils and the angles of the mouth are raised. In the depressing passions it is the reverse . . ." (p. 211). The stretching out (lengthening) of the face in joy leads to the elevation in the upper part of the face and a lowering of the jaw. "In joy the face (also) expands" (widening) (p. 211).

It is impressive to see a newborn imitating the tongue movement and the configuration of the mouth and eye area of the adult who "talks" to him or her [27]. The mother reciprocates by imitating the shape of the baby's facial expression; that gives the baby a feeling akin to pride in his or her leadership [23]. Trust is inspired by the infant's observation that there is rhythm in shape, whereby the tongue that came out goes back in, the mouth that opens will close [23, 24] and a frown will change into a smile. From the start, there is an apparatus for the recognition of the expressions of the human species to which mother and child belong. Whereas the alternation of inhaling and exhaling gives an atmosphere of confidence in one's environment, the alternation of growing and shrinking in the face creates trust in people.

To understand the interplay of mother and infant, we must keep in mind that there is a specific coordination between shape flow and tension flow, whereby widening fits well with slight changes in tension levels and narrowing with an even level of tension; lengthening fits well with low intensity and shortening with high intensity; bulging fits well with a gradual change and hollowing with an abrupt change in tension. These coordinated sets do not always work together. Mismatching of tension flow and shape flow creates clashing within the organism (i.e., future intrasystemic conflict between affects and relatedness [13, 19]). Clashing and matching have rhythms of their own; they recur periodically in everybody and are not pathological, provided that harmony prevails. For example, growing via lengthening with high intensity in bound flow gives the individual a feeling of oppression at the same time that he or she is seeking out the environment in a trusting manner. His or her inhalation is impeded, and he or she feels that something is going wrong. By using lengthening, which is an expression of comfort, the individual gives false cues to the onlooker who will not come to the rescue. If, however, the individual chooses to exhale and shorten, whereby the harmonious matching between tension and shape is restored, the cues become understandable. Conversely, the individual may reduce his or her intensity, reinstate free flow, and thus no longer feel that something is wrong. Another irregularity arises when a person uses more growing than shrinking and vice versa. In the first instance, he or she is continually seeking contact in a clinging manner, never showing neediness. In the second instance, he or she is signaling neediness incessantly, but is not able to receive comfort.

Balanced breath gives support to our actions, and we have to feel well supported to breathe in a eutonic, rhythmic fashion [12] in harmony with the supporter. A child's breath gives internal support, while a mother's breath supports the child from the outside. Here we must differentiate holding from supporting. Holding tightly does not give support; presenting a rhythmically falling and rising plastic mattresslike structure of the mother's body prevents the baby from falling and yet allows a freedom to breathe and support him- or herself. An example of a support failure is that of a hollow-chested mother whose baby sinks into her chest enclosure. Her chest respiration is impeded as she remains in a permanently expiratory position. The baby who harmonizes with this breathing also will become hollow chested. In this manner, the mutual adjustment in an unsupportive shape produces the effect of a pieta whereby mother and child suffer together. A baby who will support him- or herself will not lean on a hollow-chested mother or will refuse to sit on her lap.

Only under conditions of optimal internal and external support can shape changes flow in a balanced, harmonious manner through which mother and child can give each other clues that are reinforced by mutual mirroring of their facial expressions.

Failures in Empathy and Trust

Through the interplay of tension flow, our own and that of others, we acquire empathy for others and learn to intuit their needs. Through the interplay of shape flow, we acquire the ability to infer what is being conveyed to us by another person. Shape flow provides a structure for tension flow and thus gives it meaning.

A failure in empathy occurs when a person is incapable of letting tension flow pass through the body and overflow into another person. Such massive blocking is seen in total rigidity, which makes body boundaries impervious to the passage of feelings. Partial failures are ubiquitous. For instance, certain tension qualities, such as even flow or low intensity, may be rare in a person's movement repertoire, and he or she is not able to resonate well when these qualities of tension are transmitted from another person. One can compare this to a resonator that is not tuned properly to certain pitches but does well with others. An example is a mother feeding her child who brings the spoon to her child's lips abruptly while he or she is still busy chewing. The mother is unaware of their clash except that she considers the child to be a poor eater. One has to use retraining procedures to make her aware of the effect of such clashes before she can attune to the child.[6]

The most frequent cause of misattunement is improper holding by tensing the arm or shoulders, which prevents tension flow from being transmitted. In such cases attunement can be achieved by singing together and talking baby talk [27]. Retraining to learn optimal holding methods is difficult because people hold their babies in a way similar to the way their mothers held them. This maternal kinesthetic imprint is not easily relinquished.

Most misalignments in shape flow are selective rather than total. The child's and the mother's preferred shape-flow rhythms may not coincide. A forever-smiling mother, for instance, finds it difficult to imitate a baby's frown. She feels the tension in his body, but does not know how to interpret it. She may say to him smilingly: "Oh, it is not bad, it does not hurt, everything is fine." The mother who can respond with her own frown will say: "Oh, you don't feel well, baby. Let me see how I can make you more comfortable." Some caretakers fail to look at their babies'

---

[6] An example will help to clarify this point. Mrs. Buelte, the codirector of the Center, touches a mother's palms with her own, swaying with her and establishing a rhythm in which tension falls and rises gradually. Although this is not this mother's preferred rhythm, she is quite capable of maintaining it when one leads her into it. Suddenly, without warning, Mrs. Buelte moves abruptly and startles the mother. The mother catches on immediately and says, "Is that what I do to Paul? No wonder he turns away from me."

faces and do not train their children to regulate their facial expressiveness. The same mothers may adjust well by means of body contact and like to carry their children to help them. Children whose mothers do not get cues from the child's breathing behavior often prefer to sit in their teacher's lap rather than their mother's. This offends mothers — they do not know why they deserve such rejection. Fortunately, we can teach caretakers how to regulate their own breath to give support and to adjust shape flow.

Shape flow is impeded or distorted with a resulting loss of trust when a mother does not give her baby proper support. For instance, she may exhale irregularly, too slowly, or too rapidly for the child to have enough time or room to inhale during pumping of milk or to exhale when the milk is propelled toward the pharynx. When the mother fails to extend her inhalation to encompass her supporting arm, the baby's head drops, and proper breathing is prevented by the retroflexion of the neck.

Mutual gazing also gives support, so that distance imitation of breathing in facial movement can take place. When a young baby averts his or her gaze because he or she no longer can give the mother support, mother will withdraw her gaze and will cease to lean toward the baby. Instead, she resettles herself and finds new means of support for herself.

A parent who does not give support to the baby only rarely receives support from the child. Because their breaths, and consequently their shape flow, function independently, neither can trust the other. A mother can learn to give support by focusing on her own support system and by practicing new means of self-support that can be used to support a child.

Mention has been made of difficulties created if one of the partners suffers from mismatching of tension flow or shape flow. A further problem arises when the child's and the adult's tension flow and shape flow both operate in the reverse. For instance, when the child smiles with the corners of the mouth quivering through an adjustment of tension levels, the mother frowns in even flow; neither empathy nor trust can develop. Fortunately such cases are rare, but occasional estrangement occurs more frequently.

Applying our knowledge of the apparatuses for empathy and trust to psychoanalyses of mothers of young children can give us insight into the multiple reasons that underlie the lack of use or misuse of these apparatuses. In the following excerpts from an analysis of a mother with such misuse problems, only material pertinent to the topic under consideration is presented. The resulting picture of the analysis may be skewed, but the role of tension-flow and shape-flow apparatuses is highlighted.

Excerpts from the Analysis of a Young Mother

Fay came to analysis when she was in her late 20s. She spoke monotonously and seemed indifferent to most of the problems she presented, with one exception. She felt rejected by her 1-year-old daughter, Jenny, who cried for her father when Fay tried to pick her up. Fay wanted to be a good mother, but did not know how, and she often cried when Jenny pushed her away.

When Jenny was 8 months old, Fay began to study for her medical state board examinations, and she hired temporary help to take charge of Jenny. It never occurred to her that such a small child would resent her absence. From the start, Fay was uncertain about what to do with Jenny, and she was glad when her husband helped her. However, she resented the advice of her experienced sister-in-law.

Fay was surprised when I asked her how she had been raised. She thought that her mother did not want her and was partial to her two older sisters. She had been a burden to her mother because she was a month premature and cried all the time. Her mother used to tell the story that she had threatened to throw little Fay out of the window if her husband did not get up to care for her at night. Fay had some fond memories of her father and of his sister, who lived in the same house.

The family history contained many illnesses and deaths. An uncle (the father's brother-in-law) was paralyzed when Fay was young and died when she was 4 or 5; an aunt was aphasic and had a stroke and died when Fay was 8; and lastly, her father had several strokes and died when she was 9. Fay's mother resented having to take care of sick people all her life. She had been at continuous odds with Fay's aunt, who was critical of the way Fay's mother cared for her. Fay lost her mother when she was in her early 20s. Until she was married she was alone, for her two older sisters had long since moved away.

Reminiscing about her own childhood and Jenny's, Fay confessed that she had weaned Jenny from the breast because she felt all cooped up and enslaved by the breast-feeding. She did not quite know how it happened, but recently Jenny had begun to accept her. This change occurred almost as soon as Fay understood that she was reliving her own childhood by rejecting Jenny and being rejected by her. She was abashed as she confessed that she was pregnant; she had lost faith in regaining Jenny and hoped to replace her with a baby who would love her. She was now able to tolerate Jenny's rebukes when she recalled that Jenny was withdrawing from her in retaliation for what she, Fay, had done to her. She felt rewarded when Jenny began to hug her spontaneously.

After Lewis was born, Fay showed empathy for both children and enjoyed breast-feeding. Soon, however, she tired of Lewis, who began to cry day and night and had to be carried incessantly. One day Fay surprised me by bringing Lewis to the session. When Lewis was put on the floor next to the couch, he began to whimper. Without looking at him, Fay jumped up and placed him on her chest for comfort. When I suggested that Lewis might have been settling himself by moaning and groaning, Fay put him down, but was sure his crying would intensify. Lewis whimpered and squirmed, then closed his eyes and fell asleep within a few minutes. Fay was amazed: She did not think it was right to let a baby cry, but was not able to distinguish between real distress and mild complaining. From then on, she herself would moan and groan on the couch whenever she felt that she could not make her wants known. She could feel what Lewis felt, but she did not know that the sounds were expressions of relief-seeking by expelling something that had gone wrong.

When Lewis reached the age of 4 months, he became distractible during breast-feeding, a typical occurrence between the ages of 4 and 5 months. Rather than nurse him in a quiet room, Fay watched his loss of weight for a while and then discontinued breast-feeding.

Fay's feelings of rejection increased with Jenny as well. When Jenny wanted her father instead of her mother to put her coat on, Fay would say: "I will go away and never come back." To compound the family discomfort, at about 10 months of age Lewis began to bang his head in the middle of the night. He had been creeping and getting into everything, which annoyed Fay. She never knew how he got into her room and opened her drawers. It was obvious that she had neither kept her eyes on him nor baby-proofed her house.

Trying to demonstrate her problems and challenging me to help her, Fay brought both her children to the session without warning. Jenny played with my toys, and Lewis wandered around, pleased with his newly acquired erect locomotion. Every once in a while Fay glanced at him and reprimanded him because he touched something. Then she decided that he was restless because he was hungry, but was not sure whether bottle-feeding was permitted in my office. She started feeding him at the end of the session when Jenny was putting toys away. Jenny immediately dropped the toys. Fay saw no connection between Jenny's defiance and her own action. She scolded Jenny and made an abortive attempt to get up and help her. When I pointed out that Jenny was angry because mother picked up Lewis, Fay pulled the bottle out of his mouth. When Lewis cried she addressed him sympathetically (revealing that she knew how he felt), but offered no solution.

Fay's provocation of me and the children; her mistiming, postponing, interrupting, and miscueing; her ignoring of her children's feelings; and the way she disconnected her actions from their effects on the children were all taken up in the next months of analysis. The chaotic situation at home was confounded by her using the children as pawns in her spats with her sister-in-law and husband. For instance, when her husband began to toilet train Jenny, she insisted that Jenny pick up all her toys, smiled when her husband did not succeed, and asked Jenny "to go for mommy." She opposed her husband's idea that she should let Lewis bang his head and demanded that he get up at night to attend to him. Finally, I remarked that she too was banging her head against the wall trying to accomplish the impossible and battling with everyone.

Miraculously, Lewis stopped banging his head. This suggested that there was nonverbal communication between Lewis and his mother, and I could tell that she was capable of feeling for Lewis but her anger interfered with her acting in his interest. It soon became apparent that she perceived her own impulses but did not understand them. For instance, she allowed her husband to wean Lewis from the bottle without any warning. When Lewis responded by banging his head again, she ignored the connection between these two events. As soon as she was told of this connection and understood that she was acting maliciously toward her husband and child, as well as toward her analyst, she proceeded to wean Lewis gradually.

Fay began to muse about the mode of transmission of her feelings to Lewis. Each time I had pointed out how the children had reacted to her anger, she had been thinking about a supernatural extrasensory communication, but that did not seem right. She connected such a communication with previously discussed ideas that she could revive her parents, feed them inside of her, and care for them. When I asked her how the supernatural worked, she suddenly extended her arms toward me, moving her fingers back and forth in a rhythmic way. She withdrew just as quickly, and in subsequent sessions revealed that she had to hide her hands in order not to express her feelings to me.

Looking back to the beginning of Fay's treatment, I realized that she was now able to speak in a modulated voice and was also gesticulating. Fay went through a period of reminiscing about her own lonely childhood and her lack of understanding for her mother. She began to see that she criticized her sister-in-law in the same way her mother had criticized Fay's aunt. She became aware of shapes of people, and she vividly recalled the "shrunken" shape of Jenny at the age of 1 when she cowered in her crib refusing to be picked up by her mother. She now could not only feel for her but also understood what the child was expressing. She said that not knowing what a separation from the mother meant to an 8-month-old was not an excuse she would choose today. She accused herself of not understanding herself and not understanding the children. She began to observe herself and discovered that she only knew about her anger when it reached a certain height at a time when she could no longer control it. Her empathy was handicapped by her not knowing how others felt until their feelings reached a high intensity.

At this point of the analysis, Fay's position and movement on the couch became the focus of our attention. As soon as she lay down she raised one leg, placed the sole of her foot on the couch, and crossed the other leg over it. Her right hand was placed underneath her head and her left elbow rested on the backrest of the couch. Her right hand would sometimes venture out to gesticulate vividly, as did the left. However, the left would repeatedly wander off to scratch her mouth, cheek, forehead, and hair.

When I talked to Fay about her supernatural finger play, it became quite clear that she interfered with the free flow of her empathy by becoming rigid and immobilizing her hands. This blocked the path of transmission of feelings. Her facial expression was masked by a perennial smile and her shape flow underwent only a few changes.

I tried to show her how she incessantly lost the flow of communication with people and could only give in or fight to preserve her independence. More importantly, when she did perceive what other people felt, she neither knew what they wanted nor what she herself wanted to do. Thus, she had to ask me incessantly to tell her what to do, and this made her dependent on me. When I saw that Fay "did not understand" my interpretations, I began to draw her attention to her complex support system on the couch. She quickly raised her head with her supporting hand and laid them both down again. She then recalled that she had two dreams of falling. She described how she had to collapse in an easy chair at home to rest when she had taken care of the children for a while. It was hard to give them support because she needed support herself. When Lewis fell backward from a bench, she realized that she too was afraid of falling backward.

I was reminded of babies who are held with insufficient support and develop their own support system. I recalled that Fay had a problem giving or getting support from mutual gazing. She hardly looked at Lewis, responding mostly to his auditory communication. When I was silent for some time she became anxious and would barrage me with questions, seeking support in the form of explanations. At that point I was able to suggest to her that her position on the couch resembled the nursing position. She accepted this idea as if she had known it all along. She moved back and forth to allay her confusion. She did not know whether it was she who was being held for nursing or if she was holding and nursing the baby. In subsequent sessions her fingers repeatedly came close to her mouth, and several times she nibbled on her nails. She became aware of having to hold her head so it would not fall apart and empty itself. It was not until much later that Fay could again speak of support rather than holding and discovered that her fear of rejection originated in her fear of being "dropped."

With her new understanding of her need to hold and be held, Fay's empathy increased. Yet, she would frequently become rigid and inaccessible when too much closeness threatened. She had to hold herself, since no one else would. When she described how she felt, she was able to put herself in the children's positions and feel for them. However, she still veered from defensiveness to an indiscriminate attunement in her tone of voice and movement. When one of her children was angry, the anger became contagious, and she too was angry. Meeting anger with anger and joy with joy, she was incapable of understanding what the anger or joy signified. She did not know what made them want one thing and not another. As a result, she could not act in a sensible way and gave them only things she herself liked.

One of the few times Fay was able to express her grievances against me, I became aware that she still smiled in a fixed manner, although she left in anger. She was afraid that her facial expression might become uncontrollable and she would make faces at her sister-in-law, although she wanted to conceal her hatred for her. Thus, she veered from grimacing to a defensive smiling. Her aggression had very little structure unless she made faces or said something openly malicious. As a result, her family and acquaintances did not know what was bothering her. I began to talk to her about her miscueing through her facial expression, and this led us to a discovery of her imitation of the dead.

Since the beginning of her analysis, Fay complained that many important things in her life had been concealed from her. She did not know when her beloved aunt had died. Her father's hospitalization had been concealed from her; she had not been permitted to attend his funeral. She did not remember either her aunt's or her father's illnesses. I suggested that she may have been frightened by her relatives' facial expressions when they were paralyzed. This helped her to recall an incident when she was very young: she had asked why her uncle did not cut his meat. Her mother reprimanded her for asking such a question, and this strengthened her conviction that she should not understand. At that point she began to speak in a very confused way that made me think of the speech of aphasics. She consulted her older sister, who disclosed to her that the beloved aunt had indeed been aphasic long before she died. Not being able to understand her aunt had a bearing on Fay's belief that one cannot understand the babbling of small children; she believed that she could not be comfortable with them until they spoke clearly.

Previously, Fay worked through fantasies of harboring her dead inside of her and feeling dead herself. The problem of what dead people looked like became more meaningful to her when I asked whether she had ever seen a dead person. She recalled her dead mother and father in the funeral parlor, and she thought she may have seen many other dead people because so many soldiers had died in her neighborhood. She recalled with indignation that her mother's burial dress had been torn by the funeral parlor so that she was not properly attired below her waist. The coffin had a lid, consisting of two parts; only the upper lid was open. Looking at her position on the couch, I asked her whether the lower lid had been elevated; she said it was. However, she hastened to assure me that it was not elevated enough to allow the mother to bend her knees, as Fay did. I reminded her that she had told me she did not want me to see her belly, which would show more if she stretched out her legs. She began to lie with her legs outstretched and commented that she wanted to cross one over the other. Now, I could see that her breathing was shallow; she could not take enough breath to carry many of her sentences, so that they became garbled. Yet, she trusted me more and became a more trustworthy patient. There were far fewer reports of negligent behavior with the children and she was able to relinquish her support system on the couch entirely, putting her arms by her side.

As she began now to structure her aggression better, she became capable of witty, malicious repartee, which she enjoyed. However, when discouraged by a relative, she once more began to disconnect her aggression from its consequences. I could show her how she provoked her friends and her husband to pick on her and yet maintain the illusion that "all was well." As a result, the counterattacks and rejections came as a surprise to her. She thought "deceit" was a better word than "illusion," and she told many stories of the ways her mother and sisters used to deceive her. Her mother was herself deceived about the extent of her illness, and her death came as a surprise to Fay. The family was able to keep a poker face, making it impossible to infer from their faces that something was amiss. Yet the tension was there. She recognized that she was acting deceitfully to her husband and herself and that she was provoking him to dislike, reject, and abandon her.

Feeling more alive now, she became afraid of the loneliness she would feel if left alone. Her previous problems with sex resulted from her feeling dead and cautious lest she become too involved and suffer pain from losing a loved person. She became capable of making her needs known and understood, and she asked to be held without being afraid of rejection.

Fay drew my attention to the fact that she needed some contact between parts of her body. Thus, she had to cross her legs so that they would touch and hold each other, and she hid her hands under her body partially from fear of what they would do and partially from a need to hold them. Her left arm wandered away to her chest or her face. She knew now that she had to hold herself there. She thought that her husband was not affectionate and suddenly recalled (in her body) that her mother sang beautifully and was affectionate. She told me that she had to hold herself or be held to feel secure. When I inquired whether security meant support like an anchor point, she seemed baffled. She then explained how she felt and spoke of an anchored boat held securely; if it was not tied, it would "drift away" in the water. It would be lost. This time she was not afraid of falling, but afraid of being lost and losing if she was not held and holding.

FAY'S FAILURE IN EMPATHY

Fay's empathy was inhibited by her defensive binding of the flow of tension. When this defense weakened, she moved to find out whether she was holding or being held, and she was in danger of losing her boundaries. Once her flow was freed, it overflowed to the point of contagion. Others became infected by her, and she was infected by their feelings without much discrimination.

The most important source of loss of empathy came from her incorporation of the ill and the dead. This attitude expressed itself in a change of flow to a neutral state. Only some of the neutral flow had the quality of an infant's flow when drifting into sleep, especially when she scratched her head or fingered her face or mouth. The free-neutral flow into which Fay would lapse reflected her feeling of being lost in a blissful reunion with her dead, which kept her in a fluid state.

Freud [10] explained this type of behavior as resulting from an excessive mobility of the libido. He described such people as unable to maintain a relationship and as forming new ones only to give them up once more. He spoke of the impression he had when working with such patients as having "written on water." This indeed is a good description of Fay in states of drifting in free but inanimate neutral flow. I would lose her to her dead and they again would lose her when she drifted toward me or her children.

Another form of inanimateness was inertia, observable in bound-neutral flow. Freud [10] described this inertia in patients whose libido he called "adhesive" and thought of it as a fundamental condition of their mental apparatus. Fay was able to change from free-neutral to bound-neutral flow. Her thoughts would become heavy and could not be formulated. She would be tired and would have to sit down, feeling heavy. This was the most consistent form of her depression and mourning for the dead, whom she tried to retain and emulate. The states of free- and bound-neutral flow were expressions of inelasticity. She would wake herself up from these states by gesticulating and becoming aggressive.

There was always a danger that loving feelings would deteriorate into inanimateness — a communion with the dead. All three changes in tension flow, the excessive boundness, and the neutral-free and neutral-bound flow interfered with Fay's empathy. However, these tension changes alternated with normal states, so that her empathy was unpredictable. Moreover, she would lapse from a neutral state into a state of high tension and find herself all excited, whereas a minute before she had been in a sort of stuporous daze.

FAY'S FAILURE IN TRUST

From the start of her analysis, I had hoped to reawaken Fay's empathy, but her inability to infer the meaning of a person's feelings presented great difficulties. At first I had to function as her auxiliary ego, explaining what effect feelings had on her and others. Then I could analyze her defensive preoccupation with her own needs at the expense of others and help her take responsibility for her aggressive provocations of others. However, when I had to tackle her basic lack of trust in her own judgment and in the reliability of her children's expressions, I encountered what Balint [1] called a "basic fault" that contributed to Fay's low self-esteem. She did not trust me to the extent of thinking I could help her, neither could I trust her as a patient, which certainly put obstacles in the way of our therapeutic alliance.

I was faced with Fay's "deceit" and false obsequiousness, and I never knew what the next hour would bring. Her continual compliance and her insinuation of my incompetence, under the guise of feeling she was hopeless, sometimes threatened to undermine my own self-esteem. I was relieved to find Freud [10] referring to such a patient. He spoke of an attitude ". . . which can only be put down to a depletion of the plasticity, the capacity for change and further development, which we should ordinarily expect." He suggested that this attitude was due to ". . . some alterations of a rhythm of development in psychical life which we have not yet appreciated" (p. 242). It seems possible to me that Freud, a connoisseur of movement, derived his concept of lack of plasticity from his observation of defective shape-flow.

The shapelessness of a complete lack of plasticity comes from a neutral shape flow in which shape changes become indistinct or absent. Fay imitated the shapeless facial features of people with strokes and aphasics' or apractics' alterations of features. She defended herself against deanimation by aggressive outbursts and by maintaining a constant smile in high tension and in even flow. That made the smile look like a grin, and her "faces" were also of this order. Once she was able to confront her fear of falling and her need for support, she could proceed to uncover her identification with her deceiving mother and sisters. She deceived the deceivers.

HOLDING AND SUPPORT DEFICIENCIES

When Fay realized that I would uphold her and continue her treatment regardless of her behavior toward her children and me, she ceased to provoke me by being a "bad" mother. When she realized that her "bad" mothering was a replica of her own experience at the hands of her caretakers, she was able to utilize the holding environment offered to her in treatment. In this way the therapeutic process resembled that recommended by Kohut [20, 21]. My empathy for her was rewarded by an increase of her empathy for her children, but this improvement disappeared when I went on vacation.

Once Fay understood that she provoked people to reject (drop her), she was able to extend her arms to me and invite me to attune to her finger play. Eventually we discovered her great need to hold herself or be held and her inability to hold children without being held herself. When she acknowledged this need and could ask to be held, her empathy increased considerably. When she discussed the coffin that held the body of the dead, she became aware of her identification with the dead and realized that she held herself in a position of a dead person held by a coffin. On the other hand, she also held herself in the nursing position in which boundaries were loosened. Drifting away in neutral-free flow meant that she was not held at all; she had no anchor point.

Fay's need to be held was intertwined with her strong need for support so that she would not fall. Holding her head was preventing its falling apart, just as putting the sole of her foot on the couch gave her support so that she would not slide backward. When I showed understanding of her fear of falling, she was able to relinquish her special support system on the couch.

By then Fay trusted me enough so that she could expose herself to me and show me her breathing pattern. She then expressed concern over whether I would remain alive long enough to help her. The disturbance in her breathing turned out to be a basis for her inability to trust her "own words." She sometimes could not say what she wanted because her breath got stuck. At times she suffered from asthmatic wheezing. The understanding of her lack of breath control enabled her to develop an initial trusting feeling that she might be able to control her speech and her facial expression by proper breathing.

Thoughts about Etiology

No doubt, maternal deprivation of a special kind played a role in Fay's failure with empathy and trust. To understand the atmosphere in which she grew up, we have to empathize with her mother who was surrounded by disease and death. Fay's mother had lost her parents just before Fay was born, and Fay herself was endangered by her prematurity and by her mother's own wish to undo this pregnancy. Her deceit in which she tried to shield Fay from knowledge of illness and death was perhaps born out of her concern that Fay must not suffer a fate like her own.

Fay had special feelings about her own delivery, which was shrouded in mystery. No doubt her breathing was not quite regular at birth, and perhaps her crying and facial expressions were not as differentiated as in a full-term baby. Judging from observations of premature babies, they have much more neutral flow, both in tension and shape. Sometimes, we even see them hit out with an arm in what seems to be an effort to get their breath going. Fay's gesticulations, which brought her out of neutral flow, were similar to these movements of premature infants. Her difficulty in exhaling when she began to wheeze was related to her inability to give up her mother, whom she had incorporated.[7]

---

[7] Freud [8] described the ritual of the Wolf Man who had to exhale when he saw beggars, a ritual that started when he visited his sick father. The Wolf Man also inhaled to take in what he liked. Similarly, Fay began to have trouble exhaling when she was in touch with dogs. She and her mother had shared a dog who died some years after the mother's death. Fay could give up neither the mother nor the dog.

One can speculate that Fay's prematurity, her neutral tension flow and her neutral shape flow evoked negative feelings in her mother, and that a vicious circle ensued whereby Fay, predisposed to difficulties in this area, was trained to feel no pain and to ignore the meaning of death. Fay was not prepared to cope with the successive deaths in her family except by identification with the dead. It was not a simple maternal deprivation, but rather a number of factors that interfered with her empathy and trust.

Summary

A discussion of prevailing opinions about empathy has been contrasted with the view that empathy is based on the flow of tension, and trust is based on the flow of shape. These motor apparatuses, available to all living tissue, have been described, and examples were given of clashing between these apparatuses in one individual and in interaction between people. Some retraining procedures (procedures that are applied in a prevention center that the author directs) that restore harmony were discussed. Excerpts from an analysis were used to show how the observation and discussion of changes in tension and in shape of the body and face can enrich the analytic process and bring out feelings that stem from early infancy and childhood about lack of proper holding and proper support.

By separating empathy from trust, it is possible to treat a failure in each separately and then pay attention to the manner in which they are coordinated or isolated from one another. The free flow of empathy is related to the growing trust and trustworthiness, and the binding (inhibiting) of empathy is related to shrinking away from the environment and people, which is the basis for mistrust.

References

1. Balint, M. Primary narcissism and primary love. *Psychoanal. Q.* 24:6, 1960.
2. Balint, M. *The Basic Fault.* London: Tavistock Publications, 1968.
3. Buie, D. H. Empathy: Its nature and limitations. *J. Am. Psychoanal. Assoc.* 29:282, 1981.
4. Darwin, C. *The Expression of the Emotions in Man and Animals.* New York: Philosophical Library, 1955.
5. Erikson, E. H. *Childhood and Society.* New York: Norton, 1950.
6. Fenichel, O. Identification. In *Collected Papers of Otto Fenichel.* (1926) New York: Norton, 1953. Vol. I, pp. 97–112.

7. Freud, A. *Normality and Pathology in Childhood. Assessments of Development.* New York: International Universities Press, 1965.
8. Freud, S. From the History of an Infantile Neurosis (1918). In J. Strachey (Ed.), *The Standard Edition of the Complete Psychological Works of Sigmund Freud.* London: Hogarth, 1955. Vol. 17, pp. 3–124.
9. Freud, S. Group psychology and the analysis of the Ego (1921). *Standard Edition.* (1955). Vol. 18, pp. 67–144.
10. Freud, S. Analysis terminable and interminable (1937). *Standard Edition.* (1964). Vol. 22, pp. 209–254.
11. Furer, M. Some developmental aspects of the superego. *Int. J. Psychoanal.* 48:227, 1967.
12. Glaser, V. *Eutonie* (2nd ed.). Heidelberg: Haug Verlag, 1981.
13. Hartmann, H. *Ego Psychology and the Problem of Adaptation.* New York: International University Press, 1958.
14. Kestenberg, J. *The Role of Movement Patterns in Development I.* New York: Dance Notation Bureau Press, 1971.
15. Kestenberg, J. Psychoanalytic observation of children. *Int. Rev. Psychoanal.* 4:393, 1977.
16. Kestenberg, J. Pregnancy as a developmental phase. *J. Biol. Experience* 3:58, 1980.
17. Kestenberg, J., Berlowe, J., Buelte, A., et al. Development of the young child as expressed through bodily movement, I. In J. Kestenberg (Ed.), *Children and Parents. Psychoanalytic Studies in Development.* New York: Aronson. 1975. Pp. 195–210.
18. Kestenberg, J., and Buelte, A. Prevention, infant therapy, and the treatment of adults I and II. *Int. J. Psychoanal. Psychother.* 7:339, 1977.
19. Kestenberg, J., and Sossin, M. *The Role of Movement Patterns in Development II.* New York: Dance Notation Bureau Press, 1979.
20. Kohut, H. Forms and transformations of narcissism. *J. Am. Psychoanal. Assoc.* 14:243, 1966.
21. Kohut, H. *The Analysis of the Self.* New York: International Universities Press, 1971.
22. Mahler, M. S., Pine, F., and Bergman, A. *The Psychological Birth of the Human Infant. Symbiosis and Individuation.* New York: Basic Books, 1975.
23. Papousek, H., and Papousek, M. Mothering and the Cognitive Head Start: Psychological Considerations. In H. R. Schaffer (Ed.), *Studies in Mother-Infant-Interaction.* New York: Academic Press, 1977.
24. Piaget, J. Les trois structures fondamentales de la vie psychique: rythme, regulation et groupement. *Schweiz. Z. Psychol.* 1:9, 1942.
25. Rice, R. D. The effects of the rice infant sensorimotor stimulation treatment on the development of high-risk infants. *Birth Defects: Original Article Series* 15:7, 1979.
26. Shapiro, T. The development and distortions of empathy. *Psychoanal. Q.* 43:4, 1974.
27. Stern, D. The First Relationship. Infant and Mother. In J. Bruner, M. Cole,

and B. Lloyd (Eds.), *The Developing Child Series.* Cambridge, Mass.: Harvard University Press, 1977.

28. Vennard, W. *Singing. The Mechanism and the Technic.* New York: Carl Fischer, Inc., 1962.
29. Verny, T. R., and Kelly, J. *The Secret Life of the Unborn Child.* New York: Summit Books, 1981.
30. Winnicott, D. W. *The Ordinary Devoted Mother and Her Baby.* London: Privately printed, 1949.
31. Winnicott, D. W. Transitional objects and transitional phenomena. *Int. J. Psychoanal.* 34:89, 1953.
32. Winnicott, D. W. *The Maturational Processes and the Facilitating Environment.* New York: International Universities Press, 1965.

Glossary

empathy   An inborn capacity to know another person's inner feelings, based on sensory experiences [3]. In my view, it does not include comprehending, understanding, or inferring the significance of these feelings. Empathy utilizes attunement in tension flow, which is based on kinesthetic identification with the tension changes of another person [18]. Failure of empathy is frequently based on an inhibition of rhythms of tension flow.

shape flow   A succession of changes in the shape of the body. The basic rhythm of shape flow is an alternation of growing (as in inhalation and smiling) and shrinking (as in exhalation or frowning). The respiratory rhythm is the core mechanism that gives shape to the body. The rhythm begins to operate immediately after birth when relatedness to the environment and objects begins to be established. Expressive movements are based on derivatives or direct expressions of changes in breathing (e.g., smiling is normally done in inhalation, frowning in exhalation). Growing fosters intake of environmental substances, and shrinking fosters their expulsion. Through the repetition of breathing, the baby learns to expect that discomfort is followed by comfort. Because his or her mother is the primary regulator of his or her breathing rhythm and thus of comfort and discomfort, she is the recipient of the baby's trust. A parent's inability to regulate the baby's comfort and discomfort (e.g., in premature babies) creates a lack of trust. Changes in the dimensions of shape are narrowing and widening; lengthening and shortening; hollowing and bulging. The range of trust and mistrust is based on taking in what is good and ejecting what is bad. The proper balance between the two engenders the feeling of trustworthiness in the self and others. Failures of mirroring identification in shape flow (leading to failures in trust) are based on: an imbalance between growing and shrinking, which engenders gullibility or suspiciousness; and loss of plasticity, whereby changes in expressiveness are lacking and a neutral shape flow predominates.

tension flow A succession of changes in the tension of the body. The basic rhythm of tension flow is an alternation of free and bound flow of tension, which reflects the facilitation and inhibition of nervous impulses. Attributes of tension are remaining at the same level or changing levels of tension; high or low intensity of tension; abrupt or gradual change of tension. Attunement in tension flow occurs when tension-flow changes in one person lead to similar changes in the other person. Empathy is based on the perception of tension changes. Failures in transmission of tension changes leading to failures in empathy are based on binding of flow to block its continuity and preventing free flow from occurring; and loss of elasticity, whereby neutral flow prevails, leading to inanimateness such as fluidity or inertia.

transsensus The primary outgoingness or basic relatedness of people to the world and to each other [12]. In deep inhalation, transsensus creates the illusion of receiving another person into one's own body image. That can be accomplished only when we trust that person to introduce good substances into our body.

trust Basic trust is the "ontological source of faith and hope" [5]. It is composed of ". . . an essential trustfulness of others as well as a fundamental sense of one's own trustworthiness" (p. 96). "Mistrust is experienced whenever the world of expectations has been shaken" (p. 83). Trust utilizes an adjustment in shape flow that is based on a mirroring identification with the shape changes in another person.

5

The mother's experience during the earliest phases of infant development

Anni Bergman

When I nurse her, she and I look at each other and she'll smile and sometimes stroke my breast that's not being used. At those times, M seems so happy and at peace with the world. It is often contagious because I feel the same way. Often it seems like we are the only people in this world. It is an ego booster to have M smile and look at me as though I was the only important person in this world.

These are the words of one mother, beautifully describing her experience with her 3-month-old infant. When we look at the mother-infant dyad, we deal with two human beings engaged in a relationship of utmost intimacy and intensity. Mother and infant form a psychobiological unit in which only one of the partners has words with which to describe the experience. Yet, the intrapsychic experience of the mother during the early months of her child's life is not easy to capture. Benedek [1] observes that we generally know much more about the child than about the parents' intrapsychic reactions to the child. She feels that this is because the parents happily accept the omnipotent and idealizing fantasies of the child.

The child's fantasies, unknown by the parent, yet perceived through his play actions, reactivate in the parent the omnipotent fantasies of his own childhood; in addition, the parent identifying with the fantasies of the child accepts the role of omnipotence attributed to him. The normal parent, in spite of his insight into his realistic limitations, embraces the gratifying role of omnipotence. It induces him to identify with his own parent as he had anticipated being able to do in his childhood fantasies. Whatever the real course of events was between himself and his parents, as long as the fantasies of the child do not become hostile against him, the parent derives from the process of preoedipal identifications the reassurance that he is a good parent and, even more, the hope that he is or can be better than his parents were. (P. 128)

In this chapter I will attempt to describe the experience of the mother during the early months of her infant's life. The chapter is divided into two parts. The first part, which includes a selective review of the literature, is based on my own clinical observations of mothers with whom I have had the opportunity to have in-depth discussions. It is my goal to

165

shed further light on the process described by Winnicott [12] as primary maternal preoccupation. I will attempt to show the diversity and richness of the experience for the mother, which depends on many variables including the mother's personality, the circumstances of birth, and the infant's personality.

The second part of the chapter is based on my participation in the research study of the separation-individuation process in normal mother-child pairs.[1] Mothers and infants were observed in a playgroundlike setting several times a week over a period of several years. In addition, mothers were seen in a weekly interview. A picture of each mother's personality and her mothering experience emerged through these observations and interviews, reflecting her ongoing relationship with the child and revealing glimpses of the mother's own past. Inferences about a mother's intrapsychic experience could not be made as they would be in the analytic situation on the basis of the transference reaction to the analyst. Rather, we used our analytic thinking to understand what we saw and heard in our daily observations and conversations [6]. I will focus on two mother-child pairs from this study. I will show the difficulties one mother had during the stage of symbiosis with her son. I will discuss the difficulties another mother had allowing for gradual disengagement from the symbiotic phase and the way the symbiotic phase for this mother-child pair was marked by the mother's abruptness and symbiotic need for her child to be part of her and stimulate her.

For both of these mother-child pairs, I will offer some material from a follow-up study conducted ten years later.[2] I believe it is relevant here: It demonstrates that the difficulties the three children had in coping later had already begun during the period of symbiosis and differentiation. It is of course impossible to say that these patterns in the child were caused by the mother's handling during the first few months of life since we cannot discount the remainder of the separation-individuation process or the subsequent developments during the oedipal phase and latency. Nevertheless, I feel that it is of interest to look at the child's preoedipal identifications with the mother that have their beginnings during the early months of life.

[1] The Study of the Separation-Individuation Process in Normal Mother-Child Pairs is based on research supported by NIMH Grant MH-08238, USPHS, Bethesda, MD and FFRP Grant 069-458, Foundation Fund for Research in Psychiatry, New Haven, CN. Margaret S. Mahler, Principal Investigator; John B. McDevitt, Co-Principal Investigator.
[2] The Follow-Up Study has been supported by The Masters Children's Center, New York, NY; The Rock Foundation, New York, NY; and the Margaret S. Mahler Research Foundation, New York, NY. Margaret S. Mahler, Consultant; John B. McDevitt, Principal Investigator; Anni Bergman, Co-Principal Investigator.

The Mother's Experience

The symbiotic phase, which lasts from about the second to the fifth month, is a blissful period for most mothers and infants. Mahler and colleagues [7] describe this period.

From the second month on, dim awareness of the need-satisfying object marks the beginning of the phase of normal symbiosis, in which the infant behaves and functions as though he and his mother were an omnipotent system—a dual unity within one common boundary. (P. 44)

The beginning of the symbiotic phase is heralded by the smiling response of the baby, and it wanes when perceptual and locomotor capacities mature to a point where the infant can encompass more and more of the outside world, a process that eventually culminates in "hatching" at around 8 months of age. In order to discuss the symbiotic phase from the point of view of the mother, it is necessary to examine both the preceding period and the period that follows.

According to Winnicott [12], the state of heightened sensitivity that characterizes primary maternal preoccupation is necessary for the mother of the neonate so the infant can achieve the capacity for "going on being" that eventually results in the capacity to "withstand impingement." These capacities characterize the baby during the symbiotic phase if all goes well. The symbiotic phase is distinctly different from the preceding phase in which the infant has to find a niche in the outside world—a phase in which he must become accustomed to the extrauterine environment. The state of maternal preoccupation, which is described by Winnicott as beginning in late pregnancy, is likened by him to an illness from which the mother has to recover. Loewald [4] explicates Winnicott by saying that the mother, during certain moments in early motherhood, functions on a level of mentation that is similar to that of the infant—a level of mentation in which there exists "only one global structure, one fleeting and very perishable mental entity that was neither ego nor object, neither self nor another." The state of the mother, I feel, can best be described as a regression in the service of the baby, and it relies on a number of complex capacities. The mother needs to be secure enough within her own self to be able to "lose" herself in the process of achieving empathy and intimacy with her infant.

Mothers, when they become aware of the way in which they may temporarily lose themselves in the baby, describe loss of the usual sense of time while they are watching their infants. They also describe loss of their usual interest in other relationships or events. Although Winnicott refers to this state as a state approximating illness, we might think of it, rather, as potential illness — an illness that occurs if the mother lacks the ability to freely move in and out of the state of loss of self. Winnicott points out that a mother must be healthy in order to achieve this state, that it is not possible for every mother to achieve it, and that a mother may be able to do so with one child and not with another. Brazelton [3], I believe, describes a process of achieving this state.

In order to produce [infant's] optimal responsiveness, I had to make myself available to them with a sensitivity to their need for control over motor activity and a sensitivity to their "states." I could feel, anticipate, and respond to subtle responses that allowed me to shape my behavior to them so that they could produce their optimal responses. Joint regulation of adult and infant, then, becomes the necessary base for such responsiveness . . . The feeling of mutuality, of identification with "the other," must be at the base of successful interaction between parent and infant. (P. 42)

Sander [9] sees this early phase as the one during which mutuality is established. According to him, it requires the mother's capacity to maintain a balance between her empathy with what she feels the child needs and her capacity to view him objectively. Thus, what would be required is not only identification but also the capacity to emerge from the identified state and observe the infant with some distance. Winnicott [13] states that it is the mother's adaptive behavior that makes it possible for the baby to find that which is needed and expected outside the self. By means of the experience of "good-enough" mothering, the baby moves into objective perception. He or she is able to do this because he or she has been given perceptual equipment, an inherited tendency, and opportunity. Winnicott foreshadowed what infant observers in recent years have emphasized — namely that the baby, from the beginning, has the perceptual capacity for differentiating self from other [11].

Mothers vary in their ability to achieve the complex state of regression in the service of the baby. Life circumstances, the birth experience itself, and the experience immediately following the birth are of great importance. One mother whose child was delivered by cesarean section at first felt estranged from her infant and felt a sense of emptiness and loss. However, through the process of physical care for the infant and breast-feeding, she quickly achieved a sense of giving herself up to him: "I gave him my body. It didn't belong to me anymore."

By contrast, another mother, after the easy, natural birth of her first child in the presence of the father (who was allowed to stay in the hospital with her overnight so she was not separated from either her baby or him) felt that her connectedness with the infant was immediate. When asked to describe it she said, "I don't know what to say. It was just like being in love." This mother did not seem to feel an early stage of anxiety, insecurity, or loss. She said the infant was immediately familiar to her and that she connected what she saw now with the earlier sensations of his movements in utero: "I saw him move just as I had felt it when he was inside of me. It was an amazing feeling."

In each case, the description that the mother gave of her experience was determined in part by the circumstances of the birth but also fit well with the particular mother's personality. In the first case, what seemed to be an outstanding personality characteristic was a capacity for total devotion and temporary surrender of self-interest. In the case of the second mother, what was characteristic was a kind of calm self-possession that seems to have easily included her newborn infant. The first mother was intensely aware of having given herself over to her son during the early phase. He was an energetic little boy who nursed so vigorously that his mother's nipples often bled. The mother experienced the symbiotic phase and breast-feeding as a blissful period in her life to which she gave all her energies. She weaned her son when he began to walk at the age of about 8 months. The joy in the exclusive symbiotic attachment gave way easily and naturally to the child's needs for distancing and exploration of the world and resulted in the mother's vicarious pleasure and some relief about being able to return to her own life, which she did gradually.

The second mother did not experience a break at birth but felt immediate connection. However, her experience of the early phase was not one of giving herself up to the baby's care; she had an experience of awe and wonder that very quickly became one of exquisite intimacy. She, too, was breast-feeding and especially enjoyed the night feedings when she and her baby were alone together. She felt early on that her baby responded to her in a unique way. She focused more on the earliest signs of interaction and differentiation than on the aspect of oneness with the infant.

For both these mothers, the experience of the early love for and intimacy with their babies and the early experiences of mutuality and reciprocity were satisfying. Both mothers were able to achieve the mixture of identification and objectivity vis-à-vis the infant that, according to Sander [9], is optimal for the early phase.

In contrast to both these mothers is a third mother. She also had a baby born by cesarean section and described her earliest feelings following birth as feelings of intense excitement and happiness. This feeling lasted while she was in the hospital. However, once she brought the baby home she felt extremely overwhelmed. Her baby was difficult to care for at first. He was colicky, and she felt herself to be in the throes of strong but conflicting feelings. She described her state as one of disequilibrium. On one hand, she had strong feelings for her baby and felt his presence to be a wonderful miracle. On the other hand, she felt distant, isolated, trapped, and very frightened by his dependency on her. She missed the fact that she had no family nearby, and she had a strong sense of loss of self in surrendering all her needs to his. By the time the baby was 6 weeks old and began to sleep for longer periods, she began to integrate him into her life. It was very important to her to begin to resume some of her own activities and go back to work part time. By the time he was 2½ months old and beginning to smile, she began to enjoy him fully. However, she described how it was difficult for her to find herself again. She said: "I had lost myself to an extraordinary extent. I felt I was sacrificing myself, my self-regulation. I had lost my self-feeling. I didn't know when I was hungry or tired. I was up and down with him." When he began to smile and seemed less vulnerable, she began to see him as a person rather than "that alien thing."

This mother vividly manifests the illness aspect of primary maternal preoccupation. She was, however, able to face these feelings well enough to be able to emerge from them and to achieve a pleasurable, intense symbiotic relationship with her son. Her baby, after a difficult beginning, stabilized and achieved Winnicott's capacity for "going on being."

Winnicott [13] describes play between mother and baby during symbiosis in which the baby interrupts nursing to put a finger into the mother's mouth. This, according to Winnicott, is a primitive identification of the baby with the feeding mother.

In this way we actually witness a mutuality which is the beginning of a communication between two people; this (in the baby) is a developmental achievement, one that is dependent on the baby's inherited processes leading toward emotional growth and likewise dependent on the mother and her attitude and her capacity to make real what the baby is ready to reach out for, to discover, to create. (P. 250) Consequently, whereas the mother can identify with the baby, even with a baby unborn or in process of being born, and in a highly sophisticated way, the baby brings to the situation only a developing capacity to achieve cross-identifications in the experience of mutuality that is made a fact. This mutuality belongs to the mother's capacity to adapt to the baby's needs. (P. 251)

The baby's widening repertoire of care-eliciting behaviors brings about the more fully developed mutuality that characterizes the symbiotic phase of dual unity. This is based in part on the programmed maturational achievements of the baby (i.e., smiling, nestling, and cooing), but also on the mother having provided the possibility of mutuality for the baby, which depends on her achievement of maternal preoccupation — the development of her motherliness. According to Benedek [1]:

As motherliness facilitates the normal symbiotic processes between mother and child, it supplies the matrix for the healthy development of the child; at the same time as it enables the mother to encompass the growing child in her own person ality, it also prepares her for the individuation of her child and for his separation from her. Even the normal maturation of the child represents, in every phase, a new adaptive task to parents. (P. 165)

I have tried to show how the first phase of mothering requires a mother's healthy capacity to regress and recover, to be both part of and outside the baby — to be, as it were, a transitional phenomenon, a bridge between the subjective and objective world. The mother's role during the symbiotic phase shifts; she can now feel much more definitely that the baby responds to her. Sander [9] calls the period from 2½ to 5 months the period of reciprocal exchange and sees the task of the mother to be the stimulation of reciprocity. This is the period of bliss that has been described so richly in recent years by Stern [10] in his description of mother-infant games and by Brazelton [3] in the development of his ideas on feedback loops within the envelope of mother-infant interaction.

Mahler [5] has called the period of dual unity in which mother and infant are as within a common membrane the symbiotic phase. This comprises much more than oneness and the sense of lack of differentiation and separateness. Pine [8] has emphasized that merging during the symbiotic phase refers to moments of high intensity rather than to a continuous state, and Mahler has repeatedly stressed that during normal symbiosis a complex interaction between baby and mother takes place. In Winnicott's [12] terms, the baby has achieved the capacity for "going on being" and for withstanding impingement and the threat of disintegration. During this period, mothers often describe their babies as delightful, enchanting, and sweet. The baby no longer seems so fragile or helpless, and the mother can proudly reap the rewards of her earlier period of primary maternal preoccupation.

Mahler postulated that the beginning of the separation-individuation process occurs at the height of symbiosis at around 4 to 5 months. At this time, interest in the outside, nonmother world gains a great deal of momentum, and the exclusive, intense involvement with mother lessens. Whereas during the symbiotic phase a mother often describes how her infant stops nursing in order to smile, coo, and interact with her, the infant, during the differentiation subphase, often stops nursing and begins to look around at other phenomena in the environment. Brazelton [3] describes this process: "When the mother can allow for this and even foster it, she and the infant become aware of his burgeoning autonomy." Sander [9] calls this period, which we refer to as the differentiation subphase (the first subphase of the separation-individuation process), the period of early directed activity of the infant. He sees this stage as one in which the infant becomes more active in establishing reciprocity with the mother. If the infant can feel successful in initiating smiling play with mother, he or she learns to anticipate her response and can reproduce some of the joyful excitement by activities associated with his anticipation. As Sander [9] says:

The period from 6 to 9 months is a time which demands of the mother a certain keenness in reading and appreciating the cues of her child. It further demands that she respond as appropriately as in the initial period of adaptation. (P. 140)

This is the period of selective cueing. Not only is it necessary for the mother to have heightened sensitivity in reading the infant's cues for interacting, she must also be sensitive to the infant's cues for wishing to interact with others, to cathect the nonmother world [2]. The need to distance from mother becomes even clearer and more pronounced during the practicing subphase from 9 to 15 months. Sander [9] sees this as a time when the infant's demands on the mother become more intense and unremitting. He describes what he believes are necessary qualities of the mother during this period: She needs to be secure in her sense of identity as a mother; this enables her to be flexibly available, protecting the infant from dangers engendered during his or her explorations and occasionally from strong fear of strangers.

The smooth and satisfactory negotiation seems to depend on the mother's availability to yield or to compromise by keeping the baby in her awareness while she pursues her own interests . . . The mother who is secure enough in herself and has confidence in the ultimate separateness and integrity of her child can enjoy and yield to this possession by him. When she does so, preserving areas of reciprocity with her child, she acts as a stable base of operations for him as his growing motility and inevitable curiosity carry him away from her. (P. 142)

Sander feels that it is particularly important during this period that the baby be allowed to develop certainty about being the focus of mother's attention. Otherwise, he argues, the baby will be faced with a difficult asynchrony during the second year of life caused by the contradictory needs to assert him- or herself in relation to mother while at the same time still seeking assurance in relation to her.

From the point of view of separation-individuation theory, we feel, similarly to Sander, that it is of utmost importance for the baby to be allowed to take mother for granted, even to the extent where he or she seems oblivious of her separateness, which as yet he or she does not fully comprehend. The child during this period often uses the mother's body as if it were an object to climb on or to lean on, seemingly without any wish for interaction. Mother is not only a home base to which to return periodically for "refueling," she is also supposed to be a passive facilitator. From the point of view of separation-individuation, however, we are equally sensitive to the mother's ability to be available as we are to her ability to let go and even to provide a "gentle push" to the outside world. This is a delicate moment indeed. A mother who unnecessarily retaliates by becoming unavailable, aloof, or uninterested or a mother who continues to draw the child back into her own orbit does not provide the optimal environment for the unfolding of the child's separate self.

A mother who seemed equally sensitive to her child's needs for closeness and for distance described his emergence from a very happy symbiotic period. During the period of differentiation, he went through a difficult time. Old ways of comforting him by rocking and singing did not seem to work any longer. The baby woke up crying at night. When mother picked him up, he wanted to be put down. When she put him down, he wanted to be picked up. His mood changed from even-tempered happiness to crankiness. However, as his motility increased and he entered the early practicing subphase, he once again became much more joyful, and he was now able to let his mother know that he had outgrown the old kind of closeness. She noticed that when he was ready to go to sleep and she tried to hold and rock him, he began to pull away from her and to look at his crib. When she put him into the crib he seemed content. He began to "sing" himself to sleep as she used to do for him before that. She was both wistful and pleased as she told of his growing up.

In this section, I have tried to describe both clinically and theoretically the experience of the mother during the first year of her infant's life. During this time, she needs to go through a process in which at first she is able to relinquish her usual ways of functioning in the interest of helping her infant achieve regulation and establish reciprocity. As the infant's world widens during the second half of the first year, it becomes the mother's task to repossess her own life in such a way that room is made for the gradual achievement of separateness for the infant. As the infant's world widens, so does the world between the mother and infant. Mothers vary in how they are able to make this transition, which in turn has some influence on how the baby experiences his or her needs for autonomy and intimacy. I will illustrate this with some vignettes from the separation-individuation studies.

The Separation-Individuation Process in Normal Mother-Child Pairs

In the following vignettes, I shall describe mothers whose apparently insufficiently resolved issues of autonomy and separation-individuation in their own lives seemed to be related to difficulties in mothering their infants. The material for these vignettes was gathered in informal interviews and participant observations of the mothers in the group of mothers and infants in our study.

MRS. A

Mrs. A was an intelligent young woman who was understated, self-deprecating, and complained of being disorganized. She attended our nursery at any possible opportunity, and it seemed quite clear that it was a home away from home for her, a longed-for home that she had difficulty in establishing herself. She was the oldest of three daughters and strongly attached to her father. Her perfectionistic goals, which she was never able to live up to, were connected with her father. She said that her father had always expected his daughters to be perfect.

In connection with the father's profession, Mrs. A's family had traveled quite a bit during her childhood and adolescence. She had always been a good student and in that way had lived up to her father's expectations. While she was in college, her family once again moved, this time a considerable distance away. Mrs. A decided to stay in college and not move away with her family. However, she lost interest in her studies, and her grades deteriorated.

Mrs. A graduated from college but did not pursue any further studies and quickly married. It seemed that the marriage offered her some protection and comfort but not very much pleasure or excitement. In her present family, her emphasis was not on her relationship to her husband or their life together but rather on herself and her relationship to her children. From all this information, we might hypothesize that Mrs. A prematurely turned away from her mother and identified with her father, perhaps in connection with the birth of her siblings. Longings for closeness with mother were defended against, and a depressive mood prevailed.

The relationship to her oldest child, a girl, was central in Mrs. A's emotional life. She described the symbiotic phase with this baby as having been blissful for herself and the child. It seemed that by way of caring for her girl child she had been able to experience a pleasure in femininity that she otherwise denied. She took great pride and pleasure in her daughter's prettiness and dressed her exquisitely. When they entered our nursery, the daughter was 1 year old and quickly took possession of the nursery by way of her precocity and charm. Her mother took great pleasure and pride in her and was quite tolerant of difficulties the little girl experienced during the rapprochement subphase.

When her second child, a boy, was born, Mrs. A seemed to experience a great deal of pain and anxiety around separation from her daughter, who was then entering nursery school. Mrs. A's primary maternal preoccupation with her son (Nicholas) was a painful one. She never seemed to know what her infant son wanted or needed. She prolonged feedings endlessly, jiggling him to keep him awake while bottle-feeding him. The baby was difficult—unusually fussy and uncomfortable. Using Winnicott's concept, one could describe him as a baby who did not attain a state of "going on being"; he did not learn to withstand impingement during the early phase. Although there was some improvement in his state during the symbiotic phase and a certain amount of reciprocity became established between mother and infant, there remained a sense of fragility in the baby and in the mother-child relationship. His frequent illnesses and several hospitalizations disrupted what sense of safety and well-being could be established. Nevertheless, Nicholas developed quite satisfactorily during the separation-individuation period. His mother was particularly skillful in reading the cues that indicated his increasing competence and ability to cathect the outside world. She was able to support his separation-individuation process and took pride and pleasure in his good intelligence and his achievements.

For Mrs. A there seems to have been an important difference in mothering a boy and mothering a girl. We might hypothesize that she experienced her girl child as a narcissistic enhancement, an opportunity to take pleasure in femininity that she could not otherwise allow herself. She had experienced the girl child as perfect and herself as the perfect mother for the child. Thus, in caring for her perfect little baby girl, Mrs. A could meet her father's wish for a perfect daughter. The perfection began to crumble as the little girl had to face the outside world (i.e., nursery school), a world that did not know of her perfection and thus did not give her the special treatment that both mother and daughter thought she deserved. The mother experienced every blow the child suffered as a blow to herself.

Mrs. A was not able to experience symbiotic bliss with her son. She often complained that she did not feel herself to be a good mother to him when he was an infant and he was not a perfect child. Nicholas was small and fragile and did not easily find his niche in the extrauterine environment. Throughout his separation-individuation process he remained fragile, and he suffered several hospitalizations.

The follow-up study of Nicholas (at 10 years of age) revealed some interesting personality characteristics harking back to his difficult beginnings. Nicholas had turned out to be an intelligent, high-achieving child. He seemed to be confident and considered himself to be the smartest boy in his class. However, his self-confidence seemed to be very dependent on high achievement. When he was tested, he suddenly became confused and panicky after he had solved a difficult problem correctly. He began to doubt his solution of the difficult problem and thought of several incorrect alternatives. This pointed to a problem in Nicholas reminiscent of that of his mother—the need to be perfect. Also, it was a problem reminiscent of his infancy—namely, the tendency to fall apart and lose his bearings when he was under pressure.

Another interesting observation noted during the follow-up study related to Nick's love for stray animals. Like his mother, he liked to take them in the house and take care of them. Here we seem to see a double identification: On one hand, he is identifying with a caretaking mother; on the other hand, he is identifying with a neglected child in need of care. The follow-up tests revealed that Nicholas is a child who strongly defends against impulses and, in particular, passive strivings. His defenses take the form of self-sufficiency and achievement orientation. Again, this was reminiscent of his mother who appeared self-sufficient and cool and had great difficulty in acknowledging her dependency needs consciously. Underneath a seemingly strong ego, one sensed fragility in Nicholas, reminiscent of his early life with mother.

MRS. B

Mrs. B was an older mother and, in many ways, the opposite of Mrs. A. If Mrs. A understated her capacities, Mrs. B overstated hers. She tried to be supermother not only to her own child but to the other mothers in our group, ever ready with good advice and knowledge of how to do things. However, underneath the bravado and apparent self-assurance of Mrs. B, observers began to notice her depressive tendencies and a strong narcissistic need for admiration. She constantly overstimulated her baby and when not in direct contact with him or when not engaged in active conversation with others, she would lapse into a somewhat withdrawn state. She described her own mother as a dominating and overly efficient person. She described that she regressed when she went home, allowing her mother to do everything.

Mrs. B's account of the way in which she had left home seemed revealing of her own difficulties in establishing her separate identity and in separating from her family. She had grown up in a small midwestern town and was still living at home after having finished college. She was then in her 20s and working in an excellent job. On the spur of the moment she decided to go to New York on a visit with a friend. To her own surprise, she found herself looking for an apartment and a job and very quickly found both. To the dismay of her parents, she decided to move to New York and felt happy and content living on her own, relieved to have escaped her mother's domination.

Mrs. B rarely talked about her father. She described him as kind and unassuming; she loved and admired him. The man Mrs. B chose to marry in no way resembled the kind, unassuming father. Quite the contrary, he was a demanding, opinionated, and erratic man. He dominated the family and decided on child-rearing methods. His most important demand was that little Seth should never be frustrated. Mrs. B went along with her husband and seemed to agree with him; she thought of herself as the embodiment of motherliness. She was quite dominating, overstimulating, and seemingly needed her child to be constantly engaged with her.

Seth developed well during the symbiotic phase. He was alert, calm, and smiling. Observers noted that early in the beginning of the differentiation subphase (at around 5 months) he began to attempt to push away from his mother's tight grip. At this time, we observed the following.

Mrs. B sits him up by holding on to his hands and pulling him up. It looked as if he would rather hold onto his mother than have her hold onto him. He continually tried to loosen his hands from her grip and tried to hold onto her himself.

At the same time, Mrs. B became concerned because Seth, at nursing time, became distractible and no longer exclusively focused on the breast. She decided that she had to nurse him in a quiet place. She could not accept his playfulness and interest in the world that was natural for his age.

Seth, in turn, preferred to be held by others, who seemed to be a kind of refuge for him. His mother's intense overstimulation of him was designed to get a response from him. I quote again from an observation.

When Mrs. B returned, she said, "Where is my baby? Hi, you don't want to see me now. He is totally unaware of me today. He is very tired." She lifted him high in the air before putting him back into the baby's section. He quickly started to fret and she picked him up at the same time that she said, "Why don't you go to sleep?" Mrs. B lifted him high up and lowered him, shook him from side to side and kissed his stomach several times.

She spent several minutes intensely overstimulating Seth with movement, tickling him, holding him high, taking him down, holding him to her face, saying he wanted to eat her up. . . . Actually, she did not notice that Seth was, for some part of the procedure at least, markedly uncomfortable, nonresponding.

Seth was delayed in locomotor development and in entering the practicing subphase. This might have been because he could not take his mother for granted—an important aspect of the mother-child relationship for the flowering of the practicing subphase. He could not take her for granted because he could not be sure whether she would suddenly overwhelm him or be quite oblivious to him. It was difficult for Mrs. B to remain in contact with her child when she was not directly engaged with him. She was abrupt in her handling of Seth, unable to modulate her own needs for closeness and distance.

Seth was 10 years old when the follow-up study was conducted. During the first follow-up interview, it was notable that Seth did not show the same reluctance to speak of himself to a stranger, the interviewer, as had most of the other children. He immediately began to talk about himself and proudly told of his accomplishments. The interviewer had the impression that she was not being related to as a person in her own right. Seth seemed to assume that the interviewer would admire him, approve of everything he said, and want to listen to him. In this way, Seth was reminiscent of his mother and the way in which she had entered our group, overly sure of herself and not taking the reactions of others into account. It would seem that in both mother and child, this seeming self-confidence had a defensive quality.

In the test report, Seth's expectation to be admired and approved of was contrasted to his extraordinary anxiety when he was asked to perform a specific task that seemed to make him feel quite helpless. The teacher's report noted that Seth was not a generous boy, that he was not responsive to the needs of others, and that he would not contribute to the group if the contribution was anonymous. Thus, the wish to be noticed and admired was paramount and defended against by taking for granted that others would be interested in him. It was also notable that Seth was rather compliant. The tester noted that he had difficulty in expressing his own wishes vis-à-vis his mother and would instead try to comply with hers. This compliance seemed like a reenactment of his situation during symbiosis and differentiation when he had been overstimulated and his autonomous wishes had not been respected.

Summary

In this chapter I have made an attempt to describe the experience of the mother as she attains primary maternal preoccupation, a state that requires an ability to lose oneself in the other and emerge again. I have called this transient loss of self regression in the service of the baby. It is this ability in the mother that sets the stage for the attainment of reciprocity during the symbiotic phase.

Reciprocity, or symbiosis, denotes a state of mutuality and homeostasis, a state during which the unique bond to the love object becomes established for the baby and a sense of unique caregiving becomes established for the mother. Reciprocity is a state of balance between two separate beings — the mother and the baby — that creates the sense of oneness and blissfulness characteristic of the symbiotic phase. During the subphases of differentiation and early practicing, a gradual process of letting go is required of the mother. As she lets go and the infant begins to attain the capacity for distancing, mutual cueing becomes more and more important.

Mothers vary in their ability to attain primary maternal preoccupation and to emerge from it. The stage of symbiotic unity is unique in the pleasure that it provides for the mother and is a kind of reward for the dedication and loss of self that is required during the earliest period of motherhood. During the stage of symbiosis, the groundwork for further differentiation and autonomy already is laid. However, it is during the period of differentiation par excellence, beginning at 5 to 6 months, that the mother has to begin to allow the baby's interest in and relation to the outside world to begin to flourish; it is with the advent of independent locomotion and early practicing at about 9 months that the baby begins his endless explorations of the surroundings. Most mothers can facilitate or at least allow this process to happen, but difficulties in the mother may, to a greater or lesser extent, interfere with the child's unfolding of the separation-individuation process.

In examples taken from the observational study of normal mother-child pairs during the separation-individuation process, I have shown how the patterns established during symbiosis, differentiation, and early practicing become internalized by the child. I have speculated that disturbances in early mothering are connected to the mother's own difficulties, which may extend back to her own separation-individuation period. From material gathered during the follow-up study, it was possible to see how the child attempted to adapt to the difficulties in the mother and to what degree earlier patterns persisted. In the case of the first mother, Mrs. A, the difficulties were present at the very beginning in establishing a strong symbiotic relationship, and the child did not develop the capacity for "going on being." This was partly offset by the mother's excellent adaptation to the child during the separation-individuation process [6]. In the case of the second mother, Mrs. B, the difficulty was twofold: first, in the mother's need for stimulation from her infant and, second, in her difficulty in allowing him to separate and individuate and thus become a self in his own right.

Acknowledgment

The author wishes to thank David Pollens for his assistance in the preparation of this chapter.

References

1. Benedek, T. The Family as Psychological Field. In E. J. Anthony and T. Benedek (Eds.), *Parenthood: Its Psychology and Psychopathology.* Boston: Little, Brown, 1970.
2. Bergman, A. From Mother to the World Outside: The Use of Space During the Separation-Individuation Phase. In S. A. Grolnick and L. Barkin (Eds.), *Between Reality and Fantasy.* New York: Jason Aronson, 1978.
3. Brazelton, T. Precursors for the Development of Emotions in Early Infancy. In R. Plutchik and H. Kellerman (Eds.), *Emotion: Theory, Research and Experience,* Vol. 2. New York: Academic Press, 1983.
4. Loewald, H. W. Instinct Theory Object Relations and Psychic Structure Formation. In *Rapprochement: The Critical Subphase of Separation—Individuation.* New York: Jason Aronson, 1980.
5. Mahler, M. S. *The Selected Papers of Margaret S. Mahler, Vol. II, Separation-Individuation.* New York: Jason Aronson, 1979.
6. Mahler, M. S., Pine, F., and Bergman, A. The Mother's Reaction to her Toddler's Drive for Individuation. In E. J. Anthony and T. Benedek (Eds.), *Parenthood: Its Psychology and Psychopathology.* Boston: Little, Brown, 1970.

7. Mahler, M. S., Pine, F., and Bergman A. *The Psychological Birth of the Human Infant.* New York: Basic Books, 1975.
8. Pine, F. In the beginning. *International Review of Psycho-analysis* 8 : 15, 1981.
9. Sander, L. W. Issues in Early Mother-Child Interaction. In E. N. Rexford, L. W. Sander, and T. Shapiro (Eds.), *Infant Psychiatry.* New Haven: Yale University Press, 1976.
10. Stern, D. The goal and structure of mother-infant play. *J. Am. Acad. Child Psychiatry* 13 : 402, 1974.
11. Stern, D. Implications of Infancy Research for Clinical Theory and Practice, presented at the 13th Annual Margaret S. Mahler Symposium, 1982.
12. Winnicott, D. W. *D. W. Winnicott: Collected Papers.* London: Tavistock Publications, 1956.
13. Winnicott, D. W. The Mother-Infant Experience of Mutuality. In E. J. Anthony and T. Benedek (Eds.), *Parenthood: Its Psychology and Psychopathology.* Boston: Little, Brown, 1970.

6

Parenting as a function of the adult self: a psychoanalytic developmental perspective

Anna Ornstein and Paul H. Ornstein

Once human behavior became the legitimate subject of scientific inquiry around the turn of the twentieth century, infant and child development studies had become central to these research endeavors. Today, there is a great deal of literature related to the study of infants, young children, and the early phases of mothering. Indeed, the most revealing and dependable data on mothering currently available are from the burgeoning literature on infant research. The findings on parenting in these mother-infant studies, although secondary to the data from the infant studies, are of great significance because they fairly consistently support an evolutionary biological anlage for mothering. In the early phases of mothering, a biological readiness appears to complement the infant's "built-in" capacity to solicit social responses from the environment. "The mother is involved in a natural process with her baby, a process that unfolds with a fascinating intricacy and complexity for which she and her baby are well prepared by the millennia of evolution" [46].

The most persistent supporters of a biological readiness for mothering have been Klaus and Kennell [26], Ainsworth [2], and Bowlby [13]. They have maintained that only civilization and technology obscure the mother's instincts that could otherwise guide her in successful bonding and attachment to her infant. As with other mammals, these authors believe bonding and attachment have to occur at certain "critical periods" in the infant's life and that in the human these experiences have far-reaching consequences for later development, specifically for that of language and intelligence. However, this biological readiness, the capacity for bonding and attachment, remain disputed motives for parenting even during infancy and certainly beyond the earliest phases of the infant's life [15, 17, 41].

Benedek, whose studies of the development of motherliness are the most widely accepted by psychoanalysts, found that in the human female mothering behavior has two sources: one is rooted in her physiology; "the other evolved as an expression of her personality which had developed under environmental influences that could modify her motherliness" [10].

Although we agree with Benedek in the essential aspects of her observation, we wish to add that the biological roots of motherliness of the human female may not only be "modified," but may actually be outweighed or totally overshadowed by psychological factors. And while the biological and physiological factors may still be in evidence in relationship to the infant, it will be the mother's psychology, "the expression of her personality which has developed under environmental influences," that will determine her responsiveness to the increasingly more complex developmental needs of her child.

In our modern Western society, the mother (if she is to care for the child at all) may be only one member of a group of adults engaged in the care of a particular child. From the child's perspective, it may be more appropriate to speak of a "parenting unit" defined as one person (e.g., either parent) or a group of persons from whom the child can receive or extract the responses he needs for his development; to be a "mother" or a "father" is not synonymous with parenting. By introducing the notion of a "parenting unit," we do not intend to minimize the importance that the primary caretaker has in a fundamental achievement of the psyche, namely, attachment. Attachment and bonding appear to occur within the first ten days of the infant's life; within the first week, the newborn shows preference for the mother's smell, voice, and familiar appearance [33]. However, we wish to draw attention to the infant's (and child's) capacity to elicit social responsiveness from a variety of people and pets in the environment and thereby imperceptibly compensate for the unavailable primary caretaker. In this chapter, our attention is not on the disturbance in the capacity for attachment in the "primary caretaker" but on parenting in general — parenting that is not restricted to the early years of the child's life but encompasses the entire parental life cycle.

We find the concept of a parenting unit particularly useful in assessing the development of children who grow up in multiple foster homes, in divorced or "reconstituted" families, or under other unconventional circumstances. Clinicians cannot readily find an explanation for the capacity of these children not only to cope with some very obvious life stresses, but for them to continue their progressive development. Rather than attributing such resiliency to unidentified constitutional factors, although these may perhaps play a part, we are suggesting that children are able to extract developmentally needed "selfobject responses"[1] from

---

[1] The concepts of "selfobject" and "selfobject functions" will be elaborated upon later. At this time, we only want to stress that selfobject functions (e.g., the mirroring and merger with an idealized adult) are silent but active adult functions, and that the building up of

an environment that, to an external observer, may appear to have no redeeming features. And the obverse may be true as well: an environment that, to an external observer, may be "average expectable," may nevertheless not be responsive to a particular child's developmental needs. It is, therefore, understandable that no direct correlation can be made between a particular emotional illness of the parent and that parent's parental capacities or dysfunctions; however, some parental disturbances are more likely to create overt symptoms in the child, while others are more likely to create covert symptoms. Still others, under similar circumstances, may "develop a brittle normality or even super-normality" [3].

Because predictions for psychological development cannot be made by the "objective" assessment of the child's environment, it is important to make a distinction between an *etiological* and a *genetic* approach to the investigations of parenting. Data obtained from the *direct investigation* of parents in the course of psychoanalysis and psychotherapy have etiological significance for child development and psychopathology, while data regarding parenting that is obtained from the treatment of the child (or adult) are of genetic significance. Kohut [27] differentiated the etiological from the genetic approach: "The genetic approach in psychoanalysis relates to the investigation of those subjective psychological experiences of the child which usher in a chronic change in the distribution and further development of the endopsychic forces and structures. The etiological approach, on the other hand, relates to the investigation of those objectively ascertainable factors which, in interaction with the child's psyche as it is constituted at a given moment, may or may not elicit the genetically decisive experiences."

In our conceptualization of parenting, we have used both sources of information. The treatment of children and the psychoanalysis of adults have provided insight into parenting that was derived from reconstructions (the genetic approach). This has elucidated the subjective experiences of the children in relation to their parents. On the other hand, the simultaneous treatment of parents and children has provided us with a view of the "objectively ascertainable factors" of interaction (the etiological approach). It is in this latter context that we can appreciate the ongoing mutuality and reciprocity that exists between the child and his emotional environment. We have found Kohut's theory of the self and

---

psychological structures is conceptualized here as occurring through the transmuting internalization of these functions. This theory of structure formation has to be differentiated from one in which it is hypothesized that structure formation occurs through the internalization of good and bad objects.

the development of the self within an empathically responsive selfobject environment to be the most useful tool for the ordering of our data in all of these treatment modalities.

Adaptation, Development, and Pathogenesis

We are putting forward the view that parenting can only be assessed in conjunction with the assessment of a particular child, since focusing on the parent alone provides the clinician only with an etiological perspective. It is only through the immersion into the child's inner world that the clinician can also appreciate what has become genetically significant for a particular child from the many, possibly significant parental influences. Parenting is a dynamic activity; its mutuality and reciprocity with the child's inner world has thus far been encompassed by the concept of adaptation, which was articulated by Hartmann [24].

Hartmann's seminal work on "Ego Psychology and the Problem of Adaptation" [24] favored the concept of reciprocity in the process of adaptation. In psychoanalysis today, this concept has been replaced by one that considers the individual's response to the environment as either alloplastic or autoplastic. This either/or view of adaptation has been perpetuated because of the relatively rigid conceptual separation of the psychoneuroses (the result of autoplastic adaptation) from the "acting out" forms of psychopathology that have been viewed as aiming at an alloplastic adaptation. Hartmann's statement that "adaptation is primarily a *reciprocal* relationship between the organism and its environment" [24] has not remained in central focus in the subsequent psychoanalytic literature and neither has the statement he made regarding "the average *not* expectable environment": "The degree of adaptiveness can only be determined with reference to environmental situations (average expectable — i.e., typical — situations, or on the average not expectable — i.e., atypical — situations)."

It is our view that the notion of a not expectable (i.e., atypical) situation has not found its way into psychoanalytic thinking. By maintaining, at least for theoretical purposes, that the external environment is "average expectable" (i.e., invariant), analysts can focus more exclusively on what they consider to be only internal variations. This focus has undoubtedly permitted a more thorough appreciation of the internally generated, drive-related conflicts and their underlying unconscious fantasies as motives for normal development and as sources of anxiety and symptom formation. However, this sharp dichotomy between external and internal can only be maintained by the unwarranted assumption of the presence of a consensually valid external reality (at least operationally). Hartmann [24], discussing the interplay between psychological and biological factors in development, asked: "Are the exogenous factors the average expectable kind (family situation, mother-child relationship and others), or are the environmental conditions of a different sort? In other words, the question is whether, and to what extent, a certain course of development can count on average expectable stimulations (environmental releasers) and whether, and to what extent, and in what direction it will be deflected by environmental influences of a different sort."

Anthony [4] discussed the historical antecedents of the psychoanalyst's ambivalence toward the external environment, specifically the resistance to considering the importance of the family in the child's analysis. He says that to consider the family in a child's analysis "is tantamount to becoming an environmentalist, the modern equivalent of the 'wild analyst.'" In order to facilitate the psychoanalyst's treatment of the child and still take into account the child's complex experiences of his or her emotional environment, Anthony suggested that the analyst should recognize that the child constructs three forms of "families" in his psyche, to which gets added a fourth one — the one the child constructs in the course of analysis. "The various families — the intrapsychic oedipal one, the idealized representational one, the actual interpersonal one, and the analyst's hypothetical one — may all appear in symbolic play with the family figures provided by the analyst." The analyst's task is to disentangle these various "families" and to appraise the family realistically; at the same time, he or she should encourage the formation of the imaginary family via the transference.

In other words, the child analyst, by assessing the family's "reality," has to disentangle the intricate impact of the family on the child's psyche and the child's own contribution to the pathological interactions. Once this has been accomplished, the analyst is expected to help the child separate the family's real impact from his or her own oedipal wishes and fantasies. The reality of the family and its impact on the child is conceived here as something that has become "superimposed" on the unconscious oedipal fantasies, which, once exposed, becomes the legitimate subject of the analyst's interpretations.

Although this recommendation is broadly encompassing, two questions must be raised: Is the analyst in the position to appraise "the reality" of the family and is the child able to separate experientially "the interpersonal family from her internalized libidinal and ego attitudes?" [4].

The question as to what external or internal factors account for pathogenicity has been with psychoanalysts ever since Freud's time. Freud's original answer to this dilemma was the introduction of the concept of the "complemental series" [22]. This concept was to explain the pathogenesis of the adult forms of psychoneuroses; it meant that traumatic events in a child's life created libidinal fixations, which, when reactivated later in life, lead to neurotic compromise formations. Such neurotic compromises require the presence of a well-developed ego and superego. For this reason, neurotic conditions, based on the vicissitudes of the Oedipus complex, had been traditionally differentiated from "deficiency illnesses." The deficiency in the child's ego and superego structure has been related either to gross parental neglect, physical abuse, institutionalization, or other, as yet unknown, factors that have prevented children from using the environment effectively, thus possibly leading to childhood psychosis.

In clinical practice, child therapists have long recognized another group of patients — children who do not suffer from the consequences of an unresolved Oedipus complex and who do not exhibit gross structural defects because of severe parental neglect or abuse. These are children who suffer from the consequences of various degrees of discreet structural deficits that can be related to equally discreet and subtle failures in parental empathy. Kohut's discovery of the selfobject transferences has alerted child therapists to those parental functions that, because of their silent presence, by and large have been taken for granted. We are referring to the infant's and child's ongoing developmental need for validation and the need to merge first with the parents' physical strength and power and later with their moral strength and power. These parental functions do not simply "facilitate" a "drive-determined" sequence in development, but rather, they themselves are responsible for the building up of psychic structures by becoming transmutedly internalized [27, 47].

Infant research had repeatedly demonstrated that the capacity to elicit life-sustaining environmental responses that are crucial for the infant's momentary functioning and for the building up of permanent psychic structures are inborn. The infant, born with "a predictable genetic ground plan" [32], has to be assured of phase-appropriate environmental responses. These are the responses that self-psychology calls "selfobject functions." Sander [43], for example, spoke of a "fitting together" of the endogenous (infant-determined) and exogenous (caretaker-determined) influences. The fitting together is a developmental accomplishment that requires the caretaker's ability "to read" the infant's clues. The process of fitting together that Sander also conceptualized as an "interactional schema" (similar to Piaget's sensorimotor schemata) has a high level of reciprocity in the process of adaptation.

Sander [43] used the model of adaptation to account for the two major aspects of personality development: integration and differentiation. These two, seemingly opposing directions in the development of the individual, occur within the same contextual unit and, therefore, they have to be accounted for by the same theoretical model. For example, the increasing differentiation of the child's emotional, cognitive, and perceptual capacities have to become integrated into the very same system in which this differentiation has taken place in order for these capacities to achieve functional freedom. In other words, functional freedom is not achieved by the child extricating himself from "the interactive regulative system" in which he is embedded and of which he is a part, but by achieving new levels of adaptation with increasing complexity within that very same system. The sequence in this interactive regulatory system is described by Sander [43].

With one component, the infant, rapidly growing and consequently rapidly changing, new qualities and quantities of infant behavior are constantly being introduced into the content of interaction. The regulation of infant functions, based on behaviors that have become harmoniously coordinated between mother and infant, will become perturbed with the advent of each new, and usually more specifically focused and intentionally initiated activity of the growing infant. Thus adaptation or mutual modification on a new level is required. Since the behavioral innovations by the infant are often aimed at a progressive assumption of control of situations as a part of the widening of his scope of self-regulation vis-à-vis the environment (i.e., he becomes more vigorously alloplastic), these changes impinge critically on the mother's long-established strategies of self-regulation. (P. 135)

Our focus is on the parents' capacity to respond to the challenge of this impingement on their "long-established strategies of self-regulation" in relationship to the rapidly growing and, therefore, rapidly changing psychological organization of the child. This focus on parental responsiveness, however, ought not be interpreted as placing the sole responsibility of a child's development on the caretaker's capacity to pick up the growing child's clues for what should be a perfectly empathic response. We agree with Greenspan [23] that each organism has its "individual way of processing, organizing and differentiating experiences . . . and that the final common pathway is unique to each individual . . . suggesting something fundamental about the organism's manner of organizing its experience of its world, internal and external, animate and inanimate."

However, while we agree that each organism has its "individual way of processing, organizing, and differentiating experiences," we question the separation of internal from external experiences as they become integrated into a final common pathway. Rather, we suggest (in keeping with Sander's interaction schemas) that the environment's responses to the child "create" experiences that are unique not only to that child but also to that environment. The experiences that become transmutedly internalized and will constitute the relatively independent tension, affect, and self-esteem regulating systems of the self are being "created" between the infant and his emotional environment in an ongoing way.

The significance of social interaction between infant and caretaker is strongly emphasized by Stern [46]. In presenting a research tool that would measure social interactive behavior and styles, he had commented that such an instrument would have to be used in three ways [6].

The first is to identify something distinctive about particular parents and see how that factor affects their social interaction with their infants. For example, one could compare mothers who differ along an important clinical parameter such as mental illness. The second use, similarly, is to identify and compare infants as known risks for some developmental deviance. A third use is to explore the nature and ontogeny of the specific fit of particular parents and babies across time to see how they navigate the hurdles of various developmental milestones together.

Infant researchers we have cited so far and others whose work is relevant but too numerous to be quoted bring the primacy of the drives as motivators of development and as providers of psychic energy into serious question; the biological anlage for human psychological development appears to reside in the infant's capacity to elicit certain responses from the environment crucial for his development (i.e., the "selfobject functions" of self-psychology). In addition, these researchers in their careful attention to the infant's and child's emotional environment have expanded our view of development from one in which we could simply trace the acquisition of psychic functions to one in which we can also trace the source of the qualities of these functions (i.e., whether or not the acquired functions are executed with joy or only mechanically). According to Greenspan [23]: "Most importantly, under optimal circumstances we note that the toddler is capable of pleasure in a joyful manner, assertiveness and expressions of protest and anger, all tied together in complex behavioral patterns." Even though Greenspan's observations are guided by classical psychoanalytic theory, we do not believe that affects, such as self-assertiveness, anger, and joy are viewed here as drive derivatives that will have to be further modified and neutralized. Rather, these affects are seen as indicative of increased structuralization of the psyche—a developmental accomplishment that is the result of increasing differentiation of the child's affects within the selfobject matrix [7].

Greenspan's structuralist approach to the study of development is particularly useful for psychoanalysts who consider psychoanalysis as a structural psychology par excellence as did Kohut.[2] Greenspan's findings [23] confirm Kohut's assumptions that a failure by the environment to respond to the infant's cues leaves defects behind in the psyche that get "filled in" with defensive and negativistic behavior in order for the infant to remain in contact with his or her life-sustaining environment.

If emerging capacities for contingent interactions in sensorimotor and affective areas are not systematically responded to, developmental progress in the most vulnerable areas may slow down or cease, simply because there is no opportunity for repetitive action sequences or practice (i.e., there is lack of repetitive minimal stimulus nutriment necessary to consolidate these capacities) and we may observe cognitive and interpersonal delays. Secondary apathy, withdrawal, disorganization and/or other regression may follow. Also, an infant who gets no response or an inappropriate response (e.g., he is misread) to his "reaching out" cues may mobilize negativistic responses to achieve a reaction from the environment. (P. 730)

The process of "fitting together" [43], the need to maintain emotional connection between parent and child at all cost [23], and "exploring the nature and ontogeny of the specific fit of particular parents and babies across time to see how they navigate the hurdles of various developmental milestones together" [6] are not only useful conceptualizations of the complex processes of development but are fundamental to the clinician who has to understand the child's "fit," or adaptation or maladaptation, to a particular emotional environment.

The Concept of the Self, the Self-Selfobject Unit, and Parental Selfobject Functions

Kohut's developmental theory of the self is based on his description of the various forms of selfobject transferences: the mirror transference, the alter-ego or twinship transference, and the idealizing transference [27, 28]. In self-psychology, just as in classical psychoanalytic theory, hypotheses regarding development are based on the transferences that have

---

[2] For more information, see reference 5.

been observed in the psychoanalytic situation. This makes the developmental theory of the self a psychoanalytic developmental theory, and its validity, therefore, has to be established at first in the psychoanalytic situation itself. However, scientific rigor requires that validation also occur from outside the situation in which the data have originally been gathered. In psychoanalytic developmental theory, this has traditionally been done by direct observation of infants and young children and by the observation of children and their families in the offices of child analysts and child therapists. The review of current literature regarding infant research indicates a high correlation between Kohut's hypothesis regarding the structure-building function of the empathically responsive (selfobject) environment and the findings of present-day infant researchers.

Child psychotherapists have found with increasing frequency that they treat children who live under varied external circumstances, that is, in average, not expectable, environments. Under these circumstances, child therapists are confronted repeatedly with the question as to how to set up a treatment plan that will optimally address those aspects of the emotional milieu that most crucially impinge on the child's development and on the already existing symptoms. It is no longer sufficient to ask the question whether the weight of the pathology resides primarily within the child or within the environment. Rather, we now need a conceptual tool that addresses the question of the *fit* between the child and his or her emotional environment. We are suggesting that this conceptual tool is provided by the model of the *self-selfobject unit.*

Using the model of the self-selfobject unit, the clinician can conceptualize the various degrees of failures in parenting beyond the early years of the child's life since empathic selfobject responsiveness remains an essential aspect of development throughout childhood. Using this model in the clinical situation, we can either focus on the child's developing self and assess the manner in which the environment is meeting the child's selfobject needs, or we can reverse the model and determine to what extent and in what manner the parents are using the child to meet their own selfobject needs. The latter use of the model is particularly useful in determining parental self-pathology, which is the most frequent source of failures in parental empathy.

The model of the self-selfobject unit has several advantages for the organization of clinical data. It underlines the importance of having to take into consideration the infinite variations of the environment when making an in-depth psychological assessment of a child's development and/or psychopathology. That is, we now recognize that we cannot assess the state of the child's self without considering the way in which the growing self is experiencing and internalizing its emotional environment. Self and environment constitute an experiential unit; the self cannot be conceptualized without the selfobject environment, nor can the functions of the selfobjects be assessed without taking the effect that these functions have on the self into consideration.

The model of the self-selfobject as an experiential unit highlights why the process of adaptation no longer adequately characterizes human psychological development. Although the concept includes the recognition that it is not only the child's psyche that is changing, but (as a result of a high level of reciprocity) the emotional environment changes in relationship to the growing child as well; the concept of adaptation conveys the idea of two entities adjusting to each other's needs. Even when we conceive of this adjustment not only in terms of externally observable behavioral manifestations, but also in terms of the internally achieved changes, the idea of adaptation still remains the external observer's point of view of what happens between the two independent entities that are being observed. In this context the "average expectable" as well as the "average not expectable" environments are also constructed from the vantage point of the external observer. In contrast, the empathic observer attempts to see and grasp the infant's or child's experiencing of the mother or any parenting figure (i.e., the mirroring or idealized selfobject) and proceeds to describe the events between them in terms of the self-experience of each in relation to the other. A similar idea was expressed by Atwood and Stolorow [5]. "We are contending that *every* phase in a child's development is best conceptualized in terms of the unique, continuously changing psychological field constituted by the intersection of the child's evolving subjective universe with those of the caretakers . . . When the psychological organization of the parent cannot sufficiently accommodate to the changing, phase specific needs of the developing child, then the more malleable and vulnerable psychological structure of the child will accommodate to what is available" (p. 69, italics in the original).

The empathic focus on the experiencing self of the infant or child, and thus on the presence or absence of those phase-appropriate selfobject functions that it needs for its wholesome development, permits us to learn about the genetic impact of parenting on children with a variety of constitutions and special endowments. Conversely, a similar focus on the parent's experiencing of the infant or child permits us to learn about the impact that the rearing of a particular child has on the parent's adult self and on parenting capacities.

By focusing our attention on the experiencing self, the concept of the selfobject directs us to an empathic (i.e., vicariously introspective) mode of observation through which we recognize the particular roles and functions of the other for the attainment and maintenance of the cohesiveness of the self and for its vigor and vitality.[3]

Adaptation becomes a necessity on the part of the infant or growing child when the selfobject functions are unavailable or are faulty. It also is necessary when, instead of the parents being responsive to the selfobject needs of the infant or child, the infant or child needs to be responsive to the parents' own imperative needs for self-affirmation.

The model of the self-selfobject unit also helps us conceptualize the various degrees of parental dysfunctions that are related to the parent's own self-development. By focusing on the parent's self, the clinician can determine in what manner and to what extent the parent is using the child as a selfobject in order to maintain his or her fragile self and/or bolster shaky self-esteem.

The usefulness of the model is related to the fact that in the parent-child relationship, both parties, parent and child, fulfill selfobject functions for each other. While the central importance of parental selfobject functions for the child's development can readily be appreciated, the selfobject functions that children serve for the enhancement of the parent's adult self are more difficult to conceptualize. The difficulty lies in the fact that a parent's "average expectable" narcissistic investment in a child may not be readily distinguishable from the subtle ways in which a child may be used for the maintenance of the parent's self-cohesion, or more frequently, for the regulation of self-esteem.

The conception and birth of a child "reopen" adult self-development and constitute a potential for further consolidation and expansion of the adult self. This further expansion is possible because the narcissistic (selfobject) elements are inherent in the parent-child tie. The same idea was originally expressed by Benedek [12] and restated by Lax [30]. "During pregnancy a marked shift toward libidinal concentration on the self occurs. This narcissism, which cathects the expanding self-representation, enables the pregnant woman to feel that the growing body within

---

[3] What we are stating here is a considerable modification of an earlier formulation by Ornstein [38a] regarding the relationship between adaptation and the concept of the selfobject: ". . . the concept of the selfobject serves as a bridge across which intrapsychic, developmental-genetic determinants of health and illness can be integrated with the psychosocial determinants. The new integration also permits the notion of mere adjustment to external reality to be clearly differentiated from a metapsychologically sophisticated conception of *adaptation* to reality."

her constitutes an integral part of herself. In addition to this physical sense of being merged, the pregnant woman daydreams about her future child and in her fantasy molds it according to her wishes and ego-ideals."

From the time of conception, parental hopes and expectations are experienced and later unconsciously conveyed to the child, which not only shape the child's self, but simultaneously firm up the parents' sense of continuity across the generations. Erikson [19] spoke of a "procreative drive" that is part of adult generativity: ". . . generativity which is concerned with new beings as well as new products and new ideas and which, as a link between the generations, *is as indispensable for the renewal of the adult generation's own life as it is for that of the next generation.*"

If parental hopes and expectations are not conveyed with regard to the child's innate skills and talents, they do not have structure-building properties. For example, praise and enthusiasm in response to a particular behavior that is not experienced by the child as an expression of his or her nuclear self are not empathic responses; such responses are more likely expressions of the parents' own expectations than an affirmation and validation of the child's own self.

Kohut's conceptualization of the selfobject functions may be compared to Winnicott's description of the "facilitating environment" and the concept of the "good-enough mother." The empathic attunement is found repeatedly in Winnicott's work as are descriptions of interferences with the mother's mirroring functions that lead to the development of a "false self" by creating "a distortion in the ego" [49, 50]. However, although the environment facilitates an internally determined maturational process, the experiences generated by the environment are not considered to affect the processes of internalization. "The environment does not make the infant grow, nor does it determine the direction of growth. The environment, when good enough, facilitates a maturational process" [49]. Kohut, on the other hand, on the basis of his observation of the various selfobject transferences, postulated a process of transmuting internalization of the environment's empathic responses that can occur not only during infancy but throughout development. Examples of this process of internalization related to the transitional object and signal anxiety have been carefully detailed by Tolpin [47].

Since our focus is on parenting, we are only summarizing the selfobject functions that appear to be responsible for the development of a vigorous, cohesive self. From the merger experiences of infancy to the mirroring that affirms the toddler's initiative and self-assertiveness, the mirroring that validates the legitimacy of the rivalry and jealousy of the oedipal age child, the parent (ideally) continues to mirror affirmatively the adolescent's development; "divergences" and differences between parent and child put a particular strain on parental empathy. Parallel to these mirroring and validating experiences and combined with them are innumerable experiences in which the child is merged with the parents' (idealized) strength and power. The calm firmness of a parent's arms (or voice) as it calms the agitated child represents a selfobject function that, through repetition and optimal frustration, becomes the child's own ability to calm and soothe him- or herself. Repeated, innumerable merger experiences account for the development of the child's capacity to reduce tension and to tolerate anxiety. At later phases of development, these experiences concern themselves less with the child being merged with the parents' physical strength than with their moral strength and ideals.

The transformation of infantile grandiosity and exhibitionism into vigor, vitality, self-esteem (through phase-appropriate mirroring), and the establishment of valued ideals (through merger experiences with the idealized object) is not "completed" during the first few years of life. Self-assertive, grandiose, and exhibitionistic needs are in evidence throughout childhood, particularly during the oedipal phase of development; ideals and goals of the nuclear self become firmed up during adolescence. With physical growth, acquisition of new skills, and the tentative expression of innate talents, the child's growing self continually needs to be affirmed and firmed up by mirroring and idealized selfobject responses.

Parental Self-Development and Parental Empathy

Parenting, especially during infancy and the early years of the child's life, requires emotional resources that are not required by ordinary life stresses. Parents may be well-functioning adults in other ways, but discreet deficits in their own self-development may become manifest when they become parents. Specifically, it is the development of parental empathy in relationship to a particular child that most convincingly links parenting to self-development. The parent who is capable of parental attunement is one who developed an adult form of empathy — a capacity in which an adult man or woman can immerse him- or herself into the inner life of a child without this threatening his or her own sense of separateness and without the parent injecting his or her own needs into the interaction with the child. This is a more complicated and difficult task than it is generally acknowledged. The difficulty is related primarily to the determination of a small child's motives relative to a particular behavior. Virginia Demos [18] gives an example of a toddler approaching a dangerous object such as a pair of scissors accompanied by the various possible responses a caretaker can have to such a situation. In view of the danger that the scissors represent, the caretaker may have difficulty recognizing the child's motive in reaching for the scissors — namely, the wish to explore and to express curiosity. In other words, empathy involves the recognition of the child's motives for the behavior. Since in the case of a young child only the behavior is available for observation, it is more likely that this will be interpreted in terms of the meaning that it has for the caretaker rather than the meaning that the behavior has for the child. This is particularly true once the child's motive has been partially or completely ignored and the behavior has been responded to only in terms of its meaning to the caretaker. By the time the child becomes demanding, hits, or bites because his intent has originally been misinterpreted or ignored, an interaction has been set into motion that precludes the possibility of recognizing and responding to the child's original motives.

Understanding and appreciation of the child's internal state has to be distinguished from the manner in which a parent may respond to this state; "giving in" to a child is frequently mistaken for empathy. Parental responses can only be considered empathic when they encompass the child's "reality" above and beyond his momentary and, at times, imperative demands. Understanding and validating the child's inner state (i.e., appreciating his wish to explore, to touch, and to feel objects in his environment) does not exclude a response by the parent that is guided by mature judgment.

Demos [18] distinguished between six possible types of responses by caregivers. She was careful in pointing out that these responses do not represent types of caregivers but rather types of perceptions, inferences, and responses that any caregiver might employ. (1) The caregiver perceives accurately and understands the child's experience and acts so that the child's positive experiences are prolonged and enhanced, and the child's negative experiences are reduced or brought to an end. (2) The caregiver perceives accurately and understands the child's negative experiences and acts so that the child is helped to endure them and to master them. (3) The caregiver perceives accurately and understands the child's positive experiences and acts so that there is a reduction in these positive affects. (4) The caregiver perceives and understands the child's negative experiences and acts so that the child experiences an increase in negative affects. (This may be done in a nonhostile manner.) (5) The caregiver misperceives or misunderstands some or all of the child's experiences and acts according to the misperception and misunderstanding. (6) The caregiver appears not to perceive the child and acts as if the child is not present. Demos makes it clear that no single exchange has a determining impact on the child, though "each type of exchange will produce a distinctive type of experience for the child and that if such experiences become a chronic characteristic of the infant-mother system, they will begin to shape the child's developing sense of self" [18].

The question is frequently asked whether or not empathy means that a state of fusion exists between subject and object. This question appears to be related to the observation that empathy, an innate capacity of the human psyche, unfolds in the early years of psychological development. And while the infant, indeed, appears to be "fused" with the adult (e.g., the infant experiences the calmness or the anxiety of the adult as if this were his own), the requirements for empathic responsiveness to the infant's needs are the opposite of fusion. Adult empathy depends on the adult's capacity to retain his own sense of separateness. Fliess [20] spoke of "trial identification" and Schafer [44] spoke of "generative empathy" to indicate that empathy is a complex and high level of mental functioning. Norman Paul [40] is most explicit about the need for the achievement of the sense of separateness in relation to an adult, that is, in relation to parental empathy.

An empathizer, or subject, accepts for a brief period, the object's total emotional individuality, not only his simple emotions but also his whole state of being — the history of his desires, feelings, and thoughts as well as other forces and experiences that are expressed in his behavior. Empathy presupposes the existence of the object as a separate individual, entitled to his own feelings, ideas, and emotional history. The empathizer makes no judgement what the other *should* feel and, for brief periods, experiences these feelings as his own. The empathizer oscillates between such subjective involvement and a detached recognition of the shared feelings. Secure in his sense of self and his own emotional boundaries, the empathizer attempts to nurture a similar security in the other. (P. 340)

Kohut's view of the development of empathy, namely, that empathy is the product of the successful transformation of archaic narcissism into its most mature forms (along with other highly valued psychic capacities such as wisdom, humor, and the acceptance of one's own transience) is in keeping with Paul's emphasis on the empathizer's ability to feel "secure in his sense of self and his own emotional boundaries."

With each child, the parent's empathic capacities are tested anew. Each child "creates" his own mother and father as the parents' empathic responses become "dovetailed" to the specific needs of the particular child. Herein lies the essence of parental empathy. "The parents do not respond out of their own needs, nor do they respond in keeping with prescriptions as to how to be a good parent, but their responses are determined by the needs of the particular child at a particular time in the child's life" [37]. Some parents are able to be in empathic contact with young children readily, while others do not communicate meaningfully with their children until they are older or until the children reach adolescence [36]. Such variations in parental empathic capacities are generally nontraumatic, so long as other members in the parenting unit readily substitute for the temporarily unavailable one.

However, even under the most optimal circumstances, when adults become parents with a well consolidated self, the reliable, ongoing presence of their empathy still depends essentially on two major factors: (1) the support of their social milieu, and (2) the child's ability to affirm their parenting. From the moment that a mother becomes sensitive to her baby's cry — when she differentiates between the cry that signals hunger and the one that indicates general discomfort — she relies on her empathic capacity to perceive her infant's needs. But the mother's "motherliness," her capacity for empathic responsiveness, needs to be affirmed as well; feeding, cleaning, and handling that calms and comforts the baby promotes the integration of motherliness. An unhappy, discontent infant, unable to mirror the mother because of congenital or acquired disability, interferes with the integration of motherliness and with the mother's ability to be empathic over prolonged periods of time.

Impaired babies may elicit extremes in caretaker responsiveness from overprotectiveness and oversolicitousness to overt to covert rejection. Contradictory responses may occur in the same caretaker. Because of the chronic strain related to the care of an impaired baby, there are expectable lapses in the caretaker's empathy; in the empathic caretaker this creates guilt and shame that sets the stage for increased protectiveness.

In considering the impact of the impaired infant on the caretaker, we are not only referring to the cases of grossly defective or handicapped infants in which parental responsiveness is usually fairly clear-cut — namely, either increased parental compassion, love, and tolerance or obvious signs of rejection. The problem is more complicated in relationship to subtle, subliminal impairments in a child without demonstrable clinical findings. These infants, for lack of a definitive diagnosis, have been considered to be minimally brain damaged or to have immature central nervous systems. These are infants whose subtle neurological impairments interfere with the execution and mastery of their daily routines (e.g., frequent vomiting with eating, sensitivity to noise and general irritability with sleep, poor motor coordination with the phase-appropriate development of speech and locomotion). The parent, unable to feel effective in the care of the child, does not feel affirmed and experiences increasing frustration; a slow erosion of his or her empathic capacities may follow.

What needs to be emphasized is that this feedback mechanism is not restricted to infancy. The need for adequate mirroring of the parent by the child continues throughout the parents' life and becomes of particular importance to the parent with grown children. Children who have successfully mastered their various developmental tasks affirm the parents in their parenting ability and contribute to the enhancement and esteem of their adult self. The reverse is true as well: Children, who, for whatever reason, encounter difficulties in the course of their lifetime, affect their parents self-esteem to various degrees.

The parents' expectable need for affirmation of their parenting is related to the observation made by Freud: Parental love, at its roots, is "narcissistic love" [21]. It is the parent's selfobject tie (narcissistic investment) to the child that assures adequate parental care, and it is the failure of such a tie to develop that accounts for abandonment (e.g., discarding the newborn into a trash can), infanticide, or gross physical neglect.

The close tie that we are establishing between the development of the self (the transformation of archaic narcissism into its adult form, specifically into an adult form of empathy) and parenting is a departure from Benedek's conceptualization of parenting being primarily dependent on the parents' identification with their own parents. The central aspect of Benedek's [8] theory of motherliness is a double identification, one in which the mother's identification with her own mother becomes reactivated when she becomes a mother herself. As the mother identifies with the baby's regressive needs, she becomes both (i.e., her mother who has cared for her and her baby who is the recipient of this care). This concept of double identification has been useful to the clinician for the understanding of the various expressions of maternal dysfunctions. For example, when mothers make a conscious effort to care for their babies differently from the way they experienced their own mother's care, they may find that powerful unconscious identifications with their own mother interfere with their most avid conscious intent.

As useful as Benedek's theory of double identification has been, the theory has limitations as an explanatory principle both for relatively conflict-free as well as pathological forms of parenting. Identification would indicate a fixed, predictable pattern in parental responsiveness and could not account for the changes that clinicians regularly observe in parents; parents, as adults and as parents, continue to grow and develop in relationship to the same child as well as in relationship to their various children. For this reason, Brody [14] questioned the usefulness of Benedek's "identification theory" and suggested that empathy may be a better concept than identification to describe ongoing, flexible, maternal behavior. Brody's view was supported by Parens, who suggested that parenthood may not be best conceptualized as the final culmination of the psychosexual line of development. Rather, it should be considered as part of the total personality development and could best be understood as part of "the line of development pertaining to the concept of the self" [39].

As we have already indicated, we agree with this view and add that we consider parenting as one of the most important challenges to the consolidation and esteem of the adult's self. The demands of parenting will either prove to be disorganizing and fragmenting to a poorly consolidated adult self or will constitute a challenge that will bring about an enrichment and refinement to the self similar to that provided by other creative and artistic endeavors. It is in this context that we are reminded of Erikson's statement that "generativity which is concerned with new beings as well as new products and new ideas and which, as a link between the generations, is as indispensable for the renewal of the adult generations own life as it is for that of the next generation" [19].

A further question regarding the identification theory of parenting is related to the inevitability of repetition — the generation-to-generation transfer of inadequate parenting. For example, when the observation is made that abusive parents have been abused children, this does not mean that all parents who have been abused as children become abusive parents. The process that evolves between parents and children and the parents' self-development as it continues throughout their adult life is an intricate and complex process and contradicts a fixed pattern that is assumed by the theory of early identifications.

Viewing the evolution of parenting as integral to self-development shifts the emphasis from the inevitability of repetition and helps instead to conceptualize the way parenting itself provides an opportunity for furthering the development of the adult self. This is in keeping with Benedek's view that parenthood is a developmental phase [9] or rather, a developmental process [14], which implies a structural rather than simply a behavioral change. As we have indicated earlier, this developmental process is made possible because of the narcissistic investment that parents have in their children. While it is this narcissistic investment in the child that assures adequate parental care, it is also the narcissistic nature of the parent-child tie that makes parenting a vulnerable adult function and accounts for its various forms of pathology.

Parental Dysfunctions: Diagnosis and Treatment

In the clinical situation, psychotherapists are rarely consulted because of parental dysfunctions; their diagnosis and treatment becomes important when parents bring their already symptomatic children to a psychotherapist.

By the time parents seek professional help, they have recognized that they have been caught in an ever-tightening web of pathological interactions with their symptomatic child. Not understanding the nature, or rather the meaning, of the child's behavior, they react to it with anger and disappointment, which in turn create new problems that quickly cover up or accentuate the original difficulties. There occurs a "layering" of interactions between the various members of the family over time; the parents may become increasingly more rigid and punitive or appeasing and placating as they attempt to deal with the child's symptomatic behavior. Such parental attitudes are secondary: They are responses to the child's symptoms and should not be considered to be the cause of the child's original difficulties. What the professional sees at the time of the diagnostic assessment is the end product of years of pathological interactions that have had serious consequences not only for the child's development but for the parent's parenting capacities as well.

Parental dysfunctions are difficult to diagnose unless they take overt forms such as physical or sexual abuse, neglect, or abandonment. Features of parenting that we have been describing are frequently silent and usually subtle such as the proud gleam in the caretaker's eye or the tone in his or her voice. Failures in these subtle but active parental responses easily elude the clinician and are never reported because they are, more often than not, unconscious to the parents themselves. Nor are these observations readily available to the child. Caretakers, who in all other respects are attentive, may still not be able to perceive and respond to the child's developmentally determined narcissistic needs. Also, empathic failures may be "hidden" behind claims of love and material indulgences. Under these circumstances, the child finds himself emotionally trapped: He experiences his rage at the caretakers as unfounded. These children may use their own body to inflict pain on those, who, because of their inability to comprehend and respond empathically, have emotionally abandoned them. These are children who attempt or threaten to commit suicide or whose self-destructive behavior may take covert forms such as reckless driving, indiscriminate use of drugs, and running away. The self-destructive behavior represents both the expression of revenge as well as an expression of the inadequate narcissistic investment of the body: their body is not worth saving. The tragedy of this particular outcome of parental dysfunctions is that the child's rage at the parent remains largely unconscious or unacceptable, and his despair is compounded by guilt as the self-destructive behavior is considered "unexplainable." The caretaker, sensitive to the element of revenge but not able to perceive the child's pain, may experience the child's self-destructive behavior as an indictment against him- or herself.

Kohut warned that "the complexity of the pathogenic interplay between parent and child and the limitless varieties of it defy the attempt of a comprehensive description" [27]. However, in reconstructing the genesis of his patient's psychopathology, he described a spectrum of parental disturbances that "may extend from mild narcissistic fixations to latent or overt psychosis," and it was his impression that "a specific type of covert psychosis in a parent tends to produce broader and deeper fixations in the narcissistic and especially in the prenarcissistic (autoerotic) realm than does overt psychosis." Overt psychosis in the primary caretaker has its own pathogenic impact on a child. The child "adapts" to the often bizarre, frightening behavior, the repeated need for hospitalizations, and the particularly dulling effects of many of the antipsychotic medications in such a way that no symptoms may be manifested in childhood but only later in life. However, the fact that the parental disturbance is overt appears to protect the child from the kinds of internal compromises that children whose parents suffer from various degrees of discreet forms of self-pathology have to make. In the case of an overt disturbance of a caretaker, the child's own perceptions are more clearly validated and he or she can turn more freely to other members in the parenting unit to provide the developmentally crucial selfobject responses. This assures the child of adequate consolidation of his self and the capacity to be resilient to the behavior of the disturbed caretaker.

In a child therapist's everyday practice, the largest group of dysfunctional caretakers suffer from relatively discreet forms of self-pathology. These are caretakers, who, because of self-absorption, are not available to perceive their children's states of mind and who frequently project their own moods into their emotional environments. It is also the caretaker with the discreet forms of self-deficit who may selectively "overrespond" to certain aspects of the child's personality—aspects more in keeping with his or her expectations for self-enhancement than in keeping with the child's own talents and temperament.

In diagnosing the degree and nature of self-disorder that underlie the various forms of parental dysfunctions, it is useful to distinguish between caretakers who emotionally distance themselves from the child whom they can no longer fit into their self-regulatory system (especially when another child has a more successful fit) from those who insist on remaining in the center of the child's universe. This latter group of parents unconsciously create a sense of responsibility in their child for their own self-cohesion and/or for the maintenance of their own self-esteem.

Parents who "use" their children either to maintain self-cohesion or self-esteem are particularly vulnerable to rage reactions since the child is likely to frustrate their infantile, now highly intensified, selfobject needs. This explains the frequently violent attacks with which these children may be physically or verbally abused.

In relationship to physical child abuse, we found the work of Steele [45] particularly illuminating because this author had consistently used an empathic approach in his study of the child-abusing caretaker. In the psychological profiles he had sketched, we recognize people whose self-disorder had become manifest in relationship to the demand that parenthood had made on them. Steele's data support our thesis that failures in parenting are most likely to occur when parents use their children to fill their own inner emptiness or to bolster their own shaky self-esteem. The description of "the attack," the abusive act itself, helps us appreciate the imperative nature of the parent's unconscious demand to have the infant (or child) meet the caretaker's selfobject needs of the moment. The following sequence tells the story clearly. The caretaker approaches the child with a genuine intent to care for him. However, this is always accompanied by a deep, hidden yearning for the infant to respond in a highly specific way. When the infant fails to respond according to these expectations "a harsh, authoritative demand for the infant's correct response, supported by a sense of parental rightness, follows" [45]. Only when we take the imperative need for the fulfillment of the parent's selfobject need into consideration can we fully appreciate why the infant's failure to smile or otherwise express his or her appreciation for the parent's ministrations is experienced by the parent as rejection—a severe form of narcissistic injury. Steele makes it very clear that these are not ordinary, expectable parental displeasures that "can be aroused if the baby is temperamentally either very active or passive when the opposite type was hoped for." Rather, "the common denominator in the situation where abuse occurs is the innocent infant's failure to meet exaggerated, unyielding parental need" [45].

The recognition of the child-abusing caretaker as one who suffers from a form of self-pathology in which the child is expected to be responsive to an "exaggerated, unyielding parental need" can be distinguished from the caretaker who had failed to develop a selfobject tie with the child altogether. The latter form of parental dysfunction is expressed in abandonment or in chronic physical and emotional neglect. It is not the subject of this chapter to elaborate on the difference in the form that the child's psychopathology may take when he or she experiences chronic neglect rather than periodic and harsh abuse. Suffice it to say that chronic indifference is likely to result in various forms of childhood depression, low self-esteem, and lack of initiative; children who have been abused physically may be subservient to the abusing caretaker but are likely to become aggressive and provocative with younger children and/or animals.

More often than not, children perceive the parent's anxiety in relation to the parent's self-cohesion and/or self-esteem and readily comply with parental expectations at the expense of their own progressive development. This compliance is the function of the imperative developmental need to retain contact with the selfobject milieu. Winnicott called this particular form of adaptation an "impingement" on the child's psyche. "If reacting to impingements is the pattern of the infant's life, then there is a serious interference with the natural tendency that exists in the infant to become an integrated unit, able to continue to have a self with a past, present, and future" [49]. The reference here to impingements as patterns is of importance, indicating that impingements also occur with "good-enough" mothering but create distortions in the ego when they become regular or sustained and thereby constitute patterns.

In the same way that a parent may "impinge" only on certain areas of the child's development, emotional abandonment may also be restricted to a particular segment of the child's personality. Parents may affirm selectively certain of the child's physical or intellectual attributes. But as far as the child is concerned, such arbitrarily selective affirmation may be experienced as a parental failure to validate other aspects of the developing self—that is, an outright rejection of his or her total self. In his reconstructions of the wholesome development of the self, Kohut emphasized the mirroring selfobject's response to the "total self" of the infant or child as opposed to his or her isolated bodily or mental functions. A response to the whole child at first enhances the establishment of the cohesiveness of the self, and later on it contributes to the maintenance of this recently acquired and, therefore, still precarious unity of the self. "The mother's exultant response to the total child (calling him by name as she enjoys his presence and activity) supports . . . the growth of the self experience as a physical and mental unit which has cohesiveness in space and continuity in time" [27]. In a clinical example Kohut illustrates the untoward results of an arbitrarily or inappropriately selective maternal response to a body part or behavioral detail, which not only detracts attention from the child's total self, his central wish, or purpose of the moment, but is experienced by the child as a serious rejection of his whole being. "When Mr. B. would tell his mother exuberantly about some achievement or experience, she seemed not only to be cold or inattentive but, instead of responding to him and the event that he was describing, would suddenly remark critically about a detail of his appearance or current behavior: 'Don't move your hands while you are talking!' This reaction must have been experienced by the son not only as a rejection of the particular display for which he needed a confirming response but also as an active destruction of the cohesiveness of his self experience (by shifting attention to a part of his body) just at the most vulnerable moment when he was offering his total self for approval" [27]. For the child, to feel connected with and responded to by the parent is very important for survival. For this reason, infants and young children "adapt" early to parental attitudes, restrictions, and expectations that may stunt, distort, or otherwise compromise the child's developing self.

In addition to considering the various forms of self-pathology that facilitate the clinician's understanding of parental dysfunctions, it is also important to recognize how a particular developmental phase may become stressful to a particular caretaker. For this reason, we shall describe clinical situations of parental dysfunctions that correspond to various developmental phases in the child.

Clinical Examples

In terms of childhood and adult psychopathology, no other developmental phase appears to be as heavily implicated as the toddler years. Mahler, in her extensive work with toddlers and their mothers, noted that many mothers at this time "make a sharp turnabout in the overall quality of their maternal care in response to maturational events" [35]. Mahler's explanation for this sudden change in the mother's responsiveness rests on her observation that some mothers are unable to promote separation and individuation because of their own need to retain symbiotic fusion with the child. This need for symbiosis, in turn, she said, was determined by the fact that the baby frequently represented a part of the mother's body, specifically the phallus. "In our study . . . we sometimes see, in the way some of the mothers talk about the baby's body, how they hold and handle it, that the infant has the meaning of an illusory phallus for the mother." In addition to this more general meaning, each child has a more "specific meaning for the mother, according to the general and the specific fantasy connected with each child by that mother" [34].

What Mahler described here are instances in which the baby is perceived as part (or rather the missing part) of the mother's body. Physical separation under these circumstances becomes intolerable because the toddler-age child will no longer comply with the mother's wish to be held and be handled in such a way as to help the mother maintain her fantasied illusion that he or she is part of her body. Considering that such "misuse" or "misperception" of the baby may occur in a broader psychological context, we conclude that a mother who "makes a sharp turnabout" in her mothering when her baby becomes a toddler is not necessarily responding to the threat of physical separation, but rather to the baby's new demands on her, which fails to complete or enhance the mother's self in the manner in which this was possible in relationship to a younger infant.

In our view, there are various fundamental reasons that may explain why the toddler years are so heavily implicated in childhood psychopathology. The toddler's increasing self-assertiveness and autonomy as well as a more forceful introduction of individual characteristics, especially temperament, bring new qualities into the "interactive regulatory system" [43]. A new level of the infant's self-organization requires something from the environment that is very different from that of the crib infant. From the emphasis on the establishment on homeostasis in the first year of life, for which the clues may not have been easy to pick up by the environment but which, on the whole, could still be readily "accommodated" into the parent's own self-regulatory system, the toddler "demands" recognition and admiration for his or her initiative, which may dramatically confront the parent's own purposes and values. A similar form of "confrontation," though obviously on a different level of development, occurs during adolescence.

What needs to be reemphasized here is that selfobject responses, such as the validation of the child's unique way of asserting him- or herself, are active parental responses. In other words, what may function as a potentially pathogenic agent is not only the presence of an untoward response to the toddler's self-assertiveness but the *absence of a developmentally needed active response* such as the overt and enthusiastic expression of joy.

The toddler years are prime times for the experience of omnipotence and exhibitionism. Toddlers experience themselves in the center of the universe; they are now filled with a sense of initiative and healthy vigor. They want those around them to see, recognize, and acknowledge their intoxicating sense of what they have discovered to be their own powers and abilities. To an environment that is fearful of losing its control over the toddler's developmentally exaggerated sense of power, this behavior will be threatening. Under these circumstances, the environment anxiously attempts to reinforce its control, battles ensue, and a child's self-assertion disintegrates into the aimless and frequently destructive form of aggression. Children who respond to the increased control with aggression appear to maintain their self-assertiveness to a greater degree than those who give up on their initiative and become withdrawn and apathetic. This latter group of children is more likely to suffer from chronic narcissistic rage that brings about the character disorders that, at a later date, are recognized for their masochistic, paranoid, or depressive features. In other words, "the divergence" [42] or the "sharp turnabout" [35] that so commonly occurs between the toddler and his or her emotional environment may result in overt symptoms during childhood, or this divergence may remain latent and lead to some form of self-disorder later in life. In terms of overt symptoms, we witness an increase in the intensity of separation anxiety; the toddler becomes clingy and whiny and develops nightmares and other forms of sleep disturbances. Tolpin and Kohut [48] maintain that the usual childhood anxieties (e.g., fear of the dark, noise, animals, and robbers or the development of compulsive rituals) are the manifestations of "disintegration" and "depletion" anxiety created by the child feeling "unplugged" from the life-sustaining connection with his or her primary selfobject.

The following clinical example shall demonstrate a form of parental dysfunction in which the child's progressive development interfered with the mother's precariously maintained self-esteem regulation. Once the child became symptomatic, further complications ensued. The clinical example shall also permit the discussion of the implications for treatment when the nature of the parental dysfunctions are given primary consideration in the treatment of the child.

MARTIN AND HIS PARENTS

Martin was 4 years old when he was brought by his parents to a therapist, a woman, who was trained as a child analyst. The parents complained that the child was still enuretic and that in nursery school he was shy and withdrawn. This was in contrast to his provocative and "rebellious" behavior at home, especially in relationship to his mother.

Martin was the oldest of two children. His mother had him when she was 32 years old. Prior to her pregnancy she had several jobs, but none satisfied her. She described her efforts in this respect (as well as her various attempts to complete her education) as failures because of her lack of self-confidence.

The first year after Martin's birth was "blissful." Martin was a bright and responsive baby. However, battles between mother and son began in the child's second year of life; he proved to be "hard to train," and at the time of referral he was still enuretic. The father had little to do with Martin. As a young aspiring professional, he spent long hours in his office. When Martin was 2, the father became aware of the struggles between mother and son and wanted to make himself available to them. However, the mother asked that the father leave them alone and insisted that raising Martin was to be her "career."

The first two diagnostic interviews revealed an anxious little boy who was shy and very hard to engage. The therapist assessed the child as one who had "a cohesive self" with a firm hold on his object world and whose symptoms, on the basis of his play activities and associations, could be related to "phallic conflicts emanating from his emerging sexuality, castration fears, and the wish and fear to exhibit his penis and his body." Because the symptoms could be related to a structural neurotic conflict and were considered to be precipitated by the birth of his sister whom his mother "adored," the recommendation was for the child to enter psychoanalysis and for his parents to see a social worker occasionally. This latter decision was based on the fact that the parents appeared to have been "well-intended, intelligent people who were eager to cooperate in their son's treatment."

The parents agreed to the recommendation and the first six months of analysis confirmed the therapist's predictions: the child had improved considerably, except for his enuresis. The changes were most pronounced in the therapist's office. From a shy, withdrawn child, Martin changed to a vigorous and self-assertive one. The changes, the therapist felt, were directly related to her vigorous interpretations of the child's sexual and exhibitionistic wishes and his castration fears.

However, as the child improved, the mother, rather than being pleased, appeared to become increasingly more unhappy. She began to focus on Martin's enuresis and exposed the child to a series of painful physical examinations that resulted in the diagnosis of "a small urethral meatus." Only because of the therapist's interventions was surgery avoided.

At this time the parents were referred for treatment to their own therapists, and the mother spoke of Martin in extremely negative terms. In response, the therapist made great efforts to "correct" this "distorted perception" because she herself viewed Martin as a lively and engaging boy. The therapist was also "repelled" by the mother's "confession" that in spite of her friends' and doctor's advice not to yell at Martin when he wet his pants, she could not do otherwise. As the therapist reinforced the advice previously given to the mother, and as she continued to correct the mother's "distorted perception" of the child, the mother's anger increased and she abruptly terminated her own and the boy's treatment. The father continued to see the social worker for a while but he felt increasingly more helpless to do anything about the situation, and eventually he, too, discontinued treatment.

Treatment Implications

In reviewing the treatment of this child and his parents, we are not questioning the theoretical frame of reference that had guided the analyst in her interpretations of the child's fantasies and the meaning of his play activities; the child responded favorably to the therapist's interpretations of his sexual wishes and castration fears and he became vigorous and self-assertive with her. Our focus, instead, is on the treatment of the parents and the therapist's failure to have diagnosed and properly treated the self-disorder that affected the mother's parenting in the second year of the child's life. We believe that it was this that was responsible for the mother removing the child from treatment; her anger at Martin who so blatantly exposed her "inadequacy" increased with his improvement, and she had to find some explanation, other than a psychological one, for his problems.

The mother's initial insistence that the father should not participate in the child's care, that caring for him was to be her career, indicates the importance it had for the mother to experience herself as a competent, successful parent. This had particular importance to her in light of her deep sense of inadequacy in other areas of her life; the child was to help her develop a sense of perfection about herself. Martin did this as an infant but not as a toddler. The introduction of his lively temperament into "the interactive system" tested the limits of her empathic capacity. Once Martin failed to confirm the mother in the perfection of her motherliness, she increased her efforts to reestablish control over him. This resulted in the child's self-assertion degenerating into hostility and he became symptomatic, which further undermined the mother's self-esteem. When the mother insisted on a physical exploration of Martin's enuresis, she was not only trying to restitute her self-esteem but, through the painful procedure, she was also "punishing" the child for having failed her.

The importance of making the child's emotional environment an active partner in the treatment process is directly related to our use of the model of the self-selfobject unit in organizing our data and in planning the child's treatment. The child's inner world (i.e., developmental events, anxieties, and symptoms) cannot be fully understood without the environment that shapes and continually affects this intrapsychic reality. The improvement that a young child achieves in the therapist's office cannot be simply "transferred" to the home—certainly not when the parents cannot respond to the symptomatic child with the same empathic understanding as the therapist.

But how is the therapist to help a parent develop empathy toward his or her symptomatic child? We believe that a process that enhances parental empathy can be set into motion if the therapist also encompasses empathically the parents' psychic reality. While it is true that in order to know how the child experiences the parent subjectively the therapist has to immerse him- or herself empathically into the inner world of the child, such an immersion into the child's inner world does not exclude the therapist from empathically encompassing the psychic reality of the parents as well. The therapist is not asked to take sides: He or she is asked to understand and to explain.

However, in the treatment of children, this particular caveat of not taking sides appears to be particularly difficult to observe. Listening to case conferences in which families and their troubled children are being discussed, it appears to be extremely difficult for the professional not to create or reinforce guilt in the parents for their children's emotional difficulties. From the extreme of "parentectomy," the forceful separation of parent and child, to the recommendation that the parents have treatment for themselves, without which their child cannot be helped, parents are frequently treated by professionals primarily as people who can only create problems but who cannot remedy them. However, because we consider the parents' empathic responsiveness to the troubled child as one of the crucial therapeutic agents, we would suggest that therapists of children of all ages, but certainly those of young children, focus their attention on the specific features in the parents' personalities that have made the parenting of this particular child, at this particular time in the child's and the parents' lives, difficult for them. Such an approach to treatment requires that the therapist fully appreciate the child's intrapsychic state and his or her vulnerabilities, anxieties, and defenses, and, at the same time, become acquainted with the source of the parents' limitations for empathic responsiveness to a child who is manifesting various disturbing symptoms to the environment.

The parents' fear of "exposing" themselves to a professional appears to be justified. In the case of Martin's mother, for example, instead of understanding the mother's reason for viewing her child as "bad," the therapist attempted to correct this perception. Parental dysfunctions are symptoms that require exploration, understanding, and explanation as do other psychological symptoms. Martin's mother needed to find out why she felt bad about the child and what had turned this originally blissful relationship into such a difficult one. When the therapist does not appreciate the narcissistic mortification that parents experience for having a troubled child and when the parents feel further reduced in their self-esteem because they are not included into the therapeutic effort, it is then that they are most likely to remove the child from treatment or look for an explanation other than the psychological one for the child's difficulties.

When we consider the consequences of the caretaker's need to control the child's phase-appropriate curiosity, motility, and self-assertion, it is also important to recognize that, in relationship to this particular caretaker, the child has also been deprived of the affirmative responses that are essential to this phase of his development. Martin could have received these from his father who, however, could not meaningfully interact with him because of the mother's insistence that she be the only one responsible for his care. The result was that a structural deficit became manifest; in nursery school Martin was shy and withdrawn and he lacked vigor and lively interest in his surroundings.

A child such as Martin is likely to acquire necessary skills and may continue to develop but remains detached and only marginally involved with people and events around him. Greenspan [23] makes a similar point in relationship to the infant in whom the major developmental task is the establishment and maintenance of homeostasis. The optimal capacity for homeostasis, he says, involves the integration of developmentally facilitating life experiences in the *fullest sense.* It is this that assures the initiation of human relationships and interest in the environment. In other words, there is a qualitative difference between the infant who has the capacity to interact with his or her environment when homeostasis is assured by the presence of a calming "other" and the infant who has to "sacrifice" the optimal state of alertness and engagement in order to remain calm.

BOBBY AND HIS PARENTS

A brief discussion of the case reported by Burlingham and colleagues [16] should further support our thesis that the successful treatment of a child, especially that of a young child, requires that the child's emotional milieu be helped to develop the capacity to respond empathically to the symptomatic child, which would make the continuation of the child's development within the same regulative system possible.

As with the treatment of Martin, Bobby, too, was taken into analysis because he appeared to have "a good potential for improvement or even complete recovery." However, in spite of the mother's conscious efforts to cooperate in the treatment, the child's symptoms could not be fully understood until the mother was taken into analysis herself where her "unconscious fantasies and attitudes" could be explored.

This was a simultaneous analysis of mother and son. The two treatment processes, however, were kept carefully separated so as to keep "the two therapists independent and uninfluenced by the material of the other partner"; the two analysts were instructed not to communicate with each other. The mother may not have been expected to be able to appreciate the motives of the child's behavior but, importantly, the father's help was not enlisted in this effort. Bobby, like Martin, did not display any of the behavior problems related to eating and the regulation of his bowel habits with his father although he did with his mother. It would appear that the resiliency that was noted in Bobby was related to an adequate and most likely compensatory structuralization of his psyche in which the father, rather than the mother, functioned as an empathically responsive, mirroring selfobject.

Bobby's symptoms were identical to the mother's childhood symptoms, especially those concerning the withholding of feces. The authors reported that the mother, as a child, forced her own mother to remain with her during defecation: "to keep her feces inside came to represent the only means to get attention and not to feel lonely" [16]. Now, as a mother, she could not tolerate being separated from Bobby. Her need to infantilize the child and thereby keep him close to her, was interpreted as "proof of her hate for her child and her death wishes against him. When the child showed pleasure in being without her, he symbolized her own mother who had withdrawn from her" [16].

We are questioning the interpretation of the mother's separation anxiety as "proof of her hate for her child." Based on the mother's analytic material, the mother's need for the child's presence is a direct continuation of her efforts to control her own mother. She hated the child most intensely when she was not successful in this effort (i.e., "when the child showed pleasure in being without her" [16]. The rage reaction here is secondary to the frustration that the mother experienced when she could not control the responses of the selfobject child. This conceptualization affects the interpretive process. Rather than interpreting the mother's separation anxiety as the expression of her hate and death wishes toward the child, the rage would have to be interpreted as *secondary* to her efforts to control the child in order to feel affirmed by him. The mother could only feel affirmed if she could experience herself as the *only* one to whom the child responded with pleasure.

This clinical report of a simultaneous analysis of mother and child is of significance for our thesis because it confirms Kohut's (re)constructions [27] regarding the pathogenesis of failures in parental empathy. According to Burlingham [16], "Seen from the point of view of this child's analysis, we would say that, through his behavior, Bobby forced the mother to react toward him as she did. Seen from the aspect of the mother's analysis, Bobby's behavior takes on a different connotation. There is, in the mother's analytic material, ample evidence that in handling the child's feeding situation she was herself under the domination of powerful unconscious fantasies which determined her attitude. In this light the child's behavior will be seen as a reaction to the mother's provocation." However, if the two analysts could not communicate in order to remain "independent and uninfluenced by the material of the other partner," the child's analyst could not benefit from this insight and the child's behavior would be interpreted, as indeed it was, as an expression of his anal ambivalence, his death wishes, and sexual wishes toward his mother. The mother's treatment, in turn, could not benefit from the recognition that it was the mother's need to keep herself in the center of the child's universe that had perpetuated the child's psychopathology.

We have elaborated on the case of Bobby for several reasons. Along with Martin's case, Bobby's case, too, demonstrates many of the problems that are related to parental dysfunctions and their treatment. Both clinical examples highlighted the importance of involving the child's emotional environment in the treatment process in a specific way — namely, by recognizing and interpreting the specific functions that the child is serving in the parent's psychic life.

These two clinical examples also demonstrate the usefulness of the concept of the parenting unit. For both boys, the fathers apparently had fulfilled certain basic selfobject functions so that when away from their mothers, they could function adequately. Bobby's treatment team had not taken advantage of this circumstance; Martin's treatment team did but without success. We are suggesting that the successful treatment of a child is best assured when available resources are mobilized in addition to the attention given to the pathological interaction with one member of the parenting unit. The importance of such an involvement in the treatment process of members of the parenting unit who are capable of responding to the child empathically is related to the way in which we conceptualize the building up of psychological structures within the empathically responsive selfobject milieu. For a young child, everyday experiences (e.g., being fed, put to bed, sent off to school) are of "structure building" significance. When members of a parenting unit "step in" to provide the child with "average expectable" responsiveness, they not only facilitate the disengagement from a pathological enmeshment with one of its members, but they are, at the same time, providing selfobject functions that facilitate the development of compensatory structures rather than primarily defensive ones.[4] Obviously, this is only possible if

---

[4] The distinction between primary, compensatory, and defensive psychic structures is a useful one [28]. Primary structures develop in relation to optimal, phase-appropriate responses to narcissistic developmental needs. These are the structures that are responsible for the healthy functioning of the self, for the consolidation of both poles (ambitions and ideals), and the full utilization of innate skills and talents; the self is experienced as cohesive and vigorous. But if the developmental unfolding of the grandiose self meets with traumatic dysfunction of empathy on the part of the primary selfobject, the resulting defects in the self will be covered over with defensive structure that will prevent further unfolding

the member of the parenting unit who is pathologically involved with the child permits others to participate in the child's care. Martin's father, for example, was very much aware of the importance that his emotional presence had for the child. But the mother, because of her own imperative need to establish her credentials as a mother, could not allow the father to establish a meaningful contact with the boy.

The significance of the emotional presence of caretakers of both genders in the development of children of both sexes has been repeatedly asserted [1, 23, 25]. The father or another male in the parenting unit may be available as a primary selfobject when the mother's self-pathology prevents her from being optimally responsive to the infant's merger and mirroring needs. This not only provides an opportunity for the building up of compensatory psychic structures, but the child can also experience the father as strong (independent of the mother) and therefore idealizable. The developmental significance of the boy's idealization of his father can be derived from the reconstruction of transferences of adult patients as well as from the treatment of boys whose fathers have been out of the home in the early years of the child's life or emotionally not available to them [25, 29, 38].

In order to discuss further the specific importance that the idealization of the same sex parent has for a child's development, we have selected the case of a boy who was raised by his mother and who became symptomatic after a man had moved into their home. The case shall also illustrate the challenges that are faced by single parents and how "impingements" or compromises to the child's self-development that occur earlier in life may be responsible for symptoms at a later developmental phase.

DEAN AND HIS MOTHER

Dean was 9 years old when he and his mother came to the clinic. The mother complained of a major change in Dean's personality since her lover, Mr. Hillard, had moved into their home and the two had decided to get married. Dean, who up until now had been a fairly even-tempered and pleasant child, had become sullen and rebellious. His school work deteriorated rapidly and he refused to go to school on a number of occasions.

Dean was an illegitimate child. His mother was 17 years old when she became pregnant, and by then she had a history of alcohol and drug abuse. However,

---

and structuralization of the pole of the ambitions. However, if the child has an opportunity to turn to other available selfobjects, this will ensure the building up of psychic structure at either of the two poles and lead to the development of compensatory structures. If well consolidated, these structures will afford the self-sufficient functional freedom, safeguard its cohesiveness, and allow the progression of further development.

during her pregnancy she did not drink or smoke and after delivery she surprised her welfare worker with the natural competence with which she cared for the baby. The first two years the mother devoted herself completely to the care of the child. She took good care of him and their small apartment. When Dean was about 2 years old, mother took a job as a janitor in an office building. This was a night job and she took Dean with her; the child made himself at home in this environment and would easily fall asleep on one of the sofas available in these offices. With her work, mother resumed some of her drinking. She took Dean to the bar with her and the patrons there took to the bright-eyed youngster; they would take him on their laps and play with him. He was definitely the center of attention. Dean "entertained" these people to his mother's great delight. By the time Dean was 6 years old, his acting skills were considerable and his mother enrolled him in a special school where he could study acting. He liked school and did well in all his subjects but particularly in acting, securing parts in school plays and some TV commercials for which he was paid. The only thing that indicated that not all was well was Dean's shoplifting behavior. He took small items his mother could easily have afforded. Otherwise, his engaging manner and polite behavior did not reveal that the child was suffering from any form of childhood emotional disorder.

However, this attitude and behavior changed rather drastically when, for the first time in his life, a man moved into their small apartment. Not only had Dean's disposition changed, but so did his mother's: she demanded that he be nice to the man who wanted to marry her. Mr. Hillard, too, who at first took kindly to the child, began to demand that Dean show him respect by calling him "Daddy." Dean refused, insisting that since this man was not his father, he should not have to call him that. Violent fights ensued in which Dean felt betrayed by his mother, who consistently belittled and challenged him. After he ran away from home several times and threatened suicide, he was placed by the court into a group home. Here he did somewhat better, but he remained suicidal and refused to return home and to his previous school.

The most impressive feature of the joint interview with mother and son was the total absence of the mother's empathy in relation to the child's predicament. Whatever the child's motives were for feeling and behaving the way he did, the mother could not appreciate this; she could not understand why Dean wouldn't do something that was so important to her like he always did. In his own treatment, Dean spoke earnestly about suicide; the loss of interest in acting was the first sign of his depression. Acting was the major connection between him and his mother. He was no longer sure if it was he himself who wanted to go to this special school or whether it was his mother who wanted him to go into acting and he had done so only to keep her happy.

Treatment Implications

What emerged in the treatment of this very articulate little boy was a picture we see rather frequently in children who, after relatively adequate early nurturing during the first two years of life, "discover" a particular mode of behavior that secures for them the echoing and approving responses of their environment, which permits the consolidation of their self-structures at least in a narrow area. But in the case of Dean, as in children similar to him, the growing self remained vulnerable to traumatic disappointments because its consolidation was only partial and related rather rigidly to one particular segment of his personality. This segment, importantly, was one that established the connection between the child and his mother and assured adequate selfobject responsiveness from her as well as from the people at the bar.

From the time of conception, Dean fulfilled important selfobject functions for his mother. Being able to carry and give birth to a child made her feel, for the first time in her life, that she was a worthwhile human being. However, once she went back to work and began to drink again, her responsiveness to him became capricious and dependent on how well Dean was able to please her. Dean, with the hyperalertness of a child who had to extract from the environment what he needed for his emotional survival, was able to establish a workable "fit" with his mother. The mother's lack of empathy became obvious only when the demand on Dean for adaptation exceeded his psychological reserves: the child was not prepared to deal with feelings of rivalry, jealousy, and possessiveness. Because of the inadequate consolidation of his self, he experienced profound despair, disintegration anxiety, and a serious suicidal intent.

The aim of treatment was to enable the child to experience the affects that this triangular relationship demanded of him. This treatment approach was based on a self-psychological perspective on the Oedipus complex — a perspective according to which "the presence of a firm self is a precondition for the experience of the Oedipus complex. Unless the child sees himself as a delimited, abiding, independent center of initiative, he is unable to experience the object-instinctual desires that lead to the conflicts and secondary adaptations of the oedipal period" [28]. When such a self-state is not yet attained, the impact of the oedipal affects and conflicts is of a very different experiential quality. "Any person afflicted with serious threats to the continuity, the consolidation, the firmness of the self will experience the Oedipus complex, despite its anxieties and conflicts, as a joyfully accepted reality" [28]. Self-psychology emphasizes thus the positive aspects of the oedipal experience — positive features that are acquired not as a result of the resolution of the Oedipus complex, but "as a primary, intrinsic aspect of the experience itself" [28].

Dean's individual treatment began when he was still in the group home. The treatment plan included regular meetings with his mother and Mr. Hillard so that the therapist could understand them and help them understand the child in depth. In the meetings with mother and Mr. Hillard, the mother soon focused on her own childhood, especially on her adolescence when she began to drink and when she became pregnant with Dean. The mother, crying most of the time, spoke of the emptiness she felt during those years, how easy it was for her to find relief in alcohol, and how, for the first time in her life, she felt she did something worthwhile when she gave birth to her child. She felt that Dean had "cured" her; she did not need to drink — he filled her up with his smile and by being such a good baby. She did not seriously consider marriage until she met Mr. Hillard who, somewhat older than herself, was tender and affectionate toward her. And now she felt betrayed and let down by the child as he appeared to block her in her effort to make a better life for both of them.

We will not detail this family's treatment here further but wish to emphasize that it was crucial for Dean's recovery to mobilize the mother's empathy in relation to his predicament. This occurred by the therapist's appreciation of the mother's need to have Dean be responsive to her now as he had been in the past. By linking the mother's need for the child's responses to her to the emotional deprivation of her childhood, the mother was able to recognize that Dean's behavior was not in defiance of her; rather, it expressed the child's fear that unless he is the only one who can please her, he will lose her altogether. For Dean, the question was, "Up until now I was the one who made mother happy; will she still be there for me once someone else cares for her?"

Once Dean returned home, he and his stepfather got along very well. Though Dean did not call him "Dad," he enjoyed the many masculine activities that Mr. Hillard and he shared. He refused to return to the acting school and engaged in other mildly rebellious behavior. With the child's development fairly securely on its way, it was the mother who needed to continue her individual treatment.

In relation to this case, the question could be raised whether or not the child's reaction to his mother's wish to marry represented the reaction of "a cheated lover." Was Dean's reaction so devastating because he could not give up his "oedipal victory" and because Mr. Hillard's presence activated his murderous feelings toward his rival? In that case, the therapeutic work would have had to focus on helping the child "accept the reality" that he was replaced by a bigger and more successful rival rather than on the disruption that had occurred in the self-selfobject unit between mother and son with Mr. Hillard's arrival on the scene.

Since the therapist had a self-psychological perspective, the aim of her treatment was the reestablishment of the connection between mother and son. Pathological as this connection was, it was the one that assured the child's self-cohesion. It was hoped that the connection between mother and child would not have to be a pathological one. As long as the mother experienced the child's behavior as defiance, the child continued to feel threatened in his very survival. It was the therapist's empathic response to the mother's own mental state and the fairly consistent interpretation of her own sense of deprivation and need for the child's responsiveness to her that enabled the mother to be empathically accepting of the child. The mother's understanding of Dean's reasons for behaving the way he did provided the selfobject matrix that sufficiently firmed up the child's self to experience the jealousy, rivalry, and possessiveness that had previously overwhelmed him.

We are not stating here that Dean, on his return home, entered the oedipal phase of development, but that the mother's understanding and acceptance of the child's feelings made it more likely that he would be able to experience these affects without becoming overwhelmed by them. Most importantly, it appeared that Dean's relationship with Mr. Hillard promoted a disengagement from his pathological enmeshment with his mother. Thus, Dean had a chance to resume his self-development, in which oedipal experiences might play a more fundamental part in the process of recovery. In addition, Dean now had an opportunity to experience Mr. Hillard as an idealizable male, which was a necessary aspect for the development of his own masculine self.

Our clinical examples have demonstrated the expectable impact of failures in parental empathy on the child at different developmental phases in the child's life. However, there are clinical situations in which it is the parent who becomes symptomatic in response to the changes in the self-selfobject unit in which the child was serving selfobject functions for the parent. The model of the self-selfobject unit is particularly useful in understanding that period in the parents' lives when they more overtly display their expectations of their children and when these expectations are traumatically frustrated. In the early years of the children's lives, the parents' expectations are not easy to detect since these are mainly unconscious. During latency and even more during adolescence, parental expectations become more conscious and more explicit. With the increasing awareness of their expectations, the frustrations of these expectations also become more obvious to the parties involved. The most frequent symptom in the parent following a traumatic loss of the child's selfobject function is depression of varying severity.

MRS. SILVER

Mrs. Silver was 41 years old when she began treatment for symptoms of depression. For about a year she had felt increasingly more irritable, slept poorly, lost interest in many of her activities, and found herself more and more preoccupied with ordinary aches and pains. She eventually had to be hospitalized. During this period she was intensely preoccupied with her oldest son Danny, who had abruptly left law school and went to work instead. It was in the course of her treatment that Danny's vital selfobject function for the mother was recognized.

The mother herself was a promising student but had dropped out of college to marry Danny's father. During her pregnancy she continued her studies but was unable to finish college; she retained a sense of inferiority about herself in having failed to fulfill her scholarly ambitions. She was not conscious of her expectations that Danny, the oldest and the brightest of her children, would complete her own self-development in this respect. This became clear only when she developed a severe depression following the abandonment of his studies. After her recovery from her depression, Mrs. Silver again returned to college and worked very hard to prove to herself that she could excel academically. After she had done very well she gave up college and began to look for other avenues through which she could live up to the ideals of her nuclear self.[5]

Treatment Implications

The elucidation of the major acute precipitant to Mrs. Silver's depression led us to focus on the loss of her son's intellectual-professional aspirations. On the surface, this might appear to be offering a very narrow set of explanations for Mrs. Silver's depression, thus, perhaps, simplifying a much more complex web of causative factors. Certainly, her own adverse life experiences and the dynamics of her nuclear family, as well as those of her current family, were multilayered and have undoubtedly codetermined the ensuing depression. However, the treatment process was able to uncover that, for Mrs. Silver, her son represented the embodiment of the intellectual-professional ideals and aspirations of her own nuclear

---

[5] Kohut [28] speaks of the early development of a core self—the "nuclear self." "This structure is the basis for our sense of being an independent center of initiative and perception, integrated with our most central ambitions and ideals and our experience that our body and mind form a unit in space and continuum in time. This cohesive and enduring psychic configuration, in connection with a correlated set of talents and skills that it attracts to itself or that develops in response to the demands of the ambitions and ideals of the nuclear self form the central sector of the personality. The nuclear self (a bipolar structure) has three major constituents: the grandiose-exhibitionistic self at one pole and the idealized parent image at the other, with innate skills and talents between them. Once the nuclear self is established and after . . . having become independent of the genetic factors that determined its specific shape and content, strives only . . . to live out its intrinsic potentialities." These intrinsic potentialities, the "ground plan" or "life program" of the nuclear self, are central motivating structures within the bipolar self.

self—ambitions and ideals she had given up at the time of her marriage. This left her with a vulnerability related to this structural deficit in her self. Thus, she essentially failed in the pursuit and fulfillment of her own ambitions and idealized strivings and attached them to her selfobject-son, who was to pursue and attain their fulfillment for her. When her son abruptly turned back on these pursuits, she developed a depressive reaction that was based on this specific core psychopathology. When she made another major effort at turning again to these earlier abandoned intellectual pursuits, these were only partially successful because they were to repair the enfeebled and fragmentation-prone self rather than to express its consolidated ambitions and ideals.

It should be noted that whatever complex set of dynamics might be formulated to have originally caused or brought about Mrs. Silver's depression, in the subsequent period of her psychotherapy, the importance of her son as a selfobject was understood and interpreted. It was the specificity of these interpretations that had resulted in the considerable improvement of her depression.

Aging Parents and Their Children

We shall now briefly comment on the aging parent and indicate the usefulness of the model of the self-selfobject unit in this period of the life cycle. This is a period in life when the roles between parent and child are expected to be reversed; a time when it is the parent's self that is placed into the center of the unit and the grown child is expected to be empathically encompassing and be responsive to the self-state of the aging parent. However, more often than not, grown children encounter considerable difficulties in experiencing empathy toward their aging parents; the relationship instead is frequently characterized by anger, guilt, and shame. If the now grown children have experienced their parents as having frustrated their own (narcissistic) developmental needs in the past, they are not able to respond to their aging parents empathically. The aging parents' normally or excessively weakened physical and mental states make them ready targets for their grown children's unconscious need to revenge themselves for past hurts by becoming withholding and unresponsive to them. Since the parents, in many instances, are unaware of having failed their children in any way, they are at a loss to understand their children's neglectful, and at times, cruel behavior toward them. Nor are the grown children fully conscious of the source of their need for revenge, since the parents may well have been, in reality, good providers and conscientious in the physical care of their children.

But it is not only aging parents who may suffer from their children's unrelenting need for revenge. The narcissistic rage and the guilt associated with it is a psychological burden for the children as well. Fantasies of telling the parent off and of recounting their childhood hurts are efforts to lighten this burden and to justify their angry withdrawal from their aging parents. The fantasies also express the hope that the parents would accept the responsibility for their anger and by so doing, they would finally demonstrate a capacity for empathy.

MRS. KEMPER

Mrs. Kemper was 62 years old when she consulted with a psychiatrist after having had several years of psychotherapy earlier in her life with another therapist. She was a young-looking woman; her trim and muscular body indicated that she took good care of herself. Indeed, as the therapist learned later, she spent a great deal of time in various sports in which she excelled.

Mrs. Kemper presented her complaints without introduction: Her younger child and only daughter was about to have her first child and the daughter invited her mother-in-law for the postpartum period instead of her own mother. Mrs. Kemper responded to this not only with rage and indignation, but also with considerable concern fearing that this overt rejection by her daughter would result in a complete severance of their relationship. This, she said, would be a repetition of her relationship with her own mother—a circumstance that was her reason for seeking treatment some years before.

Even though Mrs. Kemper came with a problem related to her relationship with her daughter, she began by speaking about her own mother. She gave numerous examples of her mother's emotional unavailability when she was a child and how helpless and childish her mother had become after her parents divorced. As a teenager she took full responsibility for her own, her brother's, and her mother's care and she feared that her mother would pull her back into the same situation now if she did not resist it. The therapist felt that Mrs. Kemper, by focusing on her own childhood, had tried very hard to justify her refusal to visit her now aged and ailing mother. Her repeated statements that she did not feel guilty about this only indicated the considerable guilt she indeed was experiencing.

Mrs. Kemper was married to a rather well-to-do lawyer. Theirs was a proper but not a particularly intimate relationship. She felt that by bearing two children and bringing them up, she had "repaid" her husband for the emotional and financial independence she had enjoyed in their marriage. She was "a good mother," conscientious in the care of the children; she felt a great deal closer to her son than to her daughter. The daughter grew up to be a serious, studious girl, but rather inhibited in social matters. As the daughter devoted more and more time to her studies and to political and social issues, the mother felt that her daughter considered her frivolous and superficial, and the two women grew farther and farther apart. During the last few years, Mrs. Kemper frequently felt offended by her daughter's "icy attitude" toward her, but the daughter's recent request that the mother not visit her after the baby was born was a particularly heavy blow. She wanted to know what she could do to "repair" this relationship.

The manner in which Mrs. Kemper presented her problem indicated, at first, that she had some insight that there was a connection between her relationship with her mother and that with her daughter. This initial impression, however, was misleading. She continued to be preoccupied with her relationship to her mother and with the need to justify her anger and rejection of her. In relation to the daughter, too, she felt mistreated; she considered herself to have been a good mother and she felt deeply wounded by her daughter's rejection of her.

Treatment Implications

What importance does this clinical vignette have for our view of parental dysfunctions? Could we consider this to be an example of generational transmission of faulty parenting? We would regard such an answer to be too general and misleading in the treatment of our patient. The specific features of the mother's parental dysfunction could only have been assessed from the effect that this had on the daughter's development and personality organization. We had no way of assessing that impact. However, we could assess Mrs. Kemper's personality, specifically, how her own childhood experiences had limited her capacity for parental empathy. This would provide us with the understanding of the particular features of her parental dysfunctions and make our interpretations regarding these dysfunctions more specific.

In the course of Mrs. Kemper's treatment, it became clear that it was her mother's "helplessness," her emotional dependency on Mrs. Kemper, that had constituted the childhood (strain) trauma that most powerfully shaped Mrs. Kemper's adult personality. She was a precocious child and her emotional survival depended on her pseudomaturity; she valued most highly her decisiveness and emotional independence. While behaviorally this resulted in a haughty attitude, she remained an emotionally hungry little girl, particularly vulnerable to the rejection by her own children.

It was well into the second year of her treatment that Mrs. Kemper first fully understood her daughter's reason for not inviting her for the postpartum period. The daughter, she had eventually realized, needed someone with her at this time in her life who could be with her without reservations and considerations of her own needs. Mrs. Kemper had to recognize that this was not her daughter's experience with her. The daughter, by not inviting her, was protecting herself from psychic pain, which was no different from Mrs. Kemper's own efforts to protect herself when she refused to visit with her own mother. Only when she had meaningfully linked her daughter's behavior to her own childhood experiences was she able "to forgive" her mother for having failed her as a child.

Acceptance of the limitations of the parents' empathy is a capacity of the adult psyche; not to express revenge against the parents for not having been able to place the child into the center of their universe because of their own narcissistic needs is a developmental accomplishment. Mrs. Kemper was determined to achieve this in her current treatment. As her visits to her mother began to increase and she began to feel better about these, her mother suffered a stroke and had to be placed in a nursing home. In this setting she could accept her mother's helplessness, clingy, and whiny behavior. When, on one of her visits, she was actually able to embrace her mother, which she could not do before, she experienced a peculiar elation and felt that she had indeed accomplished what she wanted in her treatment.

Conceptual Advances in the Study of Parenting: A Summation

To conclude, we shall summarize the essential propositions in this chapter by highlighting the conceptual advances that have already been made on parenting, as well as those that are most likely to follow. This task calls for some broad brush strokes with which to place parenting as a developmental achievement firmly within the whole of self-development.

The nature versus nurture controversy regarding the development of the self in health and illness has also encompassed the functions and capacities of parenting. Benedek, the most widely recognized psychoanalyst who worked in this area, postulated a biological readiness for motherliness through hormonal regulation that evolves out of the experiences of pregnancy and lactation. However, while the initial impetus for mothering in the postpartum period is a hormonally determined potentiality, mothering beyond infancy could not be explained on a hormonal or biological basis, nor could the increasingly more significant functions of fathering. Parenting beyond the early phases requires the recognition of psychological mechanisms. Regarding these, Benedek [8] elaborated on the process of identification in the following way. The mother, as a caretaker, identifies with her own mother and, at the same time, she identifies with her infant's receptive needs by regressively reexperiencing her own infancy.

Benedek's theory of motherliness, evolving out of a physiological (i.e., hormonal) regulation, has found general acceptance in psychoanalysis. Her explanation as to what sustains motherliness throughout the child's development, however, has to be questioned. The assumption that identification would create fixed, unchangeable patterns of parenting was not in keeping with clinical observations. Clinical observations indicate that parenting usually undergoes necessary changes in relation to the same child and in relation to the various children of the same parents. The theory of identification also could not account for the structural changes that take place in the adult self in relation to parenting as Benedek had postulated. It is because of these structural changes that she had maintained that parenthood was a genuine developmental phase.

In this chapter, we have suggested that: (1) the observation that parental behavior is flexible (e.g., it changes in relation to the same child in terms of the child's increasingly complex and constantly changing psychic organization as well as in relation to the varied temperaments and inborn capacities of various children) can best be explained with the adults' capacity for attunement with the child (i.e., with parental empathy); and (2) the structural changes in the adult in relation to parenting are intimately related to the narcissistic (selfobject) nature of the parent-child tie.

The developmental significance of parental empathy has been confirmed by current infant research, in which it has been repeatedly demonstrated that the infant, born with "a genetic ground plan" has to be assured of phase-appropriate environmental responses if this ground-plan is to develop into a viable, vigorous, and creative human psyche. These specific phase-appropriate environmental responses are the ones that self psychology calls "selfobject functions."

Our conceptualization of parenting is based on Kohut's self-psychology, which recognizes the central importance of empathy as a mode of observation as well as an emotional nutrient and its failures in parenting to be of major pathogenic significance. In relation to empathy as a mode of observation, we have emphasized that parental empathy requires not only a temporary immersion into the inner world of the child, but a sustained capacity to perceive the child's affects and his particular manner of protecting himself from the potentially destructive (i.e., overstimulating) impact of his emotional environment. This capacity for adult empathy (i.e., when the parent, after having briefly experienced the child's affects, maintains his sense of separateness) is the hallmark of successful transformation of infantile narcissism into its adult form. The capacity for empathy is, therefore, a reliable indicator of the completion of adult self-development, which also includes the capacity for the regulation of tension, affect, and self-esteem, along with the development of other mature psychic functions such as wisdom, humor, and the ability to contemplate one's own transience. By placing the capacity for empathy into the center of parental functions, we have linked parenting inextricably to self-development.

When we consider that parental functions cannot be grafted onto the parents' personalities since these are functions of the parents' own nuclear self, we can appreciate that successful parenting depends on the parental selves being fully consolidated, that they had "formed stable patterns of ambitions and ideals," and that "the parental selves are experiencing the unrolling of the expression of these patterns along a finite life curve that leads from a preparative beginning through an active, productive, creative middle to a fulfilled end" [28].

It makes no difference at which point of the life curve the parental selves are during the oedipal phase of the child; so long as the pattern of the parental self is clearly designed and well consolidated and is in the process of expressing itself, the fulfilling peak and the fulfilled end are already implied. The oedipal child then is the beneficiary of the fact that the parents are in narcissistic balance. If the little boy feels that his father looks on him proudly as a 'chip off the old block' and allows him to merge with him and with his adult greatness, then his oedipal phase will be a decisive step in self-consolidation and self-pattern firming, including the laying down of one of the several variants of integrated maleness — despite the unavoidable frustrations of his sexual and competitive aspirations and despite the unavoidable conflicts caused by ambivalence and mutilation fears." (P. 234)

In the course of development, parental empathy will expectedly fluctuate since it is subject to ordinary life stresses.[6] However, such ordinary fluctuations in parental empathy are nontraumatic since they are part of a progressive developmental process. Only failures in parental empathy that are sustained over long periods of time indicate a defect in the parent's own self-development.

The close linkage between parenting and self-development is further justified by the narcissistic nature of the parent-child tie. The narcissistic nature of parental love assures parental care but it is also this quality of the relationship that makes parenting a particularly vulnerable adult function. In self-psychology the narcissistic nature of the parent-child tie is encompassed by the concept of the selfobject. It is this concept that

---

[6] In a small but well conceived study, Letourneau has demonstrated that, contrary to general belief, life stresses do not affect parental empathy [31].

permits a fresh approach to the study of parenting by bringing together experientially and conceptually what the extrospective observer could only regard as "internal" or "external" in relation to development and pathogenesis. Since the parent as a selfobject is always viewed from the vantage point of the experiencing self of the infant or child, the external environment may thus be consistently studied as part of the inner world of the particular child.

The significance of selfobject functions extends throughout development and is not restricted to the early years of the child's life. The transformation of infantile grandiosity and exhibitionism into vigor, vitality, and self-esteem (through phase-appropriate mirroring) and the establishment of valued ideals (through repeated merger experiences with the idealized values of the selfobjects) is not completed during the first few years of life; self-assertive, grandiose, and exhibitionistic needs are in evidence throughout childhood, and ideals and goals of the nuclear self become firmed up only during adolescence. Though the extent and nature of these selfobject functions change with increasing differentiation and structuralization of the child's psyche, with physical growth, with the acquisition of new skills and, with the tentative expression of innate talents, the child's growing self continually needs to be validated by affirmative selfobject responses. This indicates that the psyche is more appropriately viewed as an open system, retaining its capacity for structural change, though to a progressively lesser degree, over the whole of the life cycle. It is this lifelong need for empathic selfobject responsiveness that best explains the parents' own needs to be affirmed by their children in their parenting capacity. Nothing assures such affirmation better than the child's wholesome and progressive development and, conversely, nothing can "erode" the parents' empathic capacity as quickly as a child who becomes symptomatic. We have suggested that this inherent reciprocity in the relationship is most aptly expressed in the model of the self-selfobject unit. This model is useful because the clinician can either focus on the child's self and examine it in relation to the parental selfobject or he or she can focus on the parent's self in order to examine the nature of parental dysfunctions and determine the manner in which the child is being used as the parent's selfobject.

Using the self-selfobject model, we can appreciate that it is not the overt psychopathology of the parent (which is visible to the external observer and in response to which the child may find various modes of coping), but it is the more subtle, invisible deficiency or absence of certain key functions that will have pathogenic influence. The impact, for instance, of the absence of the gleam in the mother's eyes or the lack of firmness in her arms when she holds her baby can only be discovered from within the experience of the child (or, reconstructively, in the treatment of an adult patient).

It should now be evident that both "identification" and "adaptation," especially with a frustrating caretaker, are not only phenomena noted by the external observer in relation to the social interaction between parent and child, but that these are already the results of a troubled and troubling interaction. Thus, the infant's or child's identification with the aggressor impinges on self-development and necessitates the variety of compromises in relation to the potentials of the developing self. These compromises have been described as "the false self" [49], "defensive structures" [28], and assuring "adaptations" to an "average nonexpectable environment" [24]. In all instances, they serve as a shield to protect the "true self" [49] or the "nuclear self" [27].

Our clinical examples indicate only a very small fraction of the infinite variety of situations in which the model of the self-selfobject unit aids the clinician in the diagnosis and treatment of parental dysfunctions. In discussing the cases of three young children, we hoped to indicate that the interference with parental empathy may be related to various levels of self-pathology in the parent. For example, Martin's mother had hoped to make child rearing into her "career" and thereby buttress her diminishing self-esteem, while Bobby's mother used her son as a selfobject in a more fundamental way — to protect her fragile self from fragmentation.

We have demonstrated our approach to treatment with the case of Dean. In addition to the therapeutic efforts in this case, we have illustrated that a child whose self has not attained adequate consolidation is not able to experience the passions traditionally associated with the Oedipus complex, namely, rivalry, jealousy, and possessiveness, without untoward effects. We also want to emphasize that even when the child has attained adequate consolidation of the self and could experience these affects without adverse consequences, the child is still in need of the affirmative responsiveness of the parents in relation to these affects. In other words, it is not only parental seductiveness, counteraggression, or counter-rivalry that may create the pathogenic conditions: the very *absence* of affirmative acceptance of a child's rivalry and possessiveness directed at the parents is of pathogenic significance.

In connection with Mrs. Kemper, we could raise the question regarding the role identification plays in the transmission of the dysfunction of parenting. It could be argued that Mrs. Kemper's parental dysfunction was related to her identification with her own mother. However, we would maintain that such an interpretation would neither describe the process of transmission nor would it be useful in the treatment process since it would fail to take into consideration Mrs. Kemper's personality organization and the manner in which this had determined the nature of her specific parental dysfunctions. In fact, identification with the parent's own parents is an inadequate explanation of the "generational transmission" of parental dysfunctions because, when we see such transmissions in clinical practice, the nature and extent of parental dysfunctions are not identical in the two generations. In the case of Mrs. Kemper, for example, in order to diagnose the specific features of her parental dysfunctions, we had to link these to the specific features of her self-disorder; this disorder in Mrs. Kemper found a very different expression than in her mother. Mrs. Kemper's mother was a helpless woman who, unable to respond to her daughter's needs, had expected and received considerable support from her (i.e., Mrs. Kemper was a parenting child). As an adult, in order to protect herself from further traumatization, she developed a haughty, pseudoindependence as a defense. Though proper in her behavior as a mother, she remained centered on her own needs. This created a parental dysfunction very different from her own mother's: Rather than "burdening" her daughter with her selfobject needs, she remained aloof and self-centered. When the daughter did not invite Mrs. Kemper to share one of her most important life experiences with her, she (the daughter) protected herself from the hurt of her mother's aloofness and, at the same time, she expressed her rage at the mother for not having been emotionally available to her during her childhood. Since Mrs. Kemper sought help specifically related to her parental dysfunction, treatment could focus on this rather exclusively. However, whether or not she will be successful in building a new relationship with her daughter will depend on the daughter's willingness to "forgive" her mother in the manner in which Mrs. Kemper was eventually able to forgive her own mother.

References

1. Abelin, E. Some further observations and comments on the earliest role of the father. *Int. J. Psychoanal.* 56:293, 1975.
2. Ainsworth, M. The Development of Infant-Mother Attachment. In B. Caldwell and R. Ricciuti (Eds.), *Review of Child Developmental Research,* Vol. 3. Chicago: University of Chicago Press, 1973. Pp. 1–94.
3. Anthony, E. J. A clinical evaluation of children with psychotic parents. *Am. J. Psychiatry* 126:177, 1969.
4. Anthony, E. J. The family and the psychoanalytic process in children. *Psychoanal. Study Child* 35:3, 1980.

5. Atwood, G. E., and Stolorow, R. D. *Structures of Subjectivity: Explorations in Psychoanalytic Psychotherapy.* Hillsdale, New Jersey: Analytic Press, 1984.

6. Barnett, R. K., Hofer, L., and Stern, D. *Dyadic Interactive Process Profile (DIPP): A Measure of Social Interactive Behaviors and Style.* Presented to the Third International Conference on Infant Studies, Austin, Texas, March, 1982 (unpublished manuscript).

7. Basch, M. F. The concept of affect: A re-examination. *J. Am. Psychoanal. Assoc.* 24:759, 1976.

8. Benedek, T. Toward the biology of the depressive constellation. *J. Am. Psychoanal. Assoc.* 4:389, 1956.

9. Benedek, T. Parenthood as a developmental phase. *J. Am. Psychoanal. Assoc.* 7:380, 1959.

10. Benedek, T. Motherhood and Nurturing. In E. J. Anthony and T. Benedek (Eds.), *Parenthood: Its Psychology and Psychopathology.* Boston: Little, Brown, 1970.

11. Benedek, T. Parenthood During the Life Cycle. In E. J. Anthony and T. Benedek (Eds.), *Parenthood: Its Psychology and Psychopathology.* Boston: Little, Brown, 1970.

12. Benedek, T. The Psychobiology of Pregnancy. In E. J. Anthony and T. Benedek (Eds.), *Parenthood: Its Psychology and Psychopathology.* Boston: Little, Brown, 1970.

13. Bowlby, J. *Attachment and Loss,* Vol. 1. New York: Basic Books, 1969.

14. Brody, S. Continuity and Conflict in Maternal Behavior. Panel on: "Parenthood as a Developmental Phase" reported by H. Parens. *J. Am. Psychoanal. Assoc.* 23:154, 1975.

15. Brody, S. The concepts of attachment and bonding. Paper delivered at the First International Congress on Infant Psychiatry, Estoril, Portugal, May 1980.

16. Burlingham, D. T., Goldberger, A., and Lussier, A. Simultaneous analysis of mother and child. *Psychoanal. Study Child* 10:165, 1955.

17. Chess, S., and Thomas, A. Infant bonding: Mystique and reality. *Am. J. Orthopsychiatry* 52(2):213, 1982.

18. Demos, V. Empathy and Affect, Reflections on Infant Experience. In J. Lichtenberg, M. Bornstein, and D. Silver (Eds.), *Empathy II.* Hillsdale, New Jersey: Analytic Press, 1984.

19. Erikson, E. On the generational cycle: An address. *Int. J. Psychoanal.* 61:213, 1980.

20. Fliess, R. The metapsychology of the analyst. *Psychoanal. Q.* 11:211, 1942.

21. Freud, S. On narcissism: An introduction (1914). In J. Strachey (Ed.), *The Standard Edition of the Complete Psychological Works of Sigmund Freud.* London: Hogarth, 1957. Vol. 14, Pp. 67–102.

22. Freud, S. Introductory lectures on psychoanalysis (1916/17). *Standard Edition.* 1963. Vol. 16.

23. Greenspan, S. I. *Psychopathology and Adaptation in Infancy and Early Childhood:*

Principles of Clinical Diagnosis and Preventive Intervention. Clinical Infant Reports Series of the National Center for Clinical Infant Programs. No. 1, 1981.

24. Hartmann, H. *Ego Psychology and the Problem of Adaptation.* New York: International Universities Press, 1958.

25. Herzog, J. M. On Father Hunger: The Father's Role in the Modulation of Aggressive Drive and Fantasy. In S. H. Cath, A. Gurwitt, and J. M. Ross (Eds.), *Father and Child: Developmental and Clinical Perspectives.* Boston: Little, Brown, 1982.

26. Klaus, M., and Kennell, J. H. Human maternal behavior at the first contact with the young. *Pediatrics* 46:187, 1976.

27. Kohut, H. *The Analysis of the Self.* New York: International Universities Press, 1971.

28. Kohut, H. *The Restoration of the Self.* New York: International Universities Press, 1977.

29. Kohut, H. The two analyses of Mr. Z. *Int. J. Psychoanal.* 60:3, 1979.

30. Lax, R. F. Some aspects of the interaction between mother and impaired child: Mother's narcissistic trauma. *Int. J. Psychoanal.* 53:339, 1972.

31. Letourneau, C. Empathy and stress: How they affect parental aggression. *Soc. Work* 26:383, 1981.

32. Lichtenberg, J. Reflections on the first year of life. *Psychoanalytic Inquiry* 1:695, 1982.

33. Lozoff, B., Brittenham, G. M., and Trause, M. A. The mother-newborn relationship: Limits of adaptability. *J. Pediatr.* 91:1, 1977.

34. Mahler, M. S. Thoughts about development and individuation. *Psychoanal. Study Child* 18:307, 1963.

35. Mahler, M. S., Pine, F., and Bergman, A. *The Psychological Birth of the Human Infant.* New York: Basic Books, 1975.

36. Olden, C. On adult empathy with children. *Psychoanal. Study Child* 8:111, 1953.

37. Ornstein, A. Self-pathology in childhood: Developmental and clinical considerations. *Psychiatr. Clin. North Am.* 4:435, 1981.

38. Ornstein, A. An Idealizing Transference of the Oedipal Phase. In J. D. Lichenberg, and S. Kaplan (Eds.), *Reflections on Self Psychology.* Hillsdale, N.J.: Analytic Press, 1983. Pp. 135–148.

38a. Ornstein, P. H. Self Psychology and the Concept of Health. In A. Goldberg (Ed.), *Advances in Self Psychology.* New York: International Universities Press, 1980.

39. Parens, H. Panel on "Parenthood as a Developmental Phase." *J. Am. Psychoanal. Assoc.* 23:154, 1975.

40. Paul, N. L. Parental Empathy. In E. J. Anthony and T. Benedek (Eds.), *Parenthood: Its Psychology and Psychopathology.* Boston: Little, Brown, 1970.

41. Rutter, M. *Maternal Deprivation Reassessed.* Middlesex, England: Penguin Books, 1972.

42. Sander, L. Issues in early mother-child interaction. *J. Am. Acad. Child Psychiatry* 1:141, 1962.
43. Sander, L. Infant and Caretaking Environment: Investigation and Conceptualization of Adaptive Behavior in a System of Increasing Complexity. In E. J. Anthony (Ed.), *Exploration in Child Psychiatry.* New York: Plenum, 1975.
44. Schafer, R. Generative empathy in the treatment situation. *Psychoanal. Q.* 28:347, 1959.
45. Steele, B. F. Parental Abuse of Infants and Small Children. In E. J. Anthony and T. Benedek (Eds.), *Parenthood: Its Psychology and Psychopathology.* Boston: Little, Brown, 1970.
46. Stern, D. *The First Relationship: Infant and Mother.* Cambridge, Mass: Harvard University Press, 1977.
47. Tolpin, M. On the beginnings of a cohesive self: An application of the concept of transmuting internalization to the study of transitional object and signal anxiety. *Psychoanal. Study Child* 26:316, 1971.
48. Tolpin, M., and Kohut, H. The Disorders of the Self: The Psychopathology of the First Years of Life. In S. I. Greenspan and G. H. Pollock (Eds.), *The Course of Life. Psychoanalytic Contributions Toward Understanding Personality Development, Vol. I, Infancy and Early Childhood,* NIMH, 1980.
49. Winnicott, D. W. *Maturational Processes and the Facilitating Environment: Studies in the Theory of Emotional Development.* New York: International Universities Press, 1965.
50. Winnicott, D. W. *Playing and Reality.* New York: Basic Books, 1971.

III
The abandoning parent

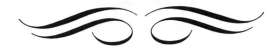

7

Mourning mothers, depressed grandmothers, guilty siblings, and identifying survivors

George H. Pollock

Some years ago on a visit to London, I came upon a small art gallery in which there was an exhibit by late nineteenth- and early twentieth-century German and Northern European painters and graphic artists. Although my interest then was mainly focused on Edvard Munch, the Norwegian artist, the prints of Kaethe Kollwitz caught my attention and I resolved to learn more about her. She intrigued me, and I felt the pattern of her life was one that was connected with my research on the mourning process. I will now begin to articulate what has been an object of my study for some time.

First, however, I must briefly describe the research program that has occupied me for nearly 30 years. The details of how this investigative work began, the various paths I have pursued in order to further understand what I have been studying, and the clinical, theoretical, and applicative details have been described in my published works. Let me summarize my conclusions without giving the evidence or the basis for them.

The mourning-liberation process is a universal transformational means of adapting to change and the loss implied in this modification of a former state. As such, this process, described by Sigmund Freud in *Mourning and Melancholia* [3], need not be connected only with loss through death. I describe such a thanatological linkage as bereavement, a subclass of the universal mourning-liberation process. My research has shown me that this mourning-liberation process has a line of development beginning in the earliest neonatal period that probably is not completed until adulthood is reached; is found in every culture and society, present and past; is intimately connected with religion, immortality beliefs, and ritual associated with change and loss; and may have four outcomes.

The first outcome is the normal process in which the result is creative

Supported in part by the Anne Pollock Lederer Research Fund of the Chicago Institute for Psychoanalysis.

235

and allows for the withdrawal of emotional investment in what no longer is and the subsequent reinvestment in what is and what can be. This creative outcome may be a product, theory, innovation, discovery, or a new and meaningful relationship to life and significant others. Joy, pleasure, satisfaction, and happiness may be as creative for a specific individual as a painting, sculpture, musical composition, or poem may be for a more gifted person. In some individuals creativity may be seen as part of the attempts to adapt. Even though the attempts may be unsuccessful, the products of such creative efforts may still have intrinsic value. Thus, creativity itself is not limited to successful mourning-liberation processes. The second outcome may be an inability to complete the mourning-liberation process because it never fully developed in childhood and adolescence. Hence there is an arrest in its development. The third outcome may be a regressive return to earlier states of the mourning process (i.e., fixation with the appearance of earlier modes of dealing with or avoiding change). Finally, the fourth outcome includes various forms of pathological-abnormal mourning processes, in which the results are not liberation and creativity, but serious psychic maladaptations that can have lethal consequences.

In attempting to discover whether the mourning-liberation process, which has various describable phases in the adult, is similar regardless of the change-loss trigger, I studied four groups of individuals whom I had personally treated or examined including adults who had lost one or both parents during childhood or adolescence; adults who had lost one or more siblings during this same period; adults who had lost a spouse; and adults who had lost a child. In all instances, I limited my study to loss through death because it was easy to establish objective times for the deaths, and all of my protocols had been collected before I became interested in this research. The same mourning-liberation process, however, occurs in change-loss situations in which there are no actual deaths.

I am now attempting to compare losses resulting from death with those due to divorce, separation, or abandonment. What I have found is a similarity of the process and its sequential phases. More recent biological research suggests that actual biochemical and endocrinologic differences occur in the phases of the adult process. If this work is confirmed and pursued, we will have biochemical correlates of the intrapsychic processes that can serve as markers of where the mourning-liberation process may be at a given time.

What I have also discovered and am pursuing now as a result of my work in life-span research are the varied meanings of "what and who" throughout the life span. For example, what is the meaning of a child throughout the life span of the mother, or what is the varied meaning of a father throughout the major life span of a child? In doing analytic work with individuals who are in their sixties, seventies, and eighties, I have been able to obtain some data and have formulated some hypotheses. I have published a paper on the normal meanings of siblings, childhood and adolescent sibling loss, and the relationship between this loss and creativity [9]. Thus, my interest in creativity has evolved from my ideas relating to the mourning-liberation process.

As the result of my working with several writers, composers, and painters, I became convinced that although the artist and his or her works are inseparable, certain life events are significant determinants of content, style, or mode of expression even though the inherent talent or genius is probably not linked with such psychosocial occurrences.[1] By being able to study the sequence of creative works or outcomes along with the conscious and unconscious emotional and mental processes of the creator, it was possible to note the temporal correlates and connections among cognitive, expressive, interpretative, psychological, and original generative activities. In some ways the creative act mirrored in composite fashion what had been and what was going on in the artist's life.

Furthermore, I found that a significant number, especially among the writers and poets with whom I worked, had had many losses throughout their fundamental developmental periods. In studying the biographies of well-known writers, poets, composers, philosophers, political and religious leaders, visual artists, and scientists, I have found confirmations of some of my hypotheses that were originally formulated on the basis of my own clinical and introspective activity [7, 8, 10, 11, 12]. More currently, I am attempting to distinguish between the creativity of scientists and artists in the broad sense of this designation.

Now I turn my attention to visual artists. Psychoanalysts have been interested in visual artists from the earlier days of this science. Freud's essay on Leonardo da Vinci was a pioneering beginning. Subsequently we have had studies of Michelangelo, Magritte, van Gogh, and Munch, to mention a few examples.

My interest in Munch dealt with his utilization of art as a means of facilitating his mourning-liberation process. This led me to investigate the Expressionist movement. I was fortunate to become involved with Kaethe Kollwitz, whose life pattern relates to various areas of my inter-

---

[1] Of course the creative people I have studied worked very hard and studied actively to attain their artistic proficiency.

est, some of which I alluded to earlier. I might also mention that I am now studying Alfred Kubin, another artist identified with the Expressionist movement, and a very early Italian painter and muralist, Luca Signorelli.

Kaethe Kollwitz was more than a sculptress or a graphic and visual artist. She was a courageous woman who inspired many — a symbol of opposition to war, a champion of social justice and peace, and a courageous human being. Throughout her adult life, she fought for the underprivileged, oppressed, and helpless women, children, and men. She became a symbol of these values and ideals; her life became a myth. Her artwork is not only highly valued but now well known throughout the world. Her life is no myth, however. She was a devoted wife, mother, and grandmother. Her life pattern raises questions about some of the still current formulations as to why there are no great women artists who are also able to be secure in their femininity and maternity.

In this chapter, I will raise questions, share insights, and give you some of the facts of Kollwitz's life. I intend to close with a brief discussion of some of the implications of my study of Kollwitz for psychoanalysis and possibly also for artistic creativity.

Kaethe Kollwitz: The Pattern of the Creative Life

In the last few years several excellent biographies, more or less detailed accounts of the events and circumstances of Kollwitz's life, and the appearance of her own diaries, letters, and reports of close friends and family members have provided us with data for understanding the possible influences of life events on artistic themes. Even with the destruction of many documents during World War II, we still have many photos, prints, drawings, and documents.

CHILDHOOD

Kaethe Ida Schmidt was born on July 8, 1867, the fifth child of her parents. Two boys had not survived, but Kaethe had an older brother and sister. She grew up in the town of her birth, the East Prussian industrial city of Koenigsberg. She was a "high-strung" child who kept her feelings hidden. Her mother was not physically affectionate toward any of her children, although as Kaethe Kollwitz writes in her diary about her ninth birthday [4]:

I received a set of skittles as one of my birthday presents. In the afternoon, when all of the children were playing skittles, they would not let me play — I don't know why. As a result, I had one of my usual stomachaches. These stomachaches were a surrogate for all physical and mental pains . . . . I went around in misery for days at a time, my face yellow, and often lay belly down on a chair because that made me feel better. My mother knew that my stomachaches concealed small sorrows, and at such times she would let me snuggle close to her.

Kaethe seemingly regretted her mother's reserve, and except for a few instances fixed in her memory because of their emotional significance, she remembered little about her mother when she was very young. Katherina Schmidt was always busy as a mother and wife, devoting her life to raising Kaethe, Konrad, Julie, the then youngest Lise (born three years after Kaethe), and her husband Karl. I wonder if Katherina's undemonstrativeness was a manifestation of her underlying depression, perhaps resulting from the deaths of her two sons before Kaethe's birth.

A younger brother, Benjamin, was born. When he was 1 year old, Kaethe writes:

We were sitting at table and Mother was just ladling the soup — when the old nurse wrenched open the door and called out loudly, "He's throwing up again, he's throwing up again." Mother stood rigid for a moment and then went on ladling. I felt very keenly her agitation and her determination not to cry before all of us, for I could sense distinctly how she was suffering.

Shortly after this incident Benjamin died of meningitis, as had the Schmidt's first-born child, their son Julius. Kaethe wanted desperately to comfort her mother but could not because her mother seemed stiff and aloof with "that distant look of hers" [4]. The theme of the dead child and the living but deeply grieving mother would later permeate Kaethe Kollwitz's works.

Mother's apparent depression, or as I would call it now a deep unresolved and possibly pathological mourning process for her dead children, troubled Kaethe, who feared losing her mother [4].

I was always afraid she would come to some harm. If she were bathing, even if it were only in the tub, I feared she might drown. Once I stood at the window watching for Mother to come back, for it was time . . . . I felt the oppressive fear in my heart that she might get lost and never find her way back to us. Then I became afraid that Mother might go mad. (P. 4)

Yet Kaethe never saw her mother break down. As Kearns correctly observes [4], ". . . without self-pity, without seeking to cast blame, she endured the loss of three of the seven children she had borne" (p. 4).

In her diary Kaethe [6] notes that "although she [her mother] never surrendered to the deep sorrow of those early days of her marriage, it must have been her years of suffering that gave her forever after the remote air of a madonna." This point is further elaborated upon by Kearns [4].

While Katherina Schmidt never cried, tender hearted, nervous young Kaethe did, often and violently; some of her roaring and kicking tantrums lasted for hours . . . . Perhaps Kaethe's childhood fits were unconscious expressions of her mother's pent-up rage and grief. But in later years, Katherina Schmidt's stoicism appeared in Kaethe herself—and in her many images of mothers. (P. 4)

One might further suggest that young Kaethe was angry with her mother for not giving her the love and warmth she felt her mother had to offer. Kaethe identified strongly with her mother: Unfortunately, Kaethe Kollwitz's second son and later her first-born grandson were both killed in the two world wars. Grieving mothers, frightened children, death, and oppression were life themes that found their way into Kollwitz's art but had their roots in her life—in some way perhaps even before her birth or conception. There were many cheerless days in the early years of Kaethe Kollwitz. Her life seemingly was always related to death, mourning that was unresolved, and controlled fear.

Kaethe's mother, Katherina Rupp Schmidt, was the daughter of a nonconformist religious leader who suffered much political abuse. She grew up in a household of religious, political, and social liberality, although her own strict religious training emphasized sincerity, seriousness, and truth. Katherina also possessed artistic interests and talents, "indicated by the successful copies of old masters with which she decorated her home" [4]. Although her mother read Shakespeare, Byron, and Shelley in the original English, Kaethe rarely saw her reading and never heard her discuss what she had read. Katherina did not share her experiences; Kaethe learned about her mother from carefully observing her—a characteristic form of communication useful to the later artist.

Kaethe's father was also an unusual man. Educated in the law, he did not engage in his profession because "his political, social, and moral views made it impossible for him to serve the authoritarian Prussian State" [4], which was conservative, right wing, and under the domination of Prince Otto von Bismarck. "Discouraged with the political climate of Bismarck's Prussia, Karl Schmidt became intrigued by the ideas of Karl Marx" [4]. He joined the German Social Democratic Workers party and focused his faith on socialist ideology rather than on a spiritual religious deity. "Having joined the SPD, he knew it would be moral and political suicide to attempt to practice law in right-wing Prussia. He turned to the art of stone masonry and in time became an expert house builder" [4].

Identification with an artistic mother may have provided Kaethe Kollwitz with the model for her graphic artwork; identification with her father could have played a role in her later sculpture. The values of her father and grandfather became her political and social ideals, but mourning played a crucial role in the content of her creative activity.

Karl Schmidt, unlike many authoritarian Prussian fathers, was an idealist. He taught his children through examples and guidance rather than through force. He encouraged his three daughters to aspire to roles unrestricted to that of wife and mother, especially in artistic work in which they used their hands. Both Kaethe and her sister Lise showed gifts in drawing very early.

Kaethe had a crush on the boy upstairs and in her diary describes the "refreshment" of kissing. When her friend, Otto, unexpectedly moved away and their "love" was ended, Kaethe was quite upset. She scratched an "O" into her left wrist. Kaethe was greatly confused, like many preteenagers of her day, by sex, love, and reproduction. In these topics, her parents did not enlighten her. She went to her mother daily during this time—deliberately and timidly trying to share feelings and get answers. "But she said nothing at all, and so I too soon fell silent" [4]. Because of this silence on sex-related topics, Kaethe continued for many years to feel ignorant and guilty about her own sexuality.

Kearns suggests that Kaethe's mother's "puritanical attitude" had been fostered by her own father's strict moral teachings [4]. Julius Rupp was an idealistic, intellectual, and highly moral preacher who had been imprisoned 30 years earlier because his religious views differed from those of Friedrich Wilhelm IV. "Upon release, after two years of imprisonment, Rupp had founded a religious community called the Friends of Light, or the Free Congregation, based on the tenets of the early Christian communities" [4]. Although her grandfather's sermons were scholarly and erudite, Kaethe liked his spirit, laconic humor, willingness to give, and kindness. She remembered his beautiful, large, expressive hands. Her mother's hands resembled those of her grandfather. "A characteristic of Kaethe's pictures would be the beautiful hands of many of her subjects" [4].

Walking along the docks of the river, Kaethe and her sister carefully observed the workers loading and unloading crates. Kaethe was entranced by "their facial expressions, their sure, basic movements," their hard-worked bodies, and their plain, ageless clothes. But most of all, their lined faces held a mysterious beauty for her. Her later work dealt with the world of the workers, an interest that she felt could be traced back to "these casual expeditions through the busy commercial city teeming with work" [4].

ADOLESCENCE

At age 11 Kaethe sketched her younger sister, Lise. Her drawing "captured her sister's small, broad forehead, high cheekbones, and large, oval face with its strong Slavic character." She took it to her father, who expressed satisfaction with it and placed it in a drawer labeled "Kaethe's Work." She had earlier completed other compositions, some depicting major events in German and religious history (e.g., Luther burning the pope's edict in public, denouncing all ties with Roman Catholicism). Kaethe's parents appreciated her talents and encouraged her artwork. Her father felt she would be a successful painter but would "not be much distracted by love affairs" as she "was not a pretty girl" [4]. He was willing to support her training in art.

Encouraged by her father's interest, Kaethe worked very hard to please him. However, when he felt her younger sister Lise could soon be as good as Kaethe, Kaethe's relationship with Lise changed from one of complete love, companionship, and trust to one compounded with envy and rivalry. She did not want to compete with Lise, but she did not want Lise to replace her as family artist. The threat of Lise's ability created in Kaethe a single-mindedness that inspired her to ask for drawing lessons before Lise might think of asking [4]. Lise did not ask for art lessons for herself; instead she good-naturedly sat untiringly as a model for Kaethe.

Not all of Kaethe's development was focused on drawing. She became interested in poetry and was expecially moved by a poem by Ferdinand Freilgrath, "The Dead to the Living," in which the voices of the March 1848 Dead summon all survivors of that revolution to arm against profiteers and decadent monarchs. Like her left-wing parents, Kaethe identified with the two hundred March Dead martyrs killed by the kaiser's militia. About this time (age 11–12) Kaethe also had a series of nightmares in which she felt helpless and powerless. These followed her earlier episodes of crying tantrums and stomachaches. During these disturbances, she would become quite depressed. The depressed moods would last for hours, even days. With puberty she became further conflicted over her sexuality and feminine identification.

At age 14, Kaethe began art lessons with Rudolf Mauer, an engraver, in

Koenigsberg. She met Lisabeth and Karl Kollwitz during this period. Lisabeth and Karl were orphans living with a family in Koenigsberg. Karl, a friend of Kaethe's older brother, Konrad, was also a political supporter of the Social Democratic party. Initially an observer, Kaethe became more interested and involved in the discussions she heard about socialism, and slowly her discussions with Karl about socialism, revolution, art, medicine, free love, and marriage drew them closer.

Though at 16 Kaethe was old enough to enter Koenigsberg's Academy of Art, women were not allowed to do so. Her father arranged for her to study with a well-known Koenigsberg painter, Emile Neide. In 1883, she composed an illustration to Freilgrath's "The Emigrants," which portrayed the humble new arrivals. In the next year, her seventeenth, her grandfather died and Kaethe felt the loss deeply. However, in the same year, 1884, Karl Kollwitz, now a premedical student, made an engagement proposal to Kaethe, which she accepted. Kaethe's father, however, feared that the engagement would thwart his plans for her future as an artist and that marriage would inhibit her artistic career. He determined to send her away to art school and begged her to reconsider her engagement.

On a trip to Berlin that same year, Kaethe met Gerhart Hauptmann, a young poet and dramatist whose work would later influence her creativity. In Berlin, her brother, Konrad, who had made the acquaintance of Friedrich Engels, took her to the cemetery in which were buried the nearly two hundred workers killed on March 18, 1848. This made a silent but deep impression on Kaethe; one wonders whether, at a deeper level, the deaths of three brothers was connected with the martyrs and the 1848 attempt at revolution.

ADULTHOOD

In 1885, Kaethe began art studies in Berlin. When her professor saw her composition on "The Emigrants," he urged her to consider etching and lithography, which required the expert drawing skills she possessed. Initially she protested that she wished to paint, but her teacher kept telling her to stick to drawing. Influenced by her father's wish for her to be a painter she returned home and continued to study oils, color, and technique. In 1889 she accepted Karl's engagement ring. This so upset her father that he decided to again send her away — this time to Munich.

Munich in 1889 was sophisticated, challenging, and the cultural and academic center of the country. The Munich Academy of Art had a progressive and libertarian attitude. However, marriage was taboo to all students and celibacy was the commandment. "The women art students considered marriage an act of betrayal, for it meant abandoning their artistic work . . . . It was impossible for a woman to be married and an artist" [4]. Kaethe herself wrestled with the question of marriage *and* art versus marriage *or* art and came to no conclusion. She was not sure if her dual role would hinder her artistic work, but she hoped to manage the two lives of wife and artist, despite her father's attitude and that of the community. Slowly she was included in her classmates' way of life, and she enjoyed the new freedoms. She became interested in etching, discovering that this skill required manual dexterity, strength, patience, and intense concentration (this, I believe, was an identification with her father's artistic manual activity). Kaethe discovered that this method suited her. "Her creative process was not one of instant inspiration but of arduous technical, emotional, and intellectual labor" [4]. With the broadening of her experience, Kaethe added a feminist perspective to her socialistic one.

Still struggling with painting, yet aware of her difficulties with color use, Kaethe read an essay by Max Klinger on "Painting and Drawing" [4] in which the author indicated that drawing had a freer relationship to the representable world than did painting. Reading Klinger's ideas, Kaethe realized she was not a painter at all, and she turned all of her efforts to etching and drawing. One might ask again at this point if at a deeper level the turning from painting did not signify an attempt to give up an identification with her mother, who did paint. To buttress this suggestion, we find that coincidental with her decision regarding the art form she would pursue was the outcropping of doubts about marriage. She wondered if by binding herself with an engagement she had to give up the freer life of the artist.

Kaethe returned to Koenigsberg to find that Karl Kollwitz, finishing his medical education, decided to intern in Berlin the next year. Her father at this point said she could return to Munich, and she gladly accepted his offer. When 17 she had drawn a self-portrait that she did not complete. Now in Munich, in 1889, she returned to drawing, completing two self-portraits and continuing with self-portraits from then on. Kaethe returned to Koenigsberg; she still attempted to paint, but finally recognized this medium was not for her.

Karl Kollwitz had been offered a position in Berlin as one of the few doctors chosen to work in a new plan of social and medical insurance for workers that had been introduced by Bismarck. Karl, sincerely interested since his youth in serving people who were poor, took the position and shared his enthusiasm with his fiancée of seven years. Kaethe seemed to have accepted her classmates' belief that female artists must not marry, since few married women had succeeded as artists. Yet she did not want to stay in Koenigsberg as a single woman. Marrying Karl would in fact allow for more independence; a wife in Berlin could enjoy a more active intellectual and social life than a single woman in East Prussia. She wondered what would become of her creativity if she married Karl. Her father feared the worst for her career if she married. Her mother was very positive about marriage, believing there was little future for a husband-less woman — having a loving husband who would provide for her and allow her to care for him was the preferable state. Kaethe decided to marry. In part, Kearns suggests this was "a rebellious act necessary for her emotional and artistic growth" [4]. It was a way of freeing herself from her father, who intruded himself into her life and into her work: he still wanted her to be a painter. She was having increasing difficulty in trying to please her father and create work that expressed herself.

Thus her choice of marriage, overdetermined as such decisions are at times, seemed to offer emotional and creative freedom as well as social and economic security in an exciting city with a man whose social, political, economic, and philosophical goals and ideals she shared and valued. Similar to her father in independent spirit and in opposition to autocratic authority, she paradoxically found herself in opposition to his wishes for her regarding marriage and painting. And yet philosophically and even technically, she was like him. She herself was aware of her masculine identification and felt this helped her in her artistic work.

Kaethe Kollwitz believed that "bisexuality [was] almost a necessary factor in artistic production" [4]. For her, bisexuality seemingly influenced her creative psyche more than it affected her sexuality.

It is not known whether she ever acted on her feelings for women, whether she wanted to, or whether she would have been able to . . . but her love for women enabled her to love herself — something essential to every artist . . . her early self-portraits . . . show the artist examining herself for the sake of understanding; they are frank studies of an imperfect, struggling, finite human. It is the same with her depiction of other women . . . her portraits of working-class women show clearly that she appreciated women as whole human beings. (P. 59)

Karl knew that Kaethe would not give up her work after they married. He was a very devoted, kind, and optimistic partner and balanced Kaethe's introspective, more depressed, and assertive tendencies. Karl found a tenement flat in a working-class section of North Berlin (now in East Berlin), and on June 13, 1891 (Karl's twenty-eighth birthday), Kaethe and Karl were married. Kaethe was 24 years old.

For the next 50 years, Kaethe and Karl moved from floor to floor within this corner tenement building. From the start of their marriage, they both worked, each in their own settings and in their own professions. Kaethe would on occasion, however, go next door to draw poor women with their babies or older children as they waited to visit her husband for consultation and treatment. She fulfilled the duties of a housewife, but these did not provide her with as satisfying a sense of fulfillment as her drawings and etchings did.

During the autumn of 1891, Kaethe became pregnant. In 1892 she etched a beautiful self-portrait. In May 1892 she gave birth to a son, Hans, in her apartment while in the midst of working on a greeting etching for her husband to mark the occasion of the birth of his first child. In this picture, the only one in which she centers attention on the father, the mother hands the baby to the father with pride, joy, and gratitude. Kaethe did many drawings of her son [4].

Kaethe soon began to use little Hans as a model, sketching at least eighteen studies of her first son. Although Kaethe had to care for Hans' constant needs, Karl "did everything possible so that I would have time to work." As soon as they could afford it, a live-in housekeeper was hired to deal with the time-consuming housekeeping and child-rearing duties. (P. 64)

Kollwitz's work, dark in spirit and style, like that of Edvard Munch, is one reason for calling it either Expressionist or closely related to this movement. Her work was not accepted by the "establishment," and so she joined a group of younger artists with socialistic orientations and expressionistic views of art. She contributed two drawings and one etching to the Secession's first exhibit.

On February 28, 1893, Kaethe attended the premiere of the play, *The Weavers,* by Gerhart Hauptmann, the poet with whom she had dined in Berlin ten years before. Despite a Berlin police ban on all public performances of this play, the work was performed. The drama told the story of a group of Silesian peasants turned linen weavers, who, just 50 years earlier in 1844, had revolted because of low factory wages and wretched living conditions. Kaethe strongly identified with the emotions of the weavers and was so moved she began to work on *The Revolt of the Weavers* series. She spent the next five years creating and perfecting the six frames of the series, which are labeled (1) Poverty, (2) Death (a weaver's child dies of hunger), (3) Conspiracy (the weavers plan to avenge the child's death), (4) Weavers on the march to the factory owner's home, (5) Attack (on the owner's mansion by the weavers), and (6) The End (the revolt and the lives of some of the men are over).

This noteworthy graphic series, involving working women as well as men, presents the death of a child as the force that drove the workers to revolt. The death of a child, an artistic theme from her earliest days, had significant roots in Kaethe Kollwitz's childhood. Two of her brothers had died before her birth and her youngest brother, Benjamin, had died when she was a child. The Kleins [5] described how this affected Kaethe.

Memories of Benjamin's illness and death were deeply stamped on Kaethe's mind. As a mature woman and even in her old age she recalled how she had ached with love and pity as her reserved mother had grieved silently for Benjamin . . . Kaethe was tormented by feelings of guilt because of a strange circumstance that had occurred at the time of Benjamin's death. Her father had wanted his children to have worthwhile playthings and had given them large building blocks . . . From these Kaethe had built for her own use a temple to Venus . . . She was playing at worship in this temple when her mother and father, quietly coming into the room, had told her that Benjamin had died. Kaethe was terror-stricken. God, she thought, was punishing them for all her sacrifices to the pagan diety Venus. (P. 6)

Since Kaethe held herself responsible for Benjamin's death, one might ask if this was not also a cover for her feelings of surviving her two other brothers who died before her birth. Survivor guilt as it relates to childhood sibling loss through death is not uncommon [9].

In 1896, Kaethe bore her second son, Peter. She finished *The Revolt of the Weavers* that summer and traveled to see her sick father and show him her first graphic work, which was dedicated to him for his seventieth birthday. He was overjoyed, as was her mother, to realize how successful Kaethe had integrated the three lives of artist, wife, and mother. Kaethe Kollwitz's series was proposed for the prestigious Gold Medal award of the Great Berlin Exhibit of 1898, but Kaiser Wilhelm II vetoed the nomination, possibly because of his opposition to "socialist" art. One year later, however, she was awarded the Gold Medal, and in 1899, it was conferred on her by the King of Saxony. In her thirty-second year, Kaethe Kollwitz was one of the foremost artists of her country.

In the next few years, Kaethe Kollwitz produced various revolutionary works dealing with such themes as the French Revolution, the Peasant War of the sixteenth century, and the fights of some assertive women against tyranny.

When her eldest child Hans became seriously ill, Kaethe and Karl tended him through the night [4].

Finally in the middle of the early morning, at three A.M., my husband said, "I think we've won him back" . . . . During the night an unforgettable cold chill caught and held me: it was the terrible realization that any second this young child's life might be cut off, and the child gone forever . . . . it was the worst fear I have every known . . .

Months later, the long moments of this night would return to her; she would relive the awful knowledge of mortal-parental-helplessness. At last she confronted Hans' touch with death in the creation of *Frau mit totem Kind* [Woman with Dead Child]. Though Hans had been its inspiration, she used Peter as a model for this piece.

When he was seven years old and I was doing the etching *Mother with Dead Child,* I drew myself in the mirror while holding him in my arms. The pose was quite a strain, and I let out a groan. Then he said consolingly in his high little voice: "Don't worry, Mother, it will be beautiful too." (P. 87)

The finished etching of *Mother with Dead Child* was so expressive and painfully real that viewers seeing it felt the pain of the bereaved mother. Although she loved her sons, Kaethe was undemonstrative in her show of physical affection, just as the mother who raised her, Katherina Schmidt, had been.

Even though she was receiving acclaim from all quarters and her family was healthy and growing, Kaethe's basic concerns were ever present in her works. For example, the drawing, *Raped,* the second in *The Peasant War* series, is one of the earliest pictures in Western art to depict a female victim of sexual violence sympathetically. In *Portraits of Misery,* we find working-class women falling faint from hunger, a woman mourning an infant's death, a wife being abused, a pregnant woman knocking on a doctor's door with bowed head low in shame at her need, and a begging elderly woman. Her drawings for *Simplizissimus,* a progressive Munich monthly magazine, dealt with similar themes. In 1910 she sketched *Death, Woman, and Child*—a theme to which she kept returning even before her great tragedy of 1914. *Run Over,* done also in 1910, shows a scene of simultaneous horror and grief in which parents rush to save their baby's life. Though her technique was now perfected, the theme was still death. The tragic quality of life "gave Kollwitz her creative cutting edge" [4].

Although Kaethe worried a great deal about her sons, especially their health and future, the theme of a child's death, I feel, stems from the deaths of her brothers and her attempts to "work out" her feelings about these losses as well as the loss she experienced in relation to a mother who was filled with mourning that pervaded her entire personality.

With the death of Karl's sister Lisabeth from tuberculosis, both Kaethe and Karl became even more concerned about Peter's health. He was constantly afflicted with upper-respiratory illnesses. One winter he was sent to a sanitorium in order to help him recover or at least avoid more serious difficulties.

Creatively restless, Kollwitz now began to explore the possibilities of working with stone and clay, which marked the beginning of her experiences in sculpture. This period coincided with the time when her sons began to leave home for longer stays and her child-bearing years were coming to an end—a time to which Kaethe had looked forward to with great anticipation [4].

Menopause—or her expectations about it—affected her personality and work even more dramatically than did aging. For the first time in her career, due to irregular menstrual periods, she experienced immobilizing insecurity about her work. She recorded in her log:

"This is the second time I have destroyed work which required weeks to create. I felt almost driven to do this when I got my period and didn't know or expect I was getting it. The next day I found that menstruation had been the reason for my destructiveness. I and possibly most women suffer similar pathological pressure during menstruation."

She was used to obeying her will rather than her body . . . . She feared that the changes in her body would sap her physical energy to the point of ending her creativity. A deadening mood of futility and depression overwhelmed her. Nothing engaged her usually alert intellect and social conscience for a significant period of time. It was a damaging time, fraught with anxiety. (P. 123)

With her fear of a hysterectomy and a thyroidectomy, Kaethe found "the deep faith within myself is lacking" [4]. She believed that her sexuality, manifested in her ability to produce children, also positively influenced her artistic creativity. In contrast to some views, including those of her father and her female colleagues, Kollwitz's position seemingly was that creativity paralleled procreativity, and if the latter was impossible, it made the former impossible or difficult. Of course we cannot ignore the symbolic meaning of menopause—a stoppage of menses. It is likely that Kaethe's vulnerability to loss, change, and abnormal mourning was indeed exacerbated by the threat of the loss of her uterus, her thyroid, her ability to have children, and the slackening of the ties to her sons.

Kaethe's self-portraits of this period, her mid- and late-forties, reflect her doubt, anxiety, weariness, and grief. In one dated 1911, she appears to be in pain.

With the outbreak of war in 1914, Kaethe Kollwitz was overcome by melancholy. Hans joined the army, and Peter, barely 18, also wanted to be a soldier. After many attempts to dissuade him, the sad parents did not object to his volunteering for any service. Kaethe worked as a cook and cafeteria helper in a kitchen, feeding large numbers of the unemployed, especially destitute mothers and children. She wrote a prophetic entry in her diary about young men who will die in the war. On October 22, 1914, she received the news that Peter had been killed in Belgium. Kaethe Kollwitz never fully recovered from this loss, the ultimate culmination of her lifelong vulnerability.

Slowly, Kaethe began to achieve a partial resolution of her bereavement and sought inspiration for her new creative work from Peter's death. She summoned his presence to help her in her work — work that she felt was denied to him. After months of agony she began. "She found in Goethe's 'seed for the planting must not be ground' the moral, philosophic and emotional basis she needed as a mother and an artist to continue living and working" [4]. She asserted that there is no justification for any young volunteers, of whatever country, to be killed.

Kaethe Kollwitz began to cultivate the seeds of a talent within her that she had feared would die at her menopause. This creativity was related not only to the partial resolution of bereavement but to the liberation of "energy" through the identification with the child who might have been creative if he had lived since shortly after his eighteenth birthday, Peter had decided to continue his art lessons and become a painter. In a sense, Kaethe wanted to fulfill a promise that Peter could no longer complete himself.

Thus, by identifying with Peter, the artist who could have been, Kaethe Kollwitz was dealing with her loss in a creative fashion. In the winter following his death, Kaethe Kollwitz began to create for her dead son and in this process she memorialized Peter, allowing her own creativity to again be productive — using her art in the service of the expression of grief and pain through social consciousness. She decided to create a memorial sculpture to her fallen child as well as to all the young soldiers whose lives were sacrificed. Designing the memorial however, was easier than bringing it into being [4].

As a mourning mother she was as yet unable to make her deep private suffering public. As an artist, however, she was obliged, ultimately, to reveal her emotions — as she always had — before the eyes of strangers. As she began work on Peter's memorial, she experienced great conflict between her "self-expressive" self and her "objective" self . . . . This trial, reflecting the struggle, rather than the harmony, between her "masculine" and feminine selves: the vulnerability, the intense feeling, the passion are there, but so overwhelming that she is unable to objectify and create a work in which passion is controlled by skill. (P. 136)

In 1916 Kaethe produced one self-study, a tribute to her ability to unmask her soul. In 1916 she also drew *Anguish*. In the *Widow,* a pregnant working-class woman, gaunt and harried, stands nearly full length, her large-knuckled hands cupped to hold and embrace reaching out limply in empty space. The woman is shocked and despondent from mourning; the woman is Kaethe Kollwitz, grieving at the loss of her son—the despair is her own, and yet she bears the creative product within her ready to be delivered as one gives birth to a baby. The stimulus or father is no longer there, and he is missed.

As the war continued, the term "expressionism" in Germany came to be used broadly to apply to any artist holding nonestablishment sociopolitical views and working in a nonformalistic style. Because of this broad definition, and because she was inclined toward self-expression, Kollwitz was often incorrectly called an expressionist, though she never gave allegiance to any purely expressionist group or doctrine [4].

Throughout her life she had sought to be free of everything that obfuscated her true self. Every artist tends toward self-expression, but Kollwitz used this unusually strong tendency in herself to examine and/or resolve personal conflicts and truths. Whether as art student, wife and mother, revolutionary, adventurer, or very private artist, she regarded her work as an avenue of self-discovery. Not only did she follow her feelings; she acted upon them with conviction, for in her singular quest she often disagreed with her colleagues and her society. (P. 140)

Kaethe was highly motivated to work on Peter's memorial, which changed from a sculpture of Peter to a relief of mourning parents (herself and Karl)—a monumental headstone for the entire cemetery where Peter was buried. It was the largest work she ever planned, and she accepted the years of work that would be needed for its completion. "Constantly, she strove for greater simplicity, to distill the human form to its most basic, expressive features and lives . . . . all her working time was concentrated on the memorial, and she often prayed that she would not grow old and infirm before she finished it" [4].

The war ended, there was political turmoil in Germany, and finally in 1919, the Weimar Republic was established. Kollwitz became the first woman elected to full professorship at the Prussian Academy of Arts; this position carried with it a large, fully equipped studio with side rooms. In her new studio, Kollwitz drew a picture of huddling protective mothers who hear the death knell of poverty and war that threatens their children. The picture, *The Mothers,* shows that children are the life of their mothers and thus sustain their mothers' lives instead of vice versa. This might be considered as the pictorial representation of the process I noted above: through Peter's death, Kaethe's capacity to create once again reaffirmed itself. Nonetheless, Peter's death, her aging, and the war had changed her. She became fatigued, passive, and introspective. Her politics changed to faith in eventual change rather than violent revolutionary programs. Peter's death led her to renounce all war. "Politically, Kollwitz could be termed an independent socialist, for though she gave her artistic and emotional support to Communists in Russia and Germany, she never joined their ranks as a political advocate" [4].

Starting in 1917 Kollwitz began to produce a series of woodcuts called *War*. The seven productions were an impassioned protest against the gross senselessness of war, especially as it represents a woman's outrage. She finished the series in 1923 when inflation and hunger were rampant in Germany. This situation became the stimulus for another series of woodcuts on *Hunger, Vienna Is Dying!, Save Her Children!* and *Abolish the Abortion Law!* (a lithograph poster). In 1924 she designed *Germany's Children are Starving* and lithographed two posters, *Bread* and *Never Again War!*. The 1920s were Kollwitz's most richly productive period.

Kaethe's son Hans had married and now had a son, Peter, and twin daughters, Jordi and Jutta. Her three grandchildren were a great source of pleasure for her.

In June 1926, Kaethe and Karl Kollwitz traveled for the first time to Roggevelde, the World War I cemetery where Peter was buried. After the visit she sculpted the mother and the father for her *Memorial to the Fallen* and could visualize how they would stand in the graveyard. In 1928 Kollwitz was made the first woman department head at the Prussian Academy of Arts. She taught the master graphics class and was on full-time salary; for the first time in her life, at age 61, she would receive a regular income.

The economic crash of 1929 helped the Nazis rally over six million voters. Kollwitz was angered by the Nazis' tactics of using brute force to suppress a workers' rally. Alerted to imminent political danger, she created a drawing called *Demonstration*. Kaethe felt a sense of apprehension in the political arena, and her concerns turned to her grandson, Peter. On April 22, 1931, at the Academy, she unveiled the sculpture for the *Memorial to the Fallen*. It had been 17 years since her son Peter was killed, and in those years she was able to construct creatively while involved in a mourning-liberation process. Though she never could complete this process, her memorial was a meaningful way of not allowing Peter to be forgotten. Her memorial to her dead son involved a new art form for her — sculpture. The triumphal use of sculpture was an additional creative shift that Peter's death may have set in motion.

The memorial sculptures are powerful statements about the Kollwitz's grief and loss as well as a symbolic memorial to all victims of war. The sculptures were converted to granite after an additional year. Fearing that the right-wing party might deface the memorials, "through protracted and difficult negotiations with the German Republic, the German national railway, the Belgian government and the Brussels cemetery board, expense-free shipment of the sculptures was at last arranged. Kaethe and Karl went to Roggevelde in order to direct their placement" [4]. The figures did cast a living spell of love and grief over the German cemetery, and they indeed seemed to be silent bereaved guardians of the young soldiers lying there. At Peter's grave, Kaethe paused, but when she came to the granite mother, whose face was identical to her own, she bowed low in sadness; Kaethe wept and stroked the stone cheeks.

When the Nazis came to power in 1933 and Kaethe Kollwitz and Heinrich Mann signed a manifesto calling for unity of the parties of the left, their resignation from the Academy was demanded. Kaethe suffered governmental derogation but never outright censorship until 1936, when the Nazis ordered the closing of the last museum in which a few of her pieces could still be found. She never again saw her work on public display.

In 1934 Kaethe began a series of eight lithographs on the cycle of *Death*. Her sister Lise once said that Kaethe had carried on a dialogue with death all of her life. In this last series, the artist interpreted eight different "conversations" in profound fashion [4]. In the final work, *The Call of Death*, we see the artist herself, aging and sexually undifferentiated.

On July 13, 1936, two Gestapo officers called on Kaethe Kollwitz in connection with an article that had appeared in the Soviet periodical, *Izvestia*. She was told that if she did not furnish information and retract statements attributed to her she would be sent to a concentration camp. When another officer called the following day she decided to write a statement retracting the comments that had been quoted in *Izvestia*, but she would not give the name of the other unidentified German artist who was also quoted. Although her work was severely criticized and reviled, Kollwitz was never again threatened. After the interrogation, however, both Kaethe and Karl always carried a vial of poison in case they were incarcerated by the Nazis at a future time.

After age 70, Kaethe still worked on various sculptures, but her work was labeled "degenerate" by the Nazis and could not be displayed. She designed gravestone reliefs, and when the Nazis finally banned Karl's practice altogether, the two were quite poor. An American offered Kaethe refuge in the United States, but she declined because she did not wish to be separated from her family.

World War II began in September 1939. Karl became completely bedridden in 1940. Kaethe was his constant nurse and companion and on

July 19, 1940, he died. From that day Kaethe used a cane to help her walk [4]. She was very lonely, and her grandson Peter had now joined the army. At age 74 she executed her last graphic, *Seed for the Planting Must Not Be Ground.* In this work, the seed for planting, 16-year-old boys, are around the mother, wanting to break loose. The mother will not allow this and indicates that they must be ready for life, not for war. On October 14, 1942, Hans brought word that Peter had died in Russia. It was a terrible wrenching irony that he should have suffered the same fate as his namesake.

In 1943, Kaethe created the last of 84 self-portraits. In this work she is passive, reflective, and accepting of the forces about her; one has the impression that she is truly waiting for death. Because the bombing of Berlin became dangerous, she was evacuated to the country by some friends. Six months after she left Berlin, her tenement building was hit by bombs and it burned to the ground; a sizable amount of her work was destroyed, a final blow after earlier deliberate destructions by the Nazis. Even life in the country became difficult: no heat, very reduced food rations, and the danger of air raids. She was evacuated again by a powerful collector who was appreciative of her contributions to art; her granddaughter left with her.

On April 22, 1945, four months before the end of World War II, Kaethe Kollwitz died without worldly possessions and away from her home of over 50 years. She was a symbol to those who knew her or of her. She was an ideal and an inspiration to those who were sad and threatened. She was a creator of art, of children, and of a household in which she and her husband lived harmoniously for many years.

Effects of Depressed and Pathologically Mourning Mothers on Their Children

I have selected the life story of Kaethe Kollwitz to illustrate how significant deaths, and even other serious disrupting traumas, can affect the lives of survivors in many different ways. Kaethe Kollwitz was markedly influenced by the deaths of her siblings during her childhood and early adolescence. But what was even more distressing was the impact of these losses on her family, especially on her mother who appeared to be a chronically depressed (pathologically mourning) woman. Like Sir James Matthew Barrie's mother after her child suddenly died in an accident [9], Kaethe Kollwitz's mother could not be to her children what the children wanted and needed. James Barrie, like Kaethe Kollwitz, felt guilt and remorse over the loss of his sibling, but also added responsibility for the careful monitoring of his mother's moods and behaviors. Kaethe Koll-witz and James Barrie had to become caretakers of their mothers when they themselves needed caring.

Studying the effects of depressed parents (some of whom committed suicide) on children and adolescents, I conclude that the role reversal, the fear of abandonment, and the concerns of the child that the parent might destroy himself or herself along with the child and/or other siblings are striking and significant in the individual's later development. Parental pathology does indeed play a critical role in shaping the child's defensive and adaptive structure. For example, I have found that mothers who have verifiable obsessive-compulsive neuroses have "different" children from those who have depressive, hysteric, or borderline personalities. Research on these mothers and children can be undertaken, and follow-ups, retrospectively studied, can yield rich data on the various paths followed by the developing child in response to parental pathology.

In recently published biographies, we can learn and infer with a fair degree of probability additional evidence to support this thesis. Isak Dinesen, the fascinating writer, was markedly affected by her father [13]. He, too, was a writer and traveler. Years later, she learned that, like herself, he may have had syphilis and feared madness. She was his favorite child and confidante, and he committed suicide when she was almost 10.

John Berryman's poems, especially the "Dream Songs," are full of autobiographical incidents. Mary Ellmann [2], in a recent review of a new biography, points out how Berryman's wounds were deep and, she believes, incurable. His mother claimed his father raped her and that she felt blackmailed into marrying him. Thus, John Berryman (born John Smith) was conceived in trauma. When John, the future poet, was 12, Smith (his father) committed suicide by shooting himself while on the front porch of their home. All his life Berryman saw his father in dreams or daydreams. In Dream Song 143 he says, "That mad drive wiped out my childhood." And in Dream Song 384 he writes, "I spit upon this dreadful banker's grave, / who shot his heart out in a Florida dawn" [2]. The reason for his father's suicide was never clear to him, as is true with many children whose parents commit suicide, and Berryman tried repeatedly to find out from his mother why this tragedy occurred; he even wondered if she had killed him. "Caught between hatred of his father and curiosity about him, between love of his mother and suspicion of her, he could not free his mind of either parent. When he wrote a life of Stephen Crane, he attributed to Crane the same feelings he had himself" [2].

After her husband's death, Berryman's mother quickly married again. Her second husband's name was John Angus Berryman. She changed her son's name to John Berryman, thus obliterating the poet's paternal tie, at least nominally. The poet never seemed to accept this change emotionally or in reality. His life was predictably turbulent afterward. He made a suicidal attempt while at boarding school and he repeated the pattern many times until, at age 57, he jumped off of a bridge and killed himself.

Another example is Ernest Hemingway. His father, a physician, fatally shot himself; years later Hemingway ended his life in the same way. The point I am suggesting is that depressed and suicidal parents do spawn specific pathology in their offspring, sometimes with fatal consequences. Since depression is the most common psychiatric condition in the general population, we may speculate about the consequences this emotional disorder may have on children. We increasingly read about childhood and adolescent depression and suicidal behavior [1], and recent statistics suggest that suicide is a major cause of death among adolescents and young adults in the United States.

The high risk imposed on children and adolescents whose parents committed suicide, were seriously depressed, or were involved with pathological mourning processes is a challenge to research and a reminder of the great importance of early preventive intervention or at least benign surveillance. Therapeutic intervention can break the cycle. I have personally observed this in six individuals whom I have treated. Thousands of children and adolescents are depressed, although the symptoms may be overlooked, misunderstood, ignored, or unrecognized until it is too late or until serious pathology emerges in later adult life. The impact of divorce, separation, or death of parents or siblings that occurred when the individual was a child or adolescent may predispose to childhood, adolescent, or later serious depression.

In Kaethe Kollwitz's life, additive losses through death contributed to her lifelong, chronic, unresolved, and, at times, pathological mourning. Her reactions to the death of her grandchild seemingly were less potent than her earlier reactions to the loss of siblings and of her son. However, emotional "loss" of her mother who was chronically depressed may have been a crucial determinant in her later emotional life and in its expression in her artistic work. This was also seen in the works of Munch.

References

1. Carlson, G. C., and Cantwell, D. P. Suicidal behavior and depression in children and adolescents. *J. Am. Acad. Child Psychiatry* 21:361, 1982.
2. Ellmann, M. The dream hunter: On John Berryman. *Encounter* LX:71, 1983.
3. Freud, S. Mourning and melancholia (1917). In J. Strachey (Ed.), *The Standard Edition of the Complete Psychological Works of Sigmund Freud.* London: Hogarth, 1957. Vol. 14, pp. 237–260.
4. Kearns, M. *Kaethe Kollwitz: Woman and Artist.* Old Westbury, New York: The Feminist Press, 1976.
5. Klein, M. C., and Klein, H. A. *Kaethe Kollwitz: Life in Art.* New York: Schocken Books, 1975.
6. Kollwitz, H. (Ed.). *The Diary and Letters of Kaethe Kollwitz.* Chicago: Henry Regnery, 1955.
7. Pollock, G. H. On mourning, immortality and utopia. *J. Am. Psychoanal. Assoc.* 23:334, 1975.
8. Pollock, G. H. Mourning and memorialization through music. *The Annual of Psychoanalysis,* 3:423, 1975.
9. Pollock, G. H. On siblings, childhood sibling loss, and creativity. *The Annual of Psychoanalysis* 6:443, 1978.
10. Pollock, G. H. Process and affect: Mourning and grief. *Int. J. Psychoanal.* 59:225, 1978.
11. Pollock, G. H. Aging or Aged: Development or Pathology. In S. I. Greenspan and G. H. Pollock (Eds.), *The Course of Life: Psychoanalytic Contributions Toward Understanding Personality Development,* Washington, D.C.: U.S. Government Printing Office, 1981. Vol. 3, pp. 549–585.
12. Pollock, G. H. The mourning-liberation process and creativity: The case of Käthe Kollwitz. *The Annual of Psychoanalysis* 10:333, 1982.
13. Thurman, J. *Isak Dinesen: The Life of a Storyteller.* New York: St. Martin's Press, 1982.

8

Psychotic influences on parenting

E. James Anthony

Psychosis has been considered mainly an aberration of the brain or mind depending on whether one looks at it from an organic or psychological viewpoint. Both approaches, however, acknowledge its influence on the immediate environment to be less than favorable. It has been widely believed that individuals who have been exposed to psychosis from infancy onward tend to develop into immature and dependent people. Recent work, however, has shown that this belief has a limited generality. As Bleuler [8] has pointed out, psychotic parents cast a long shadow of suffering on all their offspring, but only a proportion of the offspring (40 – 50%) become clinically maladjusted or disordered. A small number (8 – 10%) may even seem to thrive resiliently in response to the challenge of such a disadvantage in upbringing. Both inherent and environmental factors in varying degrees dispose to these different types of epigenesis. The question that arises is whether psychoanalysis has anything explanatory to offer where the situation is predominantly environmental in its influence.

Psychoanalysis is regarded as being concerned with the inner reaches of the mind and, therefore, is disinterested not only in the environment at large but more specifically in the environmental impingements of psychosis. However, psychoanalysts have denied such charges and have drawn attention to a wide range of psychoanalytic ideas about the family and the general environment that have been accruing over the years regarding both average expectable and nonexpectable conditions [5, 6] and to the "new environmentalism" [25] that has followed the course of object relations during development. In fact, Hartmann [21] insisted that the individual's interaction with the environment is always implicit in psychoanalytic theory and certainly central to ego psychology. He postulated three groups of factors — the human environment, the nonhuman environment, and the cultural environment — that formed man "from the outside" and were as complex in their effects as those that shaped him "from the inside" [20].

Child analysts have never questioned the significance of the outer environment, especially when the inner environment becomes too disturbing and threatening. But, they have been cognizant that the outer

259

environment is never the "whole" story. As Anna Freud [14] stated: "No childhood disorder is due to environmental influence alone but always to the interaction between external and internal factors" (p. 34). The external fact can take the form of trauma and, as a general rule, the earlier that this occurs in life the greater is its pathogenicity. The traumatic influence can breach the immature stimulus barrier of the child by a reactivation of earlier traumata that may have passed unnoticed, by the repetition of seemingly minor stresses that produce a cumulative effect (Khan, [24]), or by the impact of unusual provocations [18]. Psychotic parenting can be looked upon as unusually provocative.

There are many indications that a child is being overstressed by traumatic experiences: Anxiety signals are replaced by panic, appropriate motor activity is replaced by paralysis or chaotic motility, and abreaction or working through are replaced by futile repetitiveness and psychological responses by somatization. The ego may be put out of action or function at a more regressive level [14].

Trauma that is viewed as "external" to an observer may actually be having "internal" effects on its victim: when it is overwhelming or related to love objects, it is rapidly internalized and incorporated into existing structures that link it with similar past experiences. If it cannot be gradually worked through and defused, it can become chronic and blend with other ongoing developmental conflicts. What then ensues is a neurotic-traumatic complex that is highly resistant to treatment. The psychic injury resulting from psychotic management by a parent furnishes a good example of the complex interplay between environmental stresses and evolving psychosexual crises. Before examining the intrinsic problems of psychotic parenting in depth, it might be useful to take a look at cases furnished by psychoanalytic clinicians depicting the problems that arise when psychosis afflicts the parent.

In the case of Jean Drew [14], Anna Freud called attention to the "unholy influence" on a child's development of parenting by a paranoid schizophrenic mother who could not be labeled bad "in the ordinary sense of the word" since she had good attitudes about child rearing and high moral standards. The difficulty created by this psychotic parent had to do with a negative relationship with her daughter. Her ambivalence was intense: she wanted the girl to stay with her and yet she drove her away by relentless nagging; she wanted Jean to be happy but constantly deprived her of everyday pleasures; and she wanted her daughter to be good but accused her of imagined wickedness and punished her irrationally and unmercifully.

This "incomprehensible mixture of demandingness, love, hate, and overwhelming injustice" [14] filled the daughter with very mixed feelings. Jean felt sorry for her mother, needed by her, and responsible for her, but at the same time Jean hated her, wanted never to see her again, and repeatedly ran away from home. Yet, she always returned willingly to continue the relationship. Jean was deeply ashamed of her mother's bizarre behavior but stuck with her out of loyalty and repudiated the community so that she was pushed into an unhealthy social isolation. The asymmetry of the relationship was the reverse of the usual, requiring the child to tolerate and understand the mother. The predicament of the offspring in relation to psychotic parenting was summarized by Anna Freud [14] as follows.

The ill parents whom (the children) cannot help loving, nevertheless cannot be respected by them, nor can they wish to grow up like them as children do normally. The abnormality of the parent's behavior is perceived by them, first dimly, in time sharply. In either case they are frightened by it . . . such children also are invariably at odds with the neighbors against whom the parent raves and rants in the child's hearing . . . and who retaliate as openly by branding her as crazy. (P. 445)

It seems inevitable that such parenting would result in a grossly maladjusted child and it is therefore not surprising that Jean was considered difficult, coarse, rude, noisy, and argumentative with everyone. In the evaluation, the mother was regarded as impossible to live with and her daughter was regarded as one of the unhappiest children ever to be seen at the evaluation center. Surprisingly enough, however, Jean was the president of the student body, a leader on the campus, captain of the baseball team, and the best student in geometry. There was no question that she was extremely maladjusted prior to separation from her psychotic mother, but there was equally no doubt that a remarkable change occurred when she was placed in boarding school.

How can one explain this resilience, this capacity to resume normal development once the stressor has been removed? One can only assume that in addition to potentially "good genes," enough goodness was lavished by Jean's mother to compensate for the psychotic mismanagement. It is possible that the close tie to the daughter cultivated by the mother during the earliest years became increasingly anachronistic and oppressive as Jean grew older and wished to develop a normal life of her own. The "symbiosis" gave her a good start but then closed on her development like the walls of a prison. As the symbiosis was threatened, Jean became disturbed and her mother became psychotic. The parenting was too rigid to move with development. This type of mother is only able to parent a dependent child in an anaclitic relationship to her. Jean's mother was unable to cope with the child's individuation and autonomy, feeling that she was losing an essential part of herself. As a result, she regressed and became infantile while her daughter attempted to assume the parenting role that was clearly beyond her capacity.

Keeping the young child with a psychotic parent might be good for the mother as "the last precious thread" that ties her to reality and the object world, but detrimental to the offspring, who might not show any ill effects until many years later [14]. When the mother is psychotic, there does seem to be a real danger of an inadequate or deviant type of object relationship that may lead to serious maturational reversals and psychosomatic disturbances in her children. Psychosis can remove a parent from the immediate orbit of the child more effectively than any other family predicament and the child may experience the withdrawal as a psychic loss and undergo a period of mourning [2a]. The relative weakness of secondary-process thinking in the child leads him or her to interpret such unusual parental behavior in terms of highly disturbing fantasies. His or her imaginative interpretations coupled with the parent's delusional ideas may bring about bizarre clinical reciprocities. Not only do many mothers pass on their psychopathology to their children, especially the younger ones, but the couple may act out a mutual disturbance in the form of a folie à deux [2, 9]. In some instances, the mother herself may become symptomatic with her child's symptoms. Anthony [2] pointed out that such parent-child relationships have all the characteristics of a symbiosis with the child existing almost completely within the maternal ambience with little or no intervening "placental barrier" to impede the free flow of noxious thoughts and feelings between the encapsulated pair. "The child's condition in many respects simulated that of the mother, but it could as easily be said that the mother's condition resembled that of the child" [2]. In many instances, the parent's delusional fears involve the safety of the child, but in the primitive protective response, it seems as if the mothers feel themselves to be endangered. In all such cases, the children are psychologically undifferentiated, of less than average intelligence, dependent, submissive, suggestible, and deeply involved with the ill parent and her illness. There seems to be a free interplay of delusion and fantasy conducing to a transformation of fantasy into delusion. The child's reality testing clashes with the demands of loyalty by the parent and, as a result, he or she might then learn to live by a double standard of reality incorporating both real reality and the parent's reality.

The parenting process can be affected during the prepsychotic, psychotic, and postpsychotic periods. In the more benign types of psychosis, the prepsychotic phase may furnish the child with "good enough" parenting and help to counteract some of the devastating results of the psychosis when it occurs. The degree of mutual involvement (parent with child and child with parent) may be the salient factor disturbing the child. Both Winnicott [39] and Anthony [3] agree that the more the parents are chaotically psychotic, the greater the detriment to the development of the offspring, although, paradoxically, such psychoses are often deemed less malignant than the so-called process disorders. Apart from the type of psychosis, there are many other factors significantly linked with the parent-child relationship, such as the age of the child at the onset of the parent's psychosis or the occurrence of the illness at a vulnerable phase so that a normal developmental crisis becomes profoundly transformed into a clinical catastrophe.

In the case of Esther, an 11-year-old girl described by Winnicott [39], the following question, similar to that posed by Anna Freud's Jean, is raised: How was it possible for this child of a psychotic mother to publish a poem at the age of 11 conveying a "perfect picture of home life in a happy family setting" with the family "pulsating with potential living"; at the end of the poem, night falls and the dogs and owls take over, but inside the home, all is "quiet, safe, and still"?

Esther spent the first 5 months of her life with her mother, a highly intelligent woman whose "tramp-type" life had resulted in the illegitimate birth of Esther. During these 5 months, the infant was constantly with the mother, breast-fed by her, and idolized by her with what seems to have been a total maternal preoccupation. At the end of this time, the psychotic break ruptured the "perfect environment" that had been established. After a sleepless night, the mother threw her baby into a canal that she was walking along; Esther was immediately rescued by an ex-policeman who was working alongside and within view of the mother. Esther's mother was certified as a paranoid schizophrenic and hospitalized. Thereafter, Esther had a hard time. She spent 2½ years in a nursery where she was described as "difficult." After being placed with a foster family, she again became difficult and destructive when they adopted a baby boy. Her behavior contributed to the tension between the foster parents who eventually separated after the foster father, who had developed a mothering relationship with Esther, became psychotically delusional.

Winnicott poses two questions: How did this young girl learn about the serenity of a happy family setting when her experience of parenting included a psychotic mother and a psychotic foster father? Why did her mother throw her into the canal? According to Winnicott: [39]

A very ill mother like Esther's real mother may have given her baby an exceptionally good start; this is not at all impossible. I think Esther's mother not only gave her a satisfactory breast-feeding experience, but also that ego support which babies need in the earliest stages, and which can be given only if the mother is identified with her baby. This mother was probably merged in with her baby to a high degree." (P. 71)

Winnicott believed that benign contributions also came from the foster father who was "the good or idealized mother in Esther's life" and whose relationship with his wife broke up as he became "more and more compelled to supply the mothering which this child needed"; the foster mother was forced more and more into the role of persecutor. The 5-month-old baby, at the moment of being thrown into the canal, lost an ideal mother who had not yet "become bitten, repudiated, pushed out, cracked open, stolen from, hated, as well as destructively loved; in fact an ideal mother to be preserved in idealization" (p. 71). The foster mother came into Esther's life and was immediately used for all the negative things that the baby missed: biting, repudiating, pushing out, cracking open, stealing, and hating. The foster mother had taken over a child who had lost an ideal mother and who had had a "muddled experience" from 5 months to 2½ years, and with whom, moreover, she did not have the fundamental bond derived from early infant care.

Winnicott's response as to why Esther's mother threw her into the canal is a little less plausible, although dynamically intriguing.

My guess would be that she wanted to rid herself of her baby that she had been merged in with, that she had been at one with, because she saw looming up in front of her a new phase, which she would not be able to manage, a phase in which the infant would need to become separate from her. She would not be able to follow the baby's needs in this new stage of development. She could throw her baby away but she could not separate herself from the baby. Very deep forces would be at work at such a moment, and when the woman threw the baby into the canal (first choosing a time and place that made it almost certain that the baby would be rescued), she was trying to deal with some powerful unconscious conflict; such as, for example, her fear of an impulse to eat her child at the moment of separation from her. (P. 71)

For Winnicott, being psychotic is not something very alien; psychosis does not make the process of parenting an impossible task. Psychotics can function like nonpsychotics but with greater difficulty. Psychotic patients are not diseases, but *people* "who are casualties in the human struggle for development, for adaptation, and for living." They are in many respects like us so that when we see a psychotic patient we can feel "here but for the grace of God go I."

Jean's mother, although psychotic, had provided her daughter with a base that allowed her eventually to develop successfully; Esther's mother and foster father, although psychotic, also infused her with enough sense of goodness to enable an 11-year-old to write lyrically about pleasant family life.

In order to follow Winnicott's nosological attitude, one needs to eschew, as he does, a disease model. Winnicott [39] proceeds to classify psychosis in a way that is very different from the usual diagnostic categorizations.

First, we can divide psychotic parents into fathers and mothers, for there are certain effects which concern only the mother-infant relationship, because this starts so early; or, if they concern the father, they concern him in his role of mother-substitute. It may be noted here that there is another role for a father, a more important one, in which he makes human something in the mother, and draws away from her the elements which otherwise become magical and potent and spoils the mother's motherliness. Fathers have their own illnesses, and the effects of these on the children can be studied, but naturally, such illnesses do not impinge on the child's life in earliest infancy, and first the infant must be old enough to recognize the father as a man.

What Winnicott states here is important for the psychiatrist to understand: he is making human something in the psychotic mother and draws away from the distortions that prevent us from appreciating her essential motherliness. The psychotic is a person, a parent, and a psychotic, in that order of relevance. Psychosis affects the person by contributing to feelings of persecution, hypochondriasis, unreality, and asociability; it affects the parent, contributing to difficulties in making and maintaining the parent-child relationships. Children react to deficient parenting by finding it difficult to synthesize mind and body in a smooth working partnership. For example, one woman reacted to any absence of her husband with marked depression [38]. When this occurred, her children developed anorexia as a mode of defense against "her insane need to prove her value by stuffing food into her children," and yet, at the same time, she allowed them to establish themselves as independent of her.

Different types of psychoses disturb the process of parenting in different ways and to different degrees. With the chaotic psychoses, the parent becomes severely disorganized and in such a state of disintegration that the home is made impossible to live in so that the children run away repeatedly (as with the case of Jean) rather than put up with the constant insecurity. From the point of view of parenting, this kind of illness is burdensome for the offspring since such mothers tend "constantly to break up everything into fragments, and to produce an infinite series of distractions in the children's lives" [39]. As in the case of Jean, psychotic mothers are not always bad, and sometimes they can be very good as mothers, but on the whole, they are inclined to muddle the children up through unpredictable traumatic actions and cause great havoc. Husbands of psychotic women can often hide themselves in their work, but the children are put in jeopardy because of the senseless admixture of fact, fiction, and fantasy.

Manic-depressive parents not only show swings of mood but also a great variability in their approaches to caretaking. The children learn to adjust by keeping a weather eye open and, after some experience, may learn to gauge the affective climate well enough to avoid disarray.

Winnicott concludes that the illness of the parent can be most helpfully classified in terms of the amount of parenting capacity available to the psychotic individual. He proposes four classifications: (1) too ill to take care of the children; (2) moderately ill and periodically able to function; (3) mildly ill and able to protect the children from his or her illness or seek help for them; and (4) mildly ill but too involved with the children to be able to function parentally.

In families where psychosis runs through the generations, the psychotic parents can often help their offspring therapeutically and even nurse them through the early phase of mental illness; Winnicott believes that familiarity with mental illness allows such parents to know "instinctively" what to do and how much to do before seeking help while the children get to know that their parents are ill and that they need to cope with that fact [38].

Many children of psychotic parents carry the guilty conviction that they are in some ways responsible for the parent's condition. They believe it is their provocative behavior, aggressiveness, destructiveness, and negativism that pushed the parent over the edge into insanity. At the same time, they are also afraid that they will become like their parents and eventually develop psychosis. This reciprocal theme is played out on many different levels and has been discussed fully by Searles [32] in the context of "psychosis wishes," which are analogous to "death wishes."

On several occasions, when working with patients who have had an experience, earlier in life prior to their own illness, of a parent's being hospitalized because of a psychotic illness, I have found that the patients show guilt about repressed "psychosis wishes," entirely similar to "death wishes" which are productive of guilt in persons who have lost a hated parent through death. The patients who show this guilt over "psychosis wishes" show every evidence of feeling that they were once successful in a mutual struggle with the parent, in which each was striving to drive the other crazy, and the subsequent appearance of their own psychosis seems to be attributable in part to guilt, and fear of the parent's revenge, stemming from that duel in previous years. (P. 7)

This "duel" is a reality in the families that I have examined where the sanity-insanity struggle between parent and child has a life and death quality to it. Searles describes several modes of "driving the other person crazy" and emphasizes that this is carried out predominantly at unconscious levels. The parent is not aware of wanting to make his or her child psychotic, and the child certainly has no conscious wish to unbalance the parent. The techniques employed include interactions that activate personality conflicts; that simultaneously or alternatingly stimulate and frustrate the other's needs; that request help, sympathy, and understanding and at the same time rejection; that switch from one emotional wavelength to another, and from one conversational topic to another without adjusting the feeling content; and that brainwash the other by undermining ego functioning. The children of psychotic parents experience these "double-bind" parental injunctions more grossly than children of psychotogenic parents, but the following description by Johnson, quoted by Searles, [32] pertains to both types of childhood relationships with parents.

When these children perceived the anger and hostility of a parent, as they did on many occasions, immediately the parent would deny that he was angry and would insist that the child denied too, so that the child was faced with the dilemma of whether to believe the parent or his own senses. If he believed his senses, he maintained a firm grasp on reality; if he believed the parent, he maintained the needed relationship, but distorted his perception of reality. Repeated parental denial resulted in the child's failure to develop adequate reality testing.

Why would the parent or child try to drive the other crazy? First, to externalize and thus get rid of the threatening craziness in oneself; second, to precipitate a threatening craziness that is hanging catastrophically over one's head like the sword of Damocles, creating intolerable feelings of suspense and helplessness; third, to make manifest a craziness that is maintained within the family circle as a guilt-laden secret and so broadcast the knowledge as means of sharing it with a larger community; and last, to find a soul mate to assuage unbearable loneliness.

Searles [32] offers the case of Carl to illustrate how the children of psychotic parents feel themselves manipulated by the sick parent.

He suddenly started to talk about his mother's illness. Said he envied his older sister because she didn't have to bear the brunt of his mother's illness. Said that his mother "tried out" her paranoid ideas on him. Would go around the house, pull down the blinds, check to see if anyone were near, then tell him what apparently were full-blown paranoid ideas about the neighbors and friends. (He) very philosophically announced that he felt she needed company in her illness — that she felt so lonely that she had to use him in this way. (P. 9)

A Retrospective View of Psychotic Parenting

According to Shengold [33], the mythical sphinx represents the image of the "terrible mother" who strangled and devoured those who could not answer her riddle. Sophocles spoke of the sphinx as "the bitch with hooked claws," the embodiment of all destructiveness, and Shengold considers that " in present-day reality, the figure can be approximated by a psychotic parent whose defused instincts can bring into play, in relation to the child, the intent to torture, kill, and devour and is something close to a pure culture of the death instinct" (p. 727). He offers the following vignette of how the psychotic parent appears subsequently in the analysis of the grown-up child.

A patient, remembering the childhood seductions by his psychotic mother, would describe her terrifying "transformation" into a monster, "like Dr. Jekyll and Mr. Hyde" (note the transposition of sex). The mother's facial expression would completely change — she would suddenly stare at the patient and then would seem to look through him; her face would become a feral mask, while she gnashed her teeth wildly. Sometimes baring and offering her breast, she would use her finger as a penetrative organ to invade the child's anus. This was but the most frequent of the many bizarre seductions carried out by this mother from the child's third to his sixth year. It was also through this sphinx-like mother that the child was exposed to a repeated and full exhibition of her genitals to a frightening initiation into the "mystery of the origin of children," as Freud reads the riddle of the sphinx. (P. 727)

The primal image of the bad mother of the oral-sadistic stage, devouring and cannibalistic; the image of the bad mother of the anal-sadistic stage, penetrating, intruding, and soiling; and the image of the bad mother of the phallic stage, seducing and exhibiting horrifying disclosures of concealed private parts, is the compendium that is carried, almost unchanged, into the recesses of the adult mind until reactivated by some regressive process. The image of a primordial monster with the head and the breast of a woman, the body of a lion, the wings of an eagle, and the tail of a serpent emerges. It is not only the image, but also old modes of behavior needed to cope with disturbing childhood experiences of the psychotic parent that may come to consciousness again in adult life.

Miller [29] offers a vivid example, recovered through psychoanalysis, of the way in which psychosis in a parent can influence the eventual parenting process in the child.

A father, who as a child had often been frightened by the anxiety attacks of his periodically schizophrenic mother, without ever receiving an explanation, enjoyed telling his beloved small daughter gruesome stories. He laughed at her fears and afterward always comforted her with the words: "But it is only a made-up story. You don't need to be scared, you are here with me." In this way he could manipulate his child's fears and have the feeling of being strong. His conscious wish was to give the child something valuable that he himself had been deprived of, namely, protection, comfort, and explanations. But what he unconsciously handed on was his own childhood fear, the expectation of disaster and the unanswered question (also from his childhood): Why does the person whom I love and who loves me frighten me so much? (P. 25)

In this way, the "props of the childhood drama" generated by the psychotic experience and unmastered during childhood may enter the scene again when the parent-child situation is recreated in the next generation, even though they may not have manifestly affected the adult prior to his becoming a parent. In this context, Miller quotes a remark by the great educator Pestalozzi that: "You can drive the devil out of your garden, but you will find him again in the garden of your son," or, rephrased in psychoanalytic terms, the split off of unintegrated parts of the parent are introjected by the child.

The Jekyll-Hyde transformations in the psychotic parent render all interactions unpredictable and place a heavy load of anxious apprehension on the child being parented. This is especially the case in the remitting psychoses such as manic depression or the schizoaffective disorders. The offspring gradually learn that their environment is expectably unexpectable and that they must adjust to it, and this they frequently do with extraordinary skill. As Winnicott [38] states: "It is amazing how even small children learn to gauge the parent's mood. They do this when each day starts, and sometimes they learn to keep an eye on the mother's or the father's face almost all the time. I suppose later on they look at the sky or listen to the weather forecast on the BBC." But even when they have learned to live with mood swings, it is the unpredictability of behavior and the usual routines of everyday life that may get them down. Winnicott characteristically puts an inordinate degree of confidence on the preventable potential of "good enough" parenting in the earliest stage of infancy and considers that a child with such a background "can come to terms with almost any adverse factor that remains constant or that can be predicted" (p. 76).

The consequences of psychotic parenting, as retrieved in the treatment of the adult, are nonspecific and dependent on the extent that the child's needs for security, stability, respect, mutuality, and empathic understanding are interfered with by the malignant process operating in the parent. The child may be left in a tormentingly insecure state by the intense nature of the ambivalent symbiotic relatedness that interferes radically with his or her emerging individuality and autonomy or by the systematic suppression of anxious, angry, lonely, helpless, and envious feelings he or she may develop. Miller [29] expressed this as "the art of not experiencing feelings," since feelings can only be experienced fully when there is somebody there to accept, understand, and support the child at such times. The inadequate, incompetent, psychotic parent may be driven to withdraw rather than face the demands of parenthood, and the child may have to sacrifice his or her childhood in the face of this abandonment and take over the parenting of him- or herself, the siblings, and the childlike adult parent. As a result, he or she develops a fragile precocity with a huge sense of responsibility.

Another outcome that becomes apparent in the later treatment of the adult is the appearance of an "as-if" or false personality where the "true self" is masked and in a "state of non-communicando," as Winnicott phrased it. As adults, such patients complain of a sense of emptiness and futility that had resulted when spontaneity and aliveness were cut off in childhood. In the early stages of a psychotically induced symbiosis, the lack of a significant and appropriate relationship can be remedied if adequate substitution is available. It is surprising, nevertheless, how much the child can do on his or her own behalf. If mothering is deficient, the child learns to provide with whatever means he has within his own autonomy, the complementary patterns and the complementary modes of stimulation that are of rhythmical soothing activities which the symbiotic partner fails to provide. Where psychosis is present, normal symbiosis is either poorly established, poorly maintained, and poorly resolved or excessively and suffocatingly continued beyond the developmental needs of the child. Psychosis in the parent also poses major problems of actuality on early development. As Burlingham and associates [9] noted, "the child who is seduced by the mother's fantasies only, can be freed from this grip more effectively than another who has to contend also with manifest actions on the mother's part and therefore with the actual body stimulation and excitement which are aroused by them." The big difference between actual aggression and fantasied aggression and actual seduction and fantasied seduction on the part of the parent as perceived by the child is that the individual affected by actual aggression and seduction is undeniably more difficult to reach through psychotherapy in later life.

Postpartum Psychotic Parenting

Psychoanalytic observers and investigators of infancy are in general agreement that this is a period of high vulnerability and that deprivations and traumatizations at this time are fateful for all phases of subsequent development. The postpartum psychological state of the mother has a determining effect on her parental capacity. She may be transiently depressed with the so-called "baby blues," consistently but mildly depressed thoughout the first year, which is often characterized by a history of premenstrual depressions; acutely depersonalized and disoriented with an identity diffusion and an inability to recognize or accept her own baby; psychotically elated, depressed or both resulting from a flare-up of a primary affective disorder; or schizophrenically or schizoaffectively disturbed with catatonic withdrawal or chaotic behavior. The nonpsychotic illnesses may lessen the mother's wish or competence to mother by intensifying her dependency needs, her ambivalence toward the infant, her narcissistic preoccupation with herself, and her low self-esteem. The concern of these mothers with their own imperative needs makes them insensitive to the needs manifested by the baby with whom they may even compete. The mothering tasks for the first 6 months of the baby's life demand a good deal from the mother—her total attention and interest, her provision of comfort and security, her soothing response to distress, her humanization of the infant's environment in a constant flow of communication, and her personalization of the mother-child interactions by her emphasis on the baby's uniqueness. Mothers with nonpsychotic illnesses do not hold or handle the neonate satisfactorily and there is an absence of freely flowing synchronized movement between the pair.

In the case of the psychotic mother, these features are all exaggerated: in place of a mothering mother, we find a self-absorbed, inwardly directed, hungrily demanding, and ungiving woman-infant who does not qualify to be a mother since her primary preoccupation is with herself and not with her baby. The most striking feature in many of the cases is the mother's inability to enjoy the child and the tendency for the initial detachment, which normally dissipates within a few days, to persist and increase. Whatever maternal drive there is seems to fade rapidly and a psychopathology of bonding ensues.

The postpartum psychotic mother has been described as the prototype of the rejecting mother. Almost all of these mothers have negative thoughts about their children, often expressed in a wish that the children had never been born. A psychotic mother may deny that the child is hers or even that she has given birth to the child at all. She may have delusions that the baby is dead, disfigured, or dying, and some may actually attack the child, as if all maternal feeling was lost. However, Winnicott warns us not to take such acts of violence at their face value. He believes that, psychodynamically, such apparent hostility may have other meanings within the context of the mother's psychopathology. Zilboorg [41] saw maternal rejection not as a consequence of postpartum psychosis but as a cause.

Postpartum psychotic mothers expressed a number of reactions to their motherhood: some felt they had no maternal instinct, some were indifferent to the baby, some showed aversion and even outright hate, some denied the existence of the child, some had fears that the child would be injured or killed, some had fears of hurting the child, and some had dreams of the baby dying of starvation or being murdered [37]. About half the mothers had not wanted the pregnancy.

A schizophrenic mother frequently describes a flatness and deadness of feeling and an inability to play with and respond to the baby. She is also likely to show a marked inability to organize the daily routine in a practical and competent fashion. The abnormal ideas about the infant relate to his or her physical health (e.g., baby was withering away; the baby was being poisoned), to the baby as a persecutor (e.g., the son of the devil, a vampire bat, "putting thoughts into my head"), and to hate and hostility (e.g., "he is ruining my life and I feel like killing him").

Since 1955, psychoanalysts such as Main [28] have decided that psychotic mothers and their babies should be kept together because "it seemed important that a mother should be kept in touch with her job, and the children who were part of it." Main also pointed out that "remarkably little has been written about mothering and its disturbances" and that "psychiatry needs opportunities to study severe disturbances of the mother-child relationship." There seems to be some agreement among analysts who have made efforts to repair and preserve the bond that the hostility to the baby is transferred from early infantile conflicts in the mother and that the return of these into consciousness precipitates the psychosis. They have also noted that keeping the mother and infant together promotes recovery in the mother and adjustment in the baby.

Grunebaum and associates [19], in the dynamic tradition, did not look at the mentally ill mothers as suffering from a disease but rather "as needing help in accomplishing certain tasks in living." They give the history of a 22-year-old woman who gave birth to a boy the day before she graduated from college. This was a bitter disappointment for her because she wished to continue her higher education in anthropology. As a child, she had come under strong pressure from her mother academically and grew up shy and asociable. She married her husband on the understanding that they would continue their studies. During her pregnancy, she became depressed and neglected her housework; her husband took over but became critical of her. After a difficult delivery the baby developed pyloric stenosis and was operated on successfully, but his mother became markedly depersonalized and seriously depressed with feelings of inadequacy as a wife and mother. She was admitted to the hospital with her baby. Her psychotherapy dealt with her hostility toward her son and husband, as well as her rejection of motherhood and womanhood. Watching the therapist play with her infant, she gradually began to play with him herself until they were all having "a wonderful time together." This also helped in her relationship with her husband because she came to feel that the one thing she could do better than he was to be a mother and care for the baby. The therapy was directed at the parenting process and the improvement was reflected in better parenting. There was no attempt to deal with the roots of her depression, but it is clear from the full case history provided [19] that the patient's mother had been directing her away from her feminine role since early childhood. Experience has taught that as the mother's symptoms subside, she becomes able to resume normal parental caretaking, and this almost immediately reduces both the problems of the parent-child relationship and the symptomatic behavior in the children.

For the past three decades, pregnancy has come to be regarded as a normative stress culminating in the process of parturition. In the classical psychoanalytical view, it is stressful not because of concomitant psychosocial factors but for the reason that childbirth is equated in the woman's mind with castration. Freud's view was that the feminine sexual drive is secondary to her primary penis envy; this has since been much debated. Analysts still agree that feelings of castration and loss do have a place in the minds of many parturient mothers, especially those with a strong masculine identification. However, pregnancy and childbirth as manifestations of the woman's creativity may themselves be subject to envy by others, particularly the woman's mother. Husbands may also envy this capacity so that feelings of envy contribute to the widespread practice of "pseudo-maternal couvade" [13]. Lomas [27] put forward the view that postpartum psychosis results from the demands made on the woman by pregnancy and childbirth to make changes in her defensive organization in order to meet the challenge posed by close contact with the instinctual drives of her baby. She can cope with this if certain conditions are met or have been met: if she has had a good relationship with her own mother who has mothered her well and with whom she has been able to identify; if during this time of need, she can be "held" by this mother to whom she can entrust herself with a feeling of confidence; and if her personality has developed normally and is flexible and susceptible to changes such as those brought about by parenthood. If her relationship with her mother, however, was one in which feelings of hate and envy predominated, the support of the mother will be viewed with fear and mistrust, and she will especially fear the envy aroused in her mother who is idealizing and idolizing her baby.

Nearly all the women reported by Lomas had manifestly poorer relationships with their mothers and were chronically unhappy during childhood. The usual family pattern was that of a father who was either physically absent or psychologically ineffectual, leaving the mother "lonely, bitter, possessive and envious." (Some of this anamnestic material was admittedly colored by the projection of the patient's own bitter and envious feelings.) As a result of this background, the mothers came to childbirth unable to accept support from their own mothers and unable to believe in their own maternal capacity.

Because of this fear of the envy of others, when the babies were born, these women could not feel that the babies were their own. They could not be warm and loving toward the babies when their mothers were present and might even deprecate the babies or pretend to be disinterested. They did not dare show their babies off because they had long learned to conceal what they wished so much to display. Even childbirth itself was considered embarrasingly exhibitionistic by these women. Many of these postpartum psychotic parents gave a history of childhood deprivation. Thus, the fear of their mothers' envy often led them to surrender their children masochistically to their mothers. They themselves could not become successful mothers because they would be envied, and these feelings would be reinforced by projections onto themselves of their own greedy, deprived selves.

There seem to be three dynamic factors at work in the breakdown of parental functioning during the puerperum.

1. The presence of penis envy in women, manifested in an envy of men, where the baby symbolizes the longed-for penis. Childbirth is experienced as castration and loss. The reason why such mothers are unable to recathect the baby after birth is because they are narcissistic and too fearful that a "declaration of ownership of the baby" as a stolen penis would draw the anger, envy, and retaliation of those who regarded it as their own.
2. A dread of her mother's envy that she had become a successful mother although her own mother had failed. In the regression following the postpartum breakdown, the parental image is divided into an idealized, stolen part symbolized by the baby and a deprived, envious, and retaliatory part that is either introjected or projected.
3. The appearance of moral masochism is a prominent mechanism in these breakdown cases, generating a great deal of masochistic behavior together with feelings of guilt; this is most evident in those women with a strong masculine identification and for women who sacrifice themselves by demonstrating their parental failure and by surrendering their babies to the care of others.

Douglas [11], in dealing with puerperal depression, attempted to categorize the mothers who became ill in this way: By and large, they were likable, cooperative women, capable of sustained affectionate relationships, feminine in their outlook, and looking forward to having children. They came from stable families, had parents who were concerned for them, and eventually married men whom they cared for and respected. They worked well at school and later at their jobs. Why, then, did these apparently normal women break down with childbirth? What was not immediately apparent became so with psychotherapeutic exploration. These women had unusually deep affections for their mothers, together with a strong wish to please them and to conform to their expectations. But in addition, they had accumulated a huge reservoir of criticism over the years toward their mothers for denying them access to their own true feelings, their own independent judgments, and their own autonomous activities. However, these feelings had never been expressed. The resulting ambivalence was intense. What was expected of them by their mothers was in sharp contrast with what was required of them by their babies.

During the last weeks of pregnancy and following childbirth, every woman is introspective and vulnerable. To care properly for the baby when he or she is born, she needs to use her own judgment, be in touch with her own feelings, and make decisions on what is required for the well-being of her child. All this time also, the maturational crisis of pregnancy leads to a review of old relationships, especially with the mother, with some degree of relinquishment and mourning. Only then can a woman become an independent person prepared to take on the independent care of her infant with the ability to sacrifice other interests that interfere with this maternal care. This is every woman's struggle.

In the case of postpartum illness, there may be difficulties in giving up external interests, in concentrating solely on the maternal task, and in foregoing the prolonged dependency on the mother and the compliance to her wishes. When confronted with another dependent being expecting to be cared for and screaming for attention, this type of woman becomes panic-stricken, and repressed anger against always doing another's bidding breaks through. This type of woman attacks her baby and is overwhelmed with remorse afterwards. As a rule, she remains well until she undertakes the responsibility of parenthood; then she falls ill with depression and depersonalization.

Gluck and Wrenn [17] contribute a different type of understanding of the disturbances of mothering in the puerperium. They point out that the common concept of motherhood is one of "slavish devotion, selfless love and infinite patience" and that children seem to take these standards for granted and to insist that their mothers live up to these exacting ideals. As a consequence, young parents may feel that they are failing their children in exactly the same way as their own parents failed them. They localize their symptoms in the children and talk intermittently about their difficulties in managing them. When the children appear disturbed or actually become disturbed, young mothers may experience the disturbance as something emanating from themselves and reflective of the shortcomings of themselves as parents and of their parents as parents. The authors speak of Mrs. B, a weird, psychotic personality, who suffered a depressive breakdown following the birth of her daughter. Under the stress of demands from the little girl, which she could not meet, she withdrew and adopted a kneeling posture for several hours. The unconscious meaning of this became apparent in her treatment. The kneeling represented an attempt to get in touch with her dead mother from whom she could derive strength. Her mother had these high social ambitions for herself, and in failing to achieve these, then sought them for her children. She felt that she had disappointed her mother by not becoming famous. Mrs. B's daughter now represented hope of realizing both her own and her mother's unfulfilled ambition. Later, the identification with the mother became more apparent when it was found that the mother had suffered from Parkinson's disease and that Mrs. B's appearance — her weirdness, her masklike face, and her rigidity of posture — simulated her mother's symptoms.

Mrs. B's mother had failed her and she was failing her daughter. Her method of dealing with her child's anger or distress was to leave her or put her in her room by herself until she calmed down. The child was understandably alarmed at being left alone with her own uncontrollable feelings and, although overly dependent on her mother, had no confidence in her. The girl soon began to parent her mother. When the latter became withdrawn, the child amused her by surrounding her with dolls for consolation. Through identification, the child took care of herself at the same time. She was also very aware of any other child's distress and if she heard any child crying, she usually went to him or her immediately, looking very concerned; she would hug the child and offer toys as consolation. Thus she could experience her own feelings through the other child. Her insecurity was very evident. She would project it onto her dolls and then onto other adults around her, and she would construct secret places under tables and surround herself with chairs, hedging herself and her dolls in safety from the outside world. When she sensed any danger, she would immediately withdraw to this secret retreat. Yet she remained extremely vulnerable to any attack from other children and was unable to defend herself or retaliate.

In such a case, the cross-generational effects become manifest. The mother's parenting problems were traceable to her mother, and one could already see her daughter's parenting problems in the making: she would be able to respond to the child in distress but she would not be able to offer any security, except in the form of withdrawal, or to tolerate any aggression without becoming panicked and disorganized. Parental shortcomings are inevitably passed from grandmother to mother to daughter.

What is common to both nonpsychotic and psychotic puerperal breakdowns are certain aspects of regression. Zilboorg [40, 41] came up with some striking formulations based on hypotheses of masculine identification and penis envy: the more identified the woman was with her father, the less hostility she had to her baby, and the more likely she was to become schizophrenic if her unsolved oedipal problems led to a puerperal breakdown; on the other hand, if a woman's identification with her father is only partial and her acceptance of her femininity is fluctuating, she is more likely to hate her baby (as a symbol of her husband's penis) and more likely to become depressed. In Zilboorg's clinical material, the baby is seen unconsciously as a phallus with birth as a castration or as feces. In some of the cases described by Lomas [27] women had a strong masculine identification, chose "castrated" men as husbands, and became puerperally depressed. There have thus been two main theoretical positions: the position that stresses masculine identification with the baby regarded as a stolen phallus liable to be stolen again or for which punishment was to be expected from the father and the position that emphasizes the forbidden femininity where the baby is felt to be envied by or about to be stolen back by the woman's mother. In terms of instinctual regression to phallic, anal, and oral levels, the baby is regarded unconsciously as the mother's penis, her feces, or as a mouth that devours her. At the phallic level, there is either pride of ownership or illness relating to fears that the baby will be taken away from her; at the anal level, there are anal-sadistic reactions toward the baby and attempts to control the baby rigidly; at the oral level, there are marked difficulties over feeding the baby, often accompanied by fantasies of having been partially eaten up by the baby, of eating the baby, or of being a baby. It does seem possible to correlate the presence or absence of ego distortions in puerperal breakdown with the instinctual level of the mother's fantasies about the baby and his or her birth.[1]

Normal Mothering and Fathering and Their Vicissitudes in Psychotic Parenting

Motherliness can become the major ingredient of a woman's personality, causing her to respond with immediate and vigorous care to any sign or signal of helplessness. She may be recognized as a motherly woman and treated, wherever she goes, as an ancillary mother. In contrast to her there is the woman in whom motherliness is not a salient feature or even an obvious one until there is some pressing call on her for a motherly display. While this kind of woman is caring for her children or in contact with them, she reacts with an appropriate degree of motherliness, but this does not extend into other parts of her social orbit. The attribute of motherliness can be distributed along a spectrum ranging from those who have the semblance of archetypal mothers to those who show minimal amounts of motherly behavior only in response to the pressing

---

[1] The studies by Main [28], Gluck and Wrenn [17], Lomas [27], and Tetlow [37] represent a systematic attempt to study postpartum psychotic parenting in mothers admitted to hospital in England.

exigencies of child care. The total absence of motherliness has to be regarded as a clinical state and will be discussed later in relation to psychotic parenting.

One can disentangle certain subqualities of motherliness that might be regarded as elements of womanliness (and have been so looked upon, although disputably). These subqualities appear to be utilized and transformed in the service of mothering. Normal narcissism, for example, is transferred from the ego to the child so that the mother believes herself to be absolutely and exclusively indispensable and loved by the child. The child is experienced as a narcissistic extension of the mother and she responds to the child as she would to herself. In fact, a great deal of the mother's self is infused into the child, who becomes a self-object for her. This same narcissism demands that the environment should treat her child as uniquely special. Freud [16] felt that this aspect of parenthood represented a revival and reproduction of childhood narcissism long abandoned by the parent. As a result, parents overvalue their children, ascribing every perfection to them but concealing and forgetting their shortcomings. They want their children to enjoy a better life, to fulfill their own aspirations, and to ensure the immortality of the ego. "Parental love, which is so moving and at bottom so childish, is nothing but the parents' narcissism born again" and transformed into object love. Yet, it is clear that this subquality is essential for the psychological survival and well-being of the children.

Masochism is another component associated with womanliness that is recruited in the service of mothering and is manifested in the mother's readiness for self-sacrifice in the absence of any obvious return on the part of the object. The mother is also willing to undergo pain for the sake of her child, and one sees this in the course of development when she is prepared to renounce the child's dependence on her at the time when the process of separation-individuation is being completed.

Passivity is perhaps the most debatable of the subqualities attributed to womanliness, and many are prone to view it, at the present time, as a cultural artifact induced by the dominance of males in our society and his penchant for assuming all the active roles. Whether true or not, the element of passivity does seem to play a significant part in the makeup of motherliness, particularly during the period of gestation and puerperium. The woman seems capable of waiting endlessly for the ovum to grow into a nine-month fetus. Deutsch [10] includes activity-passivity along with aggression-masochism, femininity-masculinity, and sexuality-motherliness among the polarities in constant conflict within the woman, all of them adding depth and richness to the psychology of motherhood. As a background to these personality-determining struggles, there are also the more basic antitheses of individual-species, self-preservation–reproduction, and life-death. However, whether a woman behaves more actively or more passively during pregnancy and following childbirth is also determined by the nature of her personality as a whole. She may even be passive in the reproductive area and active elsewhere. As Deutsch [10] points out: "Some women have turned all their psychic activity to other goals, so that the process of birth is for them only a biological process to which they submit passively. Conversely, women otherwise more passively disposed are thrown by the first pains into a joyful, excited state that spurs them to the greatest activity" (p. 225). For a passive and infantile woman, the act of birth may have a magic character: "She simply projects into the outside world what has been injected into her in coitus. Her ego secures freedom from fear by subordinating itself from the beginning to the pause that represents life and death" (p. 235). Other women may confuse activity with being masculine and thus inhibit their active participation in the reproductive process. The little girl's identification with her active mother is one of the sources of feminine activity and prepares her for "active motherliness" in the adult phase of her development. At first she imitates her mother in everything and, with increasing success, gradually begins to reverse the roles both in motherhood games with her mother and with her dolls. With the latter, she may succeed in gratifying some of the more aggressive "maternal" tendencies such as tormenting, beating, or breaking. In this context, she will often betray her "reversal of generation" fantasy in which she is big, caring, controlling, and aggressing while the mother is small and getting smaller all the time until she disappears entirely in the most primitively aggressive part of the fantasy. The tendency of the child (boy or girl) to develop from passivity to activity is rooted in the ego, but it receives instinctual reinforcements.

The acceptance of femininity presupposes the overcoming of the "genital wound" and penis envy; the transformation of penis wish into the wish for a child is not a substitute formation, but a biologically determined dynamic process. As part of the move toward femininity, the little girl, in fantasy, may transfer her interest from the outside to the inside of the body so that the penis is then conceived of as an internal organ and therefore identifiable with the baby inside the body. Within the scope of primary process thinking, the baby, during the childhood phase, may be regarded as a compensation for the penis, but there is no doubt that following puberty, the child acquires a new significance that comes from other sources. At all stages, nevertheless, penis, baby, feces, and breast are equivalent within the domain of the unconscious. Where envy becomes a predominant trait in a woman, it appears to be directed into a variety of areas: an envy of mothers, of pregnant women, of social success and position, of clothes, of jewelry, and even of food. It is possible that in such women there is a disposition toward the envy reaction because of the castration complex and penis envy. Whatever the roots, the lavish display of motherly interests is not synonymous with real motherliness. As we noted previously, the child for such women does seem to have more of the value of the lost male organ than anything else so that, as Zilboorg [40] put it: "Childbirth being a castration, the psychotic reaction to it is a recrudescence of the penis envy."

The major drives, sex and aggression, make important contributions to motherliness, although they undergo partial suppression in the process. The sensual aspect of the sexual drive obtains expression in tenderness, while behavioral activity is exercised by caring procedures and caresses. The limits to both are nebulously set since the strength of the incest barrier varies from family to family. Aggression manifests itself in the family's protective, nurturing, and disciplining activity, although here again what passes for normal controls in one family may be regarded as brutal in another, especially when sadomasochistic impulses also invade the situation [1].

The component instincts are also involved in the genesis of motherliness: orality, as typified by the tendency of the woman to feed the object of her solicitude, and anality that compels her to maintain a neat and clean environment to groom her young.

There are many parts to this "natural and primitive phenomenon of motherhood" [10], extending from the biological through the physiological, psychological, intrapsychic, and historical; consequently, there is much to go wrong when the complex whole is out of mesh. This can happen when either the libidinal or aggressive drives get out of hand. The struggle between motherliness and eroticism can lead to two outcomes: (1) a renunciation of the erotic life in favor of the motherly one, or (2) the atrophy of maternal feelings in certain types of narcissistic women whose total interest is in sexuality. Even within the normal range of maternal attitudes, feelings, and behavior, there is a variation of response—some women expand their egos through childbirth while others feel restricted and impoverished after childbirth. Deutsch thinks that the psychologically integrated woman can generally gratify both sexual and maternal urges through the mediation of man, but the comment seems to indicate some degree of cultural bias. In cases of "pure motherliness," all human relationships, including those with the husband and children, become an outlet for maternal activity. Such women can transform every man into a child.

While paternity generally plays a small part in the animal world, in the human family, particularly in Western societies, the father is gradually achieving for himself a significant, if not essential, role. In the postulate of the Oedipus complex, psychoanalysis put the father strongly and securely at the center of the intrapsychic life of the individual, and contemporary work has constructed a preoedipal triangulation that gives him more emotional importance than merely a support for the mother. Even though a "paternal instinct," rooted in the biological makeup of the man, cannot be identified, the psychosocial significance of the father has rarely been in doubt, and fathering is clearly an attribute that thrives on experience. Furthermore, the various polarities operating in the mothering process that create conflict are also present in fathering: activity-passivity, aggression-masochism, and masculinity-femininity also delineate the profile of the father. More basic than these in some respect are other similar polarities mentioned with respect to mothering: father-child, self-preservation–reproduction, individual-species, and life-death that conduce to conflicts of choice. Fathers learn the job of caring from their mothers and, subsequently, the job of fathering from their fathers. With these two sets of identifications firmly established, they are ready to become parents. The process, however, is vulnerable to adverse experience and, although it is difficult to find a mother totally devoid of motherlinesss, there are many fathers who could be judged as completely unfatherly.

Given the psychodynamic ingredients feeding into the process of parenting under normal conditions and circumstances, is it possible to predict how a psychotic parent, undergoing profound regression, might behave? Earlier work on the impact of parental psychosis on the child [2] focused attention on the influence of psychosis in itself on the development and behavior of the child, without considering the intermediate influence of the psychosis on the process of parenting. Neither the psychology nor the psychopathology of parenthood has been explored in a way that would throw light on the child's reactions to the type of parenting being given. Until recently, for example, when a mother became mentally disordered following the birth of a child, the questions that clinicians asked themselves were whether the stresses involved in the reproductive act were etiologically responsible and whether it was safe to leave the child with such a parent. There is no doubt that pregnancy, parturition, and child care can be regarded as normative stresses for both parents with the rider that some individuals appear to be more vulnerable than others to this kind of stressful experience. But this is only a small portion of the influences that we are presently considering. The disposition to the psychosis, the disposition to deviant parenting, and the interaction between these two are the factors that concern us, and our primary interest in the offspring will not be in relation to the effect on them but on their apperception of the psychotic parenting.

For a fuller understanding, we need to know the details of the mother's long prepsychotic history dating from infancy: her own experience of being parented, her own emergence as a functioning self following the process of separation and individuation, her own resolution of preoedipal ambivalences and oedipal conflicts, her identification with her own mother and her gradual assumption of womanliness, and finally her acceptance of intimacy associated with the generative drive. The man needs to solve his psychosexual dilemmas, to identify with the caring aspect of his mother and then the fatherliness of his father, and to overcome his envy and wish for the feminine role to the extent that it allows him to function reasonably well as a father.

With psychotic parenting, the elements of personality that generate normal parental attitudes and behavior may be exaggerated or distorted to a degree that renders the associated activity more harmful than helpful. For example, under normal circumstances, the child is incorporated into the mother's ego as an object of identification, and yet, at the same time, remains an object outside the ego and attracts both positive and negative emotional attitudes. At the beginning, he or she is surrounded by the boundless narcissistic love of both parents who, even at this point, may be looking to the child to fulfill their own unachieved ideals. At this time, even the most realistic set of parents view the child as the embodiment of all perfection and a gratifying extension of both parental egos. Certainly the most powerful source of maternal love lies in the fact that narcissism erases the boundaries between self and nonself in the mother so that the child becomes loved as part of the mother's self. Under psychotic conditions where an excessive introversion may exist, there is a double danger that the real relationship to the child as an object in the environment may be jeopardized and that the intensification of self-love may cause birth to be regarded as a painful separation from a part of ego and, hence, a destructive psychic loss. The normal maternal psyche develops mechanisms for dealing with the turning-in process away from outer reality by directing "maternal instinct" toward enhancing the infant's first environment. Paradoxically, there would seem to be both introverted and extroverted tendencies operating at the same time.

The transition of woman into mother is a complex psychological undertaking of which Freud [16] said, "In the child they (the mothers) gave birth to, they are confronted with a part of their own body, as an alien object to which they can now give full object love from their narcissism." Narcissism was originally regarded as a perversion in which the person treated his own body in the same way in which the body of a sexual object was ordinarily treated, that is, looked at, stroked, and fondled until satisfaction was obtained. The mother looks at, strokes, and fondles the body of her baby in almost the same way, gaining a great deal of personal gratification in the process.

The heightened narcissism that is encountered in psychosis, especially in certain of its forms, is one example among many of how the normal ingredients of parenthood can be affected by pathology and are open to psychoanalytic study. Deutsch [10] expresses this perspicuously when she says:

When we see the mother's relationship to her growing children under the magnifying glass of psychoanalysis, we realize that we are dealing with something unique. Some components of the maternal affective complex are familiar to us from other relationships and conditions: in being in love there is similar overvaluation of the object; in mourning there is similar restriction of all life interests; in people tormented by guilt feelings there is a like masochistic readiness for sacrifice; in melancholy we find such a far reaching identification with another person that everything imputed to him in the patient's unconscious turns against the patient's own ego. (Pp. 317–318)

We would therefore not be surprised at all to find in psychotic parents excesses of narcissism, intense preoccupation, masochism, and identification to the extent that the child becomes a delusional aspect of the maternal self.

In between psychotic episodes, there is often a plethora of narcissism that remains constantly in evidence suggesting some type of narcissistic character disorder. During such nonpsychotic phases, the mother may be anxiously apprehensive that she will be required to surrender her children in favor of their further development and may behave like someone "who must give up an important, valuable, indispensable part of his own personality together with his beloved object" (p. 318) [10]. She may talk endlessly about vague somatic complaints ascribed to the child rather like a hypochondriac, and it is often difficult to know whether she is worrying about her child or herself. The involvement of such a mother with the child tells us in many ways how little she is differentiated from him [10]:

Such a mother feels the psychic umbilical cord with particular intensity: she bears a separation from her child very badly, she must be informed of his condition at every moment of his life, and her happiness and rigidness depend completely upon him. Her psychic life is an emotional echo of his experiences. (P. 318)

This "most selfless self-love is very much in evidence in psychotic parenting" [10].

When the masochistic tendencies are in excess, the child occupies that part of his or her mother's ego that she loves because this part inflicts the suffering on the remainder of the ego. She may groan under the burden of child rearing and behave like the classical *mater dolorosa,* but the self-sacrificing can become a chronic indictment of the child. Psychotically depressed women may carry the *mater dolorosa* attitude to the extreme so that all of motherhood becomes permanently saturated with guilt feelings and a need to make reparation. For them the pains of childbirth are an atonement for unconscious sins.

In some psychotic or prepsychotic women, the demands of motherhood may create an acute bisexual conflict. The stronger the masculine component, the more difficult it is for the woman to attend to the tasks of motherhood. There may be a confusion between activity required in feeding, caring for, and training the child and the thrustfulness ascribed, especially in fantasy, to the male. The more passive, anaclitic, and masochistic the depressed woman feels, the greater is her fear of the demands made on her by the child and the underlying fear that she will become dependent on someone incapable of meeting her strong dependency needs. Zilboorg [40] had called attention to the upsurge of what he described as "masculine tendencies" following childbirth in women who had previously been unduly passive and assumed that this masculinization was in response to the fantasied dangers associated with parturition and the passive-feminine position.

Zilboorg speculated that the postpartum psychotic response and the concomitant turning to masculinity was a function of an inadequate mothering capacity, which is taxed to a greater extent when the woman has to cope with more than one child. The precarious psychic balance is destabilized when an insufficient degree of mothering has to be spread over several children. With each successive birth and the recurrent traumatic separations through birth, the woman experiences an increasing depletion of her ego.

Although the separation trauma to the woman in the process of birth is a natural and expectable experience, the anxiety may reach abnormal proportions in two opposite ways. For some women the baby is the be-all and end-all of existence, and their hypermotherliness cannot tolerate the situation of independent existence; for other women the conflict about having a child has never been resolved. In the latter case, the fury and hatred toward the undesired child may become so great that infanticide may become inevitable. In less schizoid women, the killing of the new-born may precipitate huge amounts of guilt coupled with the wish to bring the child back to life in order to make reparation. The more schizoid reaction is the total refusal to recognize the child or claim it as an offspring.

Abnormal reactions after prolonged, painful deliveries may occur in women without a predisposition to psychosis and subside at some point along the postpartum phase. Like many other events in life, depending on dispositional characteristics, early experiences, and symbolic transformations, childbirth can sometimes be therapeutic and sometimes pathogenic. For example, some compulsive states are relieved by delivery while others are worsened; some depressions are lifted while others are intensified; some incipient schizophrenias are acutely activated whereas, in other cases, a prolonged remission may set in. With our present knowledge, it is hard to predict what changes the reproductive experience will bring to the parent. As Deutsch [10] states: "Only psychoanalysis can see the experience of delivery from a distance, place it in the psychic whole, and disclose its real nature" (p. 248). Psychoanalytic observation gives meaning to many incomprehensible reactions that take place at this time in response to normal obstetrical events.

The parenting process is vulnerable to delivery-room management, especially if the labor has been exhausting and painful. If there has been a big struggle, the masochistic experience may be covered over by a great deal of aggressiveness that may be turned against the woman herself in a self-destructive fury or directed against attendants. The attitude toward the baby may be anger for its part in bringing about her agony or else she may feel a complete barrier between herself and the child. These reactions may come immediately after birth and be within the range of normality, but in psychosis, they may be grossly exaggerated and made part of a delusional response.

Under the impact of psychosis, the tender component of parenting may become flagrantly sexual and lead to incestuous approaches to the child. Even under normal circumstances, the various aspects of care, especially those concerned with the cleanliness of the urogenital and anal zones, may almost imperceptibly become erotic, inducing excitement in the child and parallel excitement in the parent. The child's responsiveness and vulnerability may arouse certain immature types of adults. The sexualization of the parenting process is associated with a broad range of genital malfunctioning such as promiscuity, prostitution, frigidity, and homosexuality. In the less grossly disturbed individual, the milder eroticisms may be associated with a great deal of guilt and anxiety and handicap the parent in all types of caring tasks. A psychotic mother may disavow her maternal role when she becomes delusionally suspicious of an incestuous relationship between her husband and adolescent daughter. In one such case, the daughter protested indignantly that the mother did not treat her like a daughter but like a rival and was viciously jealous. "How can a mother think such thoughts?" the girl asked. However, as Freud pointed out, in cases of paranoia there is no smoke without some fire, and in this case, the father had long since rejected his wife sexually because of her distressing psychotic behavior and had turned to his daughter with more than usual paternal tenderness. In another instance, the husband of a manic-depressive woman had left her "in disgust" because of her outrageous behavior.

I received a call from her 7-year old son asking me to see him along with his mother. In my office, the mother tried to keep the interview on a neutral basis but, all of a sudden, her son yelled at her: "Why don't you tell Dr. A what you did to me three nights ago!" She became confused, tremulous, and inarticulate denying that she knew what he was talking about. "Tell him how you tried to screw me in bed," he yelled, and with that, her behavior became abject. She said that she had been "out of her mind," lonely, restless, and unable "to think straight," and she had found herself sitting on her son's bed not knowing, she said, how she got there, but feeling that she wanted "loving." She thought it was "all right to fondle" her son's penis and had often washed it when he was little. She did not know what made her want to go further and hold it to her genital. She was sorry and wanted to forget all about it. He shouted at her in fury: "You can forget but I'll never forget!" She appealed to him, in a whining voice, to remember that she was his mother and that she loved him very much, but he was ruthless in his response: "Don't use the word mother to me or I'll throw up."

The amount of aggression used by a parent to discipline a child may also become exaggerated in cases of immaturity and psychosis. Parent "rights" provide many rationalizations for beating the child, and once again, his or her helplessness and weakness renders the child a likely target for the sadistic adult. In psychosis, normal parental control can change rapidly to violent abuse. In one household, the father became acutely psychotic when his wife was working a night shift. In the normal course of events, he was often left to baby-sit for his six daughters and small son. On one day, his conversation with the children had begun with an apparently innocent inquiry as to what they did in the neighborhood. They innocently answered that they played around with other children and talked with neighbors; he asked them what they talked about. He started scolding them for being indiscreet about family matters, and then he said that he suspected them, his own children, of being in league with his enemies outside. He threatened that unless they revealed to him what the conspiracy was about, he would hang them by their hair outside the second floor window. In case they thought he was joking, he proceeded to demonstrate this on one of the girls who became completely panic-stricken, afraid that he would drop her to her death. She cried pathetically to him: "I'm your daughter, Dad. I would never turn against you. You can't kill me. I'm your child." The neighbors heard the commotion and called the police; he was taken to a mental hospital. Seven years later, the daughter that he had treated so aggressively had a schizophrenic breakdown. She had had an illegitimate baby for about a year and had been very neglectful toward the baby. She was hospitalized when she began persistently to express the wish to throw her baby down the stairs in order to kill the baby. Thus, the gross parental behavior in the father had led in turn to gross parental behavior in the daughter. It was interesting that the mother had her suspicions that something was "going funny" with the father, and yet, she had gone off to work and left her children alone with him (as occurs in many cases of incest).

The oral and anal components of motherliness can also become distorted and conduce to disastrous consequences. The psychotic or prepsychotic woman may equate the small child with feces and treat it as such. In one of the cases in our series, a mother gave birth to a baby on the toilet and tried desperately to flush it down the bowl. Extraordinarily enough, the baby did not die and participated in the follow-up study. The mother, when questioned, said in a confused way that she thought it was a bowel movement and that she was not a "baby killer." From further delusional data that she offered, it became clear that her act was not simply infanticidal as in our other postpartum cases; her murderous intent stemmed from extreme hostility toward the newborn.

In a case quoted by Winnicott [38], the parents of two children, a girl and a boy, were "very ill people." The mother was "quite unsuitable for being a mother, being a hidden schizophrenic," and her husband was a manic-depressive character and a "near psychopath."

As soon as the boy was "clean" the mother could stand him; she had no use for babies. She made continuous and violent love to her boy, though not physically as far as I know, and he had a schizophrenic breakdown in adolescence. The girl was much affected by a powerful attachment to her father, and this gave her a second chance; on this basis she waited until she was forty and her parents were dead before she could break down. . . . The brother married, had a family, and then got rid of his wife so that he could mother his children, *which he did excellently*. Eventually, all the past having been blotted out, this very ill person (the sister) with a successful false self came for treatment. She came to be enabled to break down, to find her own schizophrenia, which she succeeded in doing. . . . So here was a parental psychosis working itself out in two very clever children who are now nearly 40–45. The woman may perhaps have some life to lead as a real person, I am not sure yet. (Follow-up: favorable)

Here we have an example of Winnicott's somewhat eccentric view of psychosis and its impingement on the process of parenting. As he would put it, the children subjected to such care inevitably developed a false self, and they may need to break down (with the help of treatment) before the real self can emerge. Winnicott was quite aware of the extreme nature of the statement, but he had no doubt about its truth. "It is a terrible thing, and yet it is true, that sometimes there is no hope for the children until the parents have died. Psychosis in these cases is in the parent, and its grip on the child is such that the only hope is the development of a false self; and of course the child may die first, but at any rate the child's true self has preserved its integrity, hidden away, and safe from violation" (pp. 67–68) [38].

The mother that Winnicott described was not psychologically equipped to care for infants: she considered them repulsive and disgusting because they were not toilet trained. Other psychotic women react to the demands of feeding, seem envious of the baby, and take their frustrations out on the child. Although the thesis that children of psychotic parents are disposed to develop "false selves" may be tenable, clinical and analytic evidence hardly allows us to credit Winnicott's statement that effective treatment induced the necessary "breakdown" that allowed the "true self" to show itself without danger. However, one recalls that Erikson [12] also spoke of the "radical search for the rock bottom—i.e., both the ultimate limit of regression and the only firm foundation for a renewed progression" (p. 212) in cases of severe identity diffusion.

The huge ambivalence of the psychotic mother is demonstrated in the feeding situation when acute feeding battles develop that may lead to physical abuse of the child. One gets a clear illustration of this in the case of a schizophrenic mother whom I will call Mrs. Kramer [3].

She put the baby in the high chair and started feeding it as rapidly as she had before. The baby had this dismayed look on her face. She kept feeding the baby faster and faster. As soon as she put the spoon in, she put it in again. The baby, toward the end of the feeding, began spitting up food. She started yelling at her and telling her there was no reason for her to do that. About the end of the feeding, she gave her some milk, also forcing the baby. You could hear the baby gulping the milk down. Then she sort of choked, and Mrs. Kramer made a remark like "I bet you think mother is trying to strangle you" and laughing. She thought it was very funny. At the end of the feeding, the baby threw up all over her tray. Mother was very upset about the mess and how she made a mess on her dress. She again took the baby out of the high chair without taking the tray off. The baby's foot got caught again. . . . (at another feeding) the baby was gagging and spitting the food out. She jerked her hand one time and caused Mrs. Kramer to spill it, and she said, "Now don't you do that," and she hit her. . . . Sharon's feeding was rough. It ended in Mrs. Kramer pulling her out. Everytime she takes her out of the high chair, she gets her leg caught. (Pp. 367–368)

In this case, Mrs. Kramer died and her mother took over the care of the baby and, in an uncanny way, the pattern of feeding was repeated almost identically, although the now older infant would accumulate the food in her cheeks until the grandmother would hold her nose and force her to swallow, remarking, "it's the only way to get the better of her."

Aberrant Motherliness and the Atrophy of Maternal Feelings

Biological motherhood does not lead to motherliness, as Deutsch [10] repeatedly pointed out. Erikson confirmed this and stated that "the mere fact of having or even wanting children does not achieve generativity" (p. 138) [12]. The reasons that Erikson gives for this failure of generativity are all met within psychotic and prepsychotic parents who are retarded in the ability to develop true care because they are excessively narcissistic, interpersonally impoverished, nonidentified with their parents, and incapable of transmitting anything of value to their offspring. Psychotic parents are those to whom little was given parentally; they become unable to give or willing to give parentally.

A case could be made for the thesis that extreme conditions of life, whether from psychotic care or severe deprivation, will lead to an atrophy of parental feeling. Some evidence for this viewpoint comes from the anthropological literature. Kardiner [23] spoke of women of the cannibalistic culture of the Marquesans who appeared devoid of maternal instinct. He wondered whether they had been deprived from birth onward, since he had found clinically that women who have not received maternal love in their childhood tend to be less motherly, perhaps because the rejection at the hands of their mothers inhibits their maternal feelings. (It should be mentioned that clinicians also encounter the reverse situation. For example, a woman who has been deprived by her mother may become overindulgent with her children, as if to make up for what she did not have. One encounters both situations in psychotic parents.) Marquesan women are not only unmotherly but totally inconsiderate in the feeding of their children [23], somewhat like the case of the schizophrenic Mrs. Kramer.

The feeding process was brutal. The child was laid flat on its back on the house platform while the mother stood alongside with a mixture of coconut milk and baked bread-fruit which had been made into a thin, pasty gruel. She would take a handful of this stuff, and, holding her hand over the infant's face, pour the food in its mouth. The child would gasp and sputter, and gulp down as much as possible. Then the mother would wipe off that child's face with a sweep of her hand and pour down another handful of the mixture (P. 154)

The Marquesan women studied were not only unmotherly but their whole relationship to the environment had a purely sexual character and they themselves were "the quintessence of sexuality." They seemed incapable of developing tender feelings toward their children, and in the mythology of the culture, they were represented as wild creatures who seduced men only to devour them and then to devour their children. This would suggest the hyperorality of a cannibalistic society. The emotional life of the Marquesans, as reflected in their stories, their fantasies and their religious customs, was full of orality, as might be expected of cannibals. The Marquesan woman might therefore be, according to Deutsch [10], overwhelmed by panic at the oral drive of the newborn baby and fearful that she will be devoured by it. This fear has some grounds in reality since a suckling child actually does eat a part of the mother's body. Deutsch reminds us of Max Klinger's painting of "The Mother" that shows a plump baby glowing with vitality, sitting on its mother's breast; the mother's body is emaciated and lifeless. The frightening idea is that the new life flourishes on the ruin of the old.

Extreme privations, as portrayed in the life of the Iks [36] can bring about an atrophy of parental feeling in both mothers and fathers so that children are sacrificed to the needs of the parents. Turnbull refers to them as the meanest people on the earth and produces evidence to support this, since they have absolutely no altruistic feelings. It is hard to believe that parents, even under disastrous conditions, would not struggle for the well-being of their children at their own expense, but this is characteristic of the Iks.

The parents of the Yumu, Pindupi, Ngali, and the Nambutji, who inhabit the central Australian desert, were accustomed to eating their children when the drought was severe. On the initiative of the parents, every second child was eaten by the preceding child, but the adults, when hungry, would also eat the children. In explaining how it could be possible that mothers who were caring and nourishing in the treatment of their children were also capable of killing them, Roheim felt that the answer lay in the "unorganized" character of the primitive psyche in which every trend was given complete sway at the moment of its ascendancy. Thus the parents could continue to be protective while projecting their cannibalistic and libidinal propensities onto demons. In the westernized psyche, in contrast, such activities are restricted to the realm of fantasy and may not even emerge into personal consciousness except under the conditions of psychosis. One is reminded here of a satirical essay by Jonathan Swift, who was stolen from his mother as an infant, advocating the roasting and consumption of human infants in order to meet the shortage of food!

The "bad mother" concept is often portrayed in fairy tales. The witch is the bad mother for all mankind and embodies some of the "wicked" attitudes inherent in our own primordial ambivalent conflicts with our mothers. For example, in Hänsel and Gretel, the cruel mother starved the children and threw them out into the forest where they met a witch who tried to make gingerbread out of them.

What is striking to note is that not only can the parental attributes of mothering and fathering be rapidly eroded by deprivation, psychosis, and primitivism, but that abnormal maternal and paternal images are also present in the normal psyche and receive expression in folklore, fantasy, and fairy tales, although usually in juxtaposition with images of good parents and good parenting.

A Prospective View of Psychotic Parenting

Anthony and Benedek [2] have stressed the continuous development of parental behavior throughout the life cycle, culminating in grandparenthood and terminating in nonparenthood in the final stages of life. Under psychotic, psychopathic, and primitive conditions, the atrophy of maternalism that becomes submerged under an infantile neediness has been repeatedly observed. Motherliness therefore goes through the same vicissitudes as the personality as a whole. As Deutsch [10] puts it: "As mothers they are now one, now another person [p. 328).

Until this point, we have been mainly looking at the effects of psychosis on parenting from a retrospective or cross-sectional point of view, but our intention now is to present a more developmental point of view and show how the long chain of difficulties between mother and child from birth onward are steadily aggravated by primary and secondary factors that leave the mother with grave doubts about her mothering and the child with equally profound doubts about his or her emerging self and identity. Psychotic parents certainly exploit the dependent child in a wide variety of ways to protect their own vulnerable egos, which are caught up in the process of disintegration, and the child learns intuitively to exploit the fears and anxieties of the parent to the extent that both become victims of each other. The polarities at work even in the normal woman — self-interests versus altruistic concerns for the child, symbiotic wishes for unity versus the encouragement of individuation — make the psychological process of motherhood always a difficult task, but in the psychotic parent, the polarities are amplified to the point of acute and chronic schisms that divide the parent inwardly and interfere radically with the operation of the motherly core. The psychosis attacks each area of parenting, transmuting a natural personality trait into a character disorder that is incorporated into the psychotic process and alters a normal care procedure into a gross caricature of parenting behavior. Lidz and colleagues [26] provide a striking example of the way in which extreme obsessiveness in a schizophrenic woman disjointed and disrupted her day-to-day management of twins.

Mrs. Nebb fell into violent rages because of trivia that interrupted her obsessive cleanliness but gave inordinate praise for acts that the twins knew were nonsense. The household under her domination was a crazy place, and description could not be attempted without provoking the charge of gross exaggeration. For example, both twins claim that for many years they thought that constipation meant disagreeing with Mother. Whenever one of them would argue with her, she would say they were constipated and needed an enema; both boys were then placed prone on the bathroom floor naked while the mother, in her undergarments, inserted the nozzle in each boy, fostering a contest to see which could hold out longer—the loser having to dash down to the basement lavatory. (P. 177)

Under such conditions, a *folie à famille* is established and craziness reigns unrestrained throughout the home, since the other parent is seldom realistic enough to correct the psychotic child-rearing attitudes and behavior. When they have adequate heterosexual drives, psychotic adults tend to mate homogamously, sometimes searching for the same "rock-bottom" and dilapidated qualities with which they feel comfortable. They seem less conflicted when they are not challenged on each living day with a different perspective on reality or exacting standards of rational discourse.

In a small number of infants born to our psychotic group of mothers, we were unable to observe delivery-room behavior directly, but during the neonatal phase, certain incapacities were very much in evidence.

1. An inability to bond with the baby characterized by disinterest and even aversion with sometimes increasing thoughts of violence toward the child.
2. Inability to enjoy the baby, take pleasure in interacting with him or her and to express pleasure in his or her activities.
3. Inability to protect the baby from accidents, some of which did not appear to be accidental.
4. Inability to nourish the infant leading to a "failure to thrive" that is rapidly corrected when the baby is taken out of the mother's care.
5. Inability to tolerate negative behavior, such as persistent crying, that may provoke infanticidal behavior.
6. Inability to handle the baby in such a manner as to pacify him or her and enhance his or her good feelings.
7. Inability to play constructively and pleasurably.
8. Inability to play except repetitiously, stereotypically, and monotonously without affect.
9. Inability to establish a communicative dialogue with the infant accompanied by touching and fondling. (The mothers would often speak of the babies disparagingly and with a lot of implicit or explicit hostility.)

In three cases, we were able to see a gradual deterioration of parental behavior. At first the mothers would repeatedly express concern about the baby—about his or her health or about the baby being theirs; next they complained that the baby had caused them excessive pain and that they would not have another one; still later they would no longer respond to the crying, complain that they could not cope with the baby and suggest that someone else care for him or her. They would even ask about adoption. When mothers reach this point, the postpartum psychosis really takes hold and infanticidal and delusional ideas begin to develop. Women who have had previous psychotic attacks are "at risk" for breakdowns at this time.

In the manic-depressive sample of mothers, there was (with almost all of them) a stormy neonatal phase of uncontrollable weeping, followed by episodes of elation, confusion, forgetfulness, sleeplessness, feelings of depersonalization, irritability, and negative feelings toward the baby. Mothers also reported vivid visual hallucinations in which the infant appeared with his or her features and form grossly distorted. Psychotic parents, both fathers and mothers, seem to have a special predilection for tantalizing their offspring, as if, as Searles [32] would say, they were trying to drive the child crazy. This is a type of sadism seen in both manic-depressive parents in the manic phase and in schizoaffective parents. Below is an example of a schizoaffective mother manifesting this type of behavior [3].

The baby awoke, crying, as was her custom, and the mother went to her and first requested her harshly to stop. The baby stopped for a minute, but as soon as mother had turned her back, she began crying again. The mother turned on her with rage and screamed at her to stop, but this only made the baby cry harder and in such a total way as if her inner world was falling to pieces. Mother then picked her up and the baby immediately stopped crying, with mother saying, "Good girl, Sharon." Then she put the baby down and the baby started crying again, and mother said, "Bad girl, Sharon" and picked her up, whereupon the baby again stopped crying. This was repeated over and over again with the mother enjoying it but with the baby becoming more and more upset.

What one sees here is a complete failure of empathy; one also notes how defenseless the infant is against psychotic manipulation. Schizoaffective parents seem almost totally unaware of what is happening inside the child, and even when there is some glimmer of understanding, they are unable to do anything to change it. Many of them are apparently untouched by the distressed weeping of the little child, a situation that drives most normal parents to take immediate comforting action. There is a hard narcissistic core in such adults that seems oblivious to the needs of others, even when they are weak and helpless. After a while, the child begins to respond to the mother's needs rather than to his or her own and to assume whatever part in the psychic drama that has been assigned to him or her. The parent does not understand and reflect what is going on in the child, but the child may soon become a faint echo of the psychotic reverberations taking place in the parent, sometimes to the degree of a *folie à deux*. In such cases, the child will often suppress his or her own feelings and become permanently out of touch with them.

Such types of parenting may evoke not only massive and primitive defenses that try to shut out the experience altogether, but also remarkable coping skills. The defenses of affect suppression and emotional distancing from the object leaves some of the older children relatively unruffled in the midst of a psychotic crisis, and this may be helpful to parents who are losing control and feel themselves falling to pieces. When defenses fail, children may resort to fantasy and play (usually involving some form of role reversal of parent and child) or withdraw into activities that absorb and preoccupy them. All such maneuvers tend to impede rather than foster personality development and increasing limitations are set as to what unusual circumstances can be dealt with. For example, the child may be able to cope with the irrational demands made on him or her at home but find him- or herself at a loss with the realistic expectations in the outside world or with new or different conditions of living so that he or she is altogether less autonomous than would be appropriate for his or her age.

The vagaries of parenting also interfere with the regular internalization of a moral system and the child is guided by more primitive considerations. Since the environment is far from "average" and "expectable" [21], the child does the best he or she can taking into account the developmental fact that he or she, as a small child, may be too weak to oppose this overwhelming outside world in any effective way or too psychologically ill-equipped to take flight from it or understand it. He or she is powerless to change things from a material point of view and is therefore compelled to fall back on psychic maneuvers. Because of the gravity of the impingements, these tend to be more extreme than usual.

Sandler [31] has outlined the schema embodying the concept of a representational world and the ego experience of safety [30] that is relative to the experience of the child undergoing psychotic parenting. The model has three components.

1. A representational world built up as an internal framework, partly on the basis of the child's own observations and fantasies, and partly from what is presented to him or her chiefly by his or her parents. If these sets of information are contradictory, the child may attempt to resolve this by denying the evidence of his or her own eyes. The children of psychotic parents are constantly confronted by gross incongruities of thought, affect, and communication, generating what has been referred to as "double-binding." The world picture presented by the psychotic parent is full of noncommunications, miscommunications, and paradoxical communications. The child responds not only to the confusions but also to the threats emanating from this distorting and disturbing environment. When the threats become intolerable in the production of pain, the child may withdraw into fantasy, obliterate aspects of reality, misperceive them, or reinterpret them within his or her own personal context. However, the inner fantasies constructed

by the child to replace the unpleasant outer experience may become even more frightening than the original trauma, and he or she is then inwardly compelled to retreat back to reality and to some extent detoxify it by identifying with it.

2. All these strategies are undertaken by attempts on the part of the child's threatened ego to achieve an inner feeling of safety that helps him or her, at least during periods of psychotic crisis, to weather the insecurities of the environment. Under catastrophic conditions, the only safe place to go is inward.

3. The functioning of the model has an important cognitive aspect to it related to the developmental level of the child and his or her capacity to understand, make meaningful sense of what he or she experiences, and "see the inevitable in the light of reason" [30].

Children who are placed in intolerable reality situations move developmentally "with sticky feet," which hold them up at various points.

One needs to bear in mind that the psychotic parent can present in a number of contradictory ways at different times: overstimulating and seductive, physically abusive, reasonable and rational, disorganized and unpredictable, and concerned with the tasks of parenting and the effort to accomplish them. The child may therefore be drawn toward and away from the parent like a shuttle, although with time and experience, he or she may become less susceptible to the uncertain psychotic attractions. Hurry and Sandler [22] offers two cases of children at different stages of development who are profoundly affected by psychotic parenting.

CASE 1

A 3-year-old boy was referred for treatment because of depression, withdrawal, and infantile speech. He would sit huddled in the corner of a nursery school for most of the day. His mother was a seriously depressed woman who had made several suicidal attempts and spent long periods in mental hospitals. When not in the hospital, she was often extremely withdrawn, lying on the sitting room floor, and not speaking to anyone. At other times she would resort to frantic activity, rearranging all the furniture with both radio and television turned on full blast. She herself had a very deprived childhood and had little to offer her own children. In so far as they impinged upon her or made demands, she resented and even hated them. She would shout at the little boy saying, "You make me ill; you make me want to go to the hospital"; or, "don't call me Mommy. I hate the word."

In treatment, the child's representational world gradually unfolded, together with the absence of his inner sense of safety and his outer sense of security, as well as his capacity to understand his predicament. He was both terrrified of his mother and terrified of losing her. The discovery of this bind in treatment took time because he strongly denied both his fears and the facts of his mother's illness.

The relationship with the psychotic parent was replicated in the transference. He became both terrified of the therapist and fearful of losing her. At the end of each session, he would reassure her and himself by saying, "Good-bye tables, see you tomorrow; good-bye chairs, see you tomorrow." During sessions, the therapist had to play at being very ill while he took on the role of doctor, and would shake his head saying, "I don't know what's the trouble with you." When the therapist went on vacation, he felt "lost, dropped, broken, and starved." He tried to be as close to her as possible and to be looked after and fed by her, but he kept his sadness at bay by refusing to discuss the situation. One day he sat on the floor chanting repeatedly and mechanically, "Don't cry, don't cry, don't cry." It was possible to work through his reactions to his mother's many sudden disappearances. In one situation, he played out the story of a baby lamb, dead in the snow because the mother sheep forgot it, left it alone, and did not feed it. The lamb was 4 but still needed looking after. To accept that his mother was as she was meant that he had to face the intolerable terror of having no one to look after him, of being completely lost. By his denial, he attempted to preserve some inner safety. With the threat of losing the relationship with the therapist, he was brought face-to-face with the dangers caused by his mother's unreliability. He also showed extreme guilt over his anger, his resentment, and his death wishes toward his mother and it became clear that he was blaming himself for his mother's illnesses and disappearances. The fact of his mother's condition remained a puzzling mystery to him and with no explanations available, he was left helpless and powerless to face the vagaries of chance. He could not understand the explanation given by his mother: "You make me want to go to the hospital," which reinforced his feeling that he was the one to blame. At 4 he could not understand the complexities of mental illness but he could well understand, in his own terms, that his mother had worries as he had worries, that she needed help, and that she did not choose to behave as she did or not to be able to love. He began to accept the fact that while she might wish to see him as the cause of her illness, she could also be wrong and that he was, in reality, not so dangerous and threatening to her. In this case, one can see how possible it is in the transference for even a small child to repeat those aspects of a crazy reality that have been internalized in the past.

CASE 2

An 11-year-old girl was referred with severe eating and sleeping problems, psychosomatic symptoms, and a school phobia. She had a close, clinging, and demanding relationship to her mother who had a paranoid disorder; this was the most pathogenic factor in her environment. The girl's view of herself was of someone who was totally unlovable because she was so bad, so greedy, so messy, so angry, so destructive, and so damaged. She was used by both her parents as a scapegoat and the battleground on which their conflicts were fought out.

Her mother had used projection as a major defense since childhood, and it radically interfered with her parental attitudes and behavior. During her pregnancy, she consciously felt that the unborn baby was killing her, and after its birth and early development, she felt that the child hated her and wanted to kill her. As a result of these projective ideas, she activated, intensified and drew the child's own aggressive wishes into consciousness. Both mother and child developed defenses to deal with their respective aggressions toward each other, both denied their anger, and both displaced their hate onto other objects, reactively stressing their love. She and her mother spent much of their time in mutual reassurance of love, exchanging placatory gifts and denying their aggression. Frequently, they would discuss their mutual dislike for an object upon which they had both displaced their hostility. From time to time, the underlying primitive hostility erupted but was immediately followed by an intensification of the habitual defenses. This shared defensive system served to protect each member of the family (since father also took part in the dynamics) not only from their own aggressiveness, but also from any awareness of aggression in others. As a consequence, the development of the girl's autonomy and progressive adaptation was seriously impeded.

Psychosis, with its often radical impact on the personality, can bring about strange transformations as perceived by the child, as if his or her most terrifying fantasies of the "bad" internalized parent are actually brought to life and no longer correctable by benign everyday experience.

In the retrospective viewpoint, as illustrated by Shengold [33], the psychotic mother would undergo a terrifying "transformation" in which "her face would become a feral mask, while she gnashed her teeth wildly." In prospective studies [3], the change from good parent to bad parent is as vivid and sinks deeply into the psyche to reappear in the dreams and nightmares of later life. A comment by a 9-year-old girl with a schizophrenic mother illustrates this point. "I wake up dreaming or maybe just daydreaming—I don't know what, but her face is coming toward me and she looks good, and then suddenly her face begins to change and look mean and horrible, like a monster."

It is the unpredictable and extreme nature of the change that does violence to the child's growing understanding of parental functioning.

Below are typical examples [1] of psychotic transmogrifications experienced by children where the children's most fearful fantasies become coincident with outer reality in a potent traumatic mixture that haunts the memories forever, irrespective of how competently he or she schools him- or herself to deal with the more ordinary exigencies of life. There is a stickiness about these images that stem from the continued interchange between fantasy and reality, with reality feeding into fantasy.

"You cannot believe what it is like to wake up one morning and find your mother talking gibberish."

"She is quite a nice mother really. She doesn't do anything bad. She doesn't hit or anything. She is like a kid mostly. When I give her a lot of candy, she just sucks it all up like a vacuum cleaner. She doesn't comb her hair, and her dress has spots on it. Sometimes she laughs at me and I am not making any jokes. I say, 'Mom, why are you laughing at me?' And she just laughs more. It's not like real laughing. She never used to be like this when I was little. She was ordinary."

"I was sitting at the table just eating my cereal, and as I was pouring out the milk, my hand hit his cup and it went over his lap, and he jumped up and shouted at me and said that I did it on purpose and that I was trying to kill him, and that he knew I hated him. Then he hit me on the head and said I had plans and he knew about them, and he would get me first; and I said it was an accident, but he just wouldn't listen to me. He wasn't so grouchy last year. He has become real mean."

Spitz [35] has talked of the "psychotoxic diseases" produced in infants who, while remaining under the uninterrupted care of their mothers, receive "the wrong kind of mothering," which implies the wrong kind of emotional supplies. These children are not suffering from deprivation of adequate parenting but from an overdose of affective stimulation. The problems of suffering from "too much" parenting are different from the problems generated by having "too little." With psychotic parents, we encounter both types of parental behavior. Spitz provides a model of the mother-child interaction to explicate the dynamics of the "wrong kind of mothering" and its consequences. The normal exchanges between a mother and her baby are a mutual giving and taking — an "action cycle" (primal dialogue) in which both partners take turns being active and passive. With inappropriate mothering (both quantitatively and qualitatively) "derailment" of this dialogue takes place because of a cumulation of interrupted and incompleted "action cycles." Manifestly, this results in profound changes in the child's behavior. The long-lasting overload during infancy gives rise to the "psychotoxic" conditions, while long-lasting underload produces the familiar picture of deprivation. Inappropriate mothering may take the form of overt rejection, anxious permissiveness, anxiety covering underlying hostility, rapid oscillations between pampering and hostility, cyclical alternations of mood, and consciously compensated hostility. The psychotoxic diseases (e.g., coma in the newborn, colic at 3 months, infantile neurodermatitis, rocking, fecal play, and hyperthymic aggressivity) are different from the deficiency diseases (e.g., anaclitic depression, marasmus) that result from partial or complete emotional deprivation.

Spitz's model [35] provides a good beginning to an understanding of the complex reactions and interactions that take place between a disordered mother and her infant, but the father is omitted from the picture even though his role is often crucial, either in offsetting or aggravating the inappropriate parenting of the mother. He may intervene in the frequently provocative situation between the mother and her parents and between the mother and the children, and he will often try to understand, often in a distorted fashion, what is going wrong with the mother in her illness and what is happening to their marital relationship. Here, for example, is an account of a father who is getting, according to him, more than his share of parenting because of his wife's schizophrenic illness; he resents her mothering ineptness that has brought about this onerous situation.

Mr. L is convinced that his wife's sickness is the fault of her parents (both physicians), who were constantly ill. They had inculcated her, he thought, into the culture of disease and made her dependent on doctors and constantly preoccupied with death. "She gets a pain in the back of her neck and says that a fruit fly flies out of her ears; her theory is that her ailments are due to brain damage and that someday research will vindicate her. When Mr. L married her, he knew that she was ill and had tried to break the relationship off but was never successful. This hinted at a mutually dependent but very ambivalent marriage. He complained that she was sexually passive and even frigid. She had never attached herself to anyone even in fantasy. But she enjoys being pregnant and feels better when she is. When the first baby arrived, it took her two months to accept him and she seemed to cut him off completely. He called this "the biggest busted romance I've ever seen. She is in no way a maternal person. She is easily frustrated, yells at the children, or completely ignores them. When she is sick she tells them that she is sick and that they have to keep out of her way, and the kids rapidly got to know this. I myself practice callousness as I think it is helpful to her. If I cater to her needs, she simply gets sicker. What irritates me most is that she leaves me to look after the children as if they were entirely my responsibility, and I myself have never gotten on with children." When asked to describe the children, he was unable to differentiate one from the other with regard to their developmental data and personal characteristics. He said that his own parents had been busy with their lives and had not taken much notice of him while he was growing up. Now that he was an adult, they had turned to him, and he had great pleasure in rejecting them in turn. He thought that he and his wife should never have had children since they both lacked an interest "in the species" and preferred to work at their own interests.

Both children in this case were curiously aloof, difficult to engage therapeutically, precociously autonomous, and in the household turned to each other rather than to mother and father to meet their daily needs. They described their routines as if they had established these for themselves, and spoke with little warmth about either parent. The mother described how she was always better when pregnant but fell ill three months after the babies were born. In this "illness" she felt panicky and very apprehensive, as if something terrible would happen. When talking of her pregnancy, she seemed to become confused, her affect became inappropriate, and she talked in a mechanical stereotyped way. She had also been on drugs and feared that the child within her would be damaged. In addition, she always had difficult births. She wished that she had been better able to take care of her babies. She had no knowledge about them at all. "Some women have an instinct about these things, but I only have an instinct about myself." She could not tell what she meant by this. She felt that the children made her ill, and she found their illnesses intolerable. "Stress always makes me worse." In one of the interviews, her son said that when he married, he would marry a girl but he would make sure he would marry someone who did not get sick. Father repeated that his wife turned on her illness deliberately to punish her parents or him. We see here how parental pathology not only interfered with parenting in one generation but created obvious pathology as well as parental pathology in the next.

The status of being a parent is not difficult to acquire in any culture since the manifest routines and rituals are relatively easy to follow, and significant inadequacies of motherliness and fatherliness can be disguised. Even severely psychotic parents may often pass the scrutiny of neighbors and be considered adequate parents, although as people, they may be recognized as "peculiar."

The H family was an unusual one in our series since both parents were schizophrenic. The mother became psychotic gradually over the years with schizoid characteristics that stemmed from early life, whereas the father held precariously onto reality until his increasing failure to hold down a job brought his severe paranoia into the open and led to his suicide. The seven children were parented by a mother who was abnormally shy, hypersensitive, fearful, dreamy, dependent, and submissive when she was not overtly schizophrenic and a father who was extremely nervous, rigid, suspicious, and asociable. Both parents felt that they were failures: the father believed that the world was responsible for his lack of success, while the mother was sure that she was born "to be no good at anything." They were two waifs in a storm who should never have undertaken the exacting tasks of parenting. However, they did with a vengeance and brought into being a large group of lovely children who were all maladapted, hyperexcitable or withdrawn, prone to weird symptoms, and not too well grounded in reality. The father reported that both he and his wife were the least adequate members of their respective families, and that this fact seemed to draw them to each other in some strange way. As a highly religious man, his basic thesis was that God was the best parent and that he was ready to entrust his children completely to

Him. The children therefore received an overdose of religion and an underdose of care. "They are very attached to one another and not much to us, and they have more or less brought themselves up. They know not to interfere with our lives or to disturb us when we have our work to do. I like them best when they are out of my hearing in the basement."

During a state of remission, the mother said that she had never been able to function as a wife and a mother. "I feel like a child, not a married woman. There is no real relationship between me and my husband except on a religious level. The children form some sort of bridge between him and me. He wanted ten to thirteen children and so I was always pregnant. He said that the Lord would provide, but I got more and more depressed with each child. It's nothing important but I think I may kill myself. I really feel like Alice in Wonderland, as if I was in a dream and still a child. People expect me to be grown-up and look after my children but I don't know how to be grown-up and I don't know how to look after children. The children will all become good mothers and fathers because they have had so much practice with one another." (This did not turn out to be the case: all the older children dreaded the very idea of becoming parents and were determined not to have children.) She said that she heard "voices" and these were always of the children crying, fighting, screaming, and arguing, and that she could not bear it when she heard these "voices." When asked what had interfered with her becoming a good mother, she cited a very guilty incestuous relationship with her brother after which she felt that all her female organs and femaleness were damaged. "I always felt very sorry and ashamed that I was a girl because such things could happen to you." She never felt any good at any time, but her pregnancy, she said, made her feel more real so that she no longer felt completely blank. "It almost seems as if the pregnancy makes me into a person. I don't know why." But as soon as the baby arrived, she immediately felt small and childlike herself and began to get steadily depressed. "I have always been afraid of hurting people and when these small creatures were born, I felt even more scared that I would injure them in some way. It didn't seem as if I could be any good for anyone." The only bit of parental advice she had to offer her daughters was that they should never take their underpants down for anyone: this was due to the guilty sexual play with her brother. (The middle daughter, who was closely identified with the mother in all her schizoid characteristics, despite an intense religious training by the father, allowed a boy to take her pants down for a quarter. This girl had a schizophrenic break at the age of 14.)

Some of the psychotic mothers in our sample corresponded to the narcissistic Marquesan women referred to as courtesan types by Kardiner [23] who were, according to him, "devoid of maternal instinct and whose exaggerated sexual interests led to a marked rejection of the maternal function." For example, Mrs. G was labeled a paranoid schizophrenic with a highly erotic delusional system. She presented as a masculinized woman with strong masculine interests and a disturbed menstrual function. Paradoxically, she had a strong nymphomaniacal drive that intensified with the development of psychosis. She would pester men, take to prostitution from time to time, and was constantly on the lookout for a man. "I am always looking for someone but I can never seem to find him." She developed erotic delusions that certain eminent men were in love with her and were constantly sending her messages, indicating their interests in a sexual adventure. However, she seemed quite indifferent to her children and offered them little more than routine care. She said that she disliked their greediness and spoke of them eating her "out of house and home." She had never wanted children and were it not for her husband, she would never have had children. She constantly reproached them for their gluttony and messiness. She said that she had had a very unhappy childhood with little or no relationship with her parents. An uncle had been kind to her, "perhaps a little too kind," and she recalled him making her very excited by tickling and touching her. Some people, judging from her appearance, had thought of her as homosexual but when they saw her behavior with men, they rapidly revised this viewpoint. "Men are my life; I could have sex around the clock; it's a pity that sex sometimes ends in childbirth—so much romance going down the drain." The cleavage between sexual and maternal behavior was particularly marked in her psychotic state. She was jealous of the interest shown by her husband and other men in her young daughter toward whom she occasionally had murderous fantasies. She felt certain that her children did not care for her and that they wanted to be rid of her. In one of her delusional fantasies, she saw herself being roasted alive by them and eaten as Thanksgiving dinner.

Psychosis can force people with incompatible minds and ways into marriage. For example, Mr. and Mrs. B were the most unlikely people to get together. Mr. B was an illiterate, domineering, demanding, autocratic, and foul-tempered Jewish businessman who was a complete workaholic; Mrs. B was quiet, unobtrusive, compliant, highly subdued, academically strong with a good college degree, and Episcopalian. She never knew what it was to have a mother since her mother died when she was very young. She felt that her children had "wildly mixed up genes."

My husband is like an angry dynamo while I am easygoing, lacking in energy, and ready to do what I am told. It is because I spend so much time in such a relaxed state that I imagine things and that is what led me to become crazy. People like me, who spend so much time in their own heads, should never have children. We make terrible parents because we don't live in the real world, and children have to live in a real world if they are to grow up normal. Having a baby is like having a bucket of cold water poured over you; it's meant to bring you to your senses but in fact it drives you further into your own thoughts. I became very disturbed after the birth of each one of my three children. It is not surprising that they have all had problems. Their father forces them to work "voluntarily" in his business to give them "a sense of reality" while I constantly wonder what's going on in their heads and give them no sense of reality whatsoever. When I thought that I was responsible for dropping the atom bomb on Japan, I felt that the Japanese in St. Louis would find out and destroy each of my children. As a result, I did not bother to do anything for them in the way of bringing them up properly: all I was concerned with was keeping them safe from being murdered. It was not maternal protection as they write about it in books. It was just stark craziness, and it raised three very frightened children who did not know what they were frightened about. The children must have been very confused since I lived a dream life and their father lived a very matter-of-fact life. I was so concerned about the atom bomb business that I did not teach my kids anything about everyday living.

Mrs. B's teenage daughter remarked: "She worries about the dropping of many atom bombs and the killing of millions of people, but at the same time, she seems hardly concerned at all about her own kids. She is worried about the world but not about us, and she feels guilty about not saving the world, but not at all guilty about us becoming so maladjusted. She is everybody's parent and nobody's parent." All three children were victims of postpartum psychosis in addition to the chronic schizophrenia that invaded their lives. The absence of early bonding was apparent in the looseness and tenuousness of their subsequent object relationships. None of them were able to keep friends. None of them wanted to become parents because, as the daughter put it, "We don't know what it means." None of them wanted to get married because, as the daughter said, "Men and women are really too different for them to be able to live together without driving the other crazy."

Another example of disturbed parenting is Mrs. P. Mrs. P married into an Italian "clan" and it was "like hell on earth." Mr. P gave his weekly pay packet to his mother. Mrs. P was the odd person out. She had very much wanted to have a family of her own because she had been brought up without parents — both of hers had died when she was very small. "I thought that I could learn to become a parent from books, but there was always something missing inside me. I always felt that I did not want to be a parent; I wanted to have a parent. I thought that I would have gained parents when I entered this Italian family but I was never allowed to become one of them and so I learned nothing about being a parent." When she became psychotic, she refused to have anything more to do with her husband because he behaved like a son and not a father, and she wanted a father for her children. "And yet when he gave them love, I immediately felt jealous and deprived. I realized, when I was sane again, that I was competing for my husband's fathering with my own children."

Still another case of disturbed parenting is observed with Mr. O. Mr. O had a very strict upbringing ("no sex, no swearing, no vulgarity, and absolutely no aggression"). He was the youngest of four sons, and his mother had a psychotic depression when he was an infant. He grew up quiet, shy, dependent, reserved, and isolated. He felt "terribly repressed" and every now and then a wildness surged out of him and he would become maniacal. "During my quiet times, I think that I am a good parent although, if the children are noisy, they quickly get on my nerves. But when I am in a manic phase, I am just too foolish to be a decent father. You need to be stable and sensible, and I am rushing around everywhere like a cat on hot bricks." Although Mr. O had very little psychological insight, he was aware that his illness caused the children to react. His wife, who was a psychologist, said that he lacked all empathy, especially parental empathy. He had no idea how to make contact with his children, how to communicate with them meaningfully, how to handle their problems, and how to handle them consistently. The fact that he was so unpredictable led to a great insecurity in the other members of the family, and they learned very rapidly not to rely on him for anything. Below, Mr. O's 9-year old son is talking about his sick father.

He said that his father had a nervous breakdown and had become real nervy, couldn't control himself, and had to go to the hospital to have shock treatment. He could not tell the other kids about this at school because he felt very ashamed. "When you get nervous like this, it's because God has made you like that and you can't do anything about it." He wondered why God chose to make some people like that. He first knew that his daddy was sick when he was 7 years old and heard him say all sorts of bad and mean things. "He starts to hit everybody and bawls everyone out. My mom says he does it because he thinks he is going to get someplace, but he won't get anywhere by screaming at anyone. He thinks he is a real big person and my mom thinks he isn't. He's only just another person in the house. He bawls me out for things I don't do and then I get some terrible thoughts myself, such as running away from home and bad angry thoughts about him. My dad gets bad thoughts because he can't control his nerves and sometimes

I cause him to become sick by not obeying him. When he is sick, my mom also gets angry and has bad thoughts about going away and leaving us. I then leave them and go to my room where I think a lot."

The glamour of grandiosity is highly seductive for the developing child, but this represents only one of the many deficits that affects the developing life of the child exposed to bipolar disorders [4].

As a parent, the manic-depressive is loaded with damaging deficiencies: he takes but refuses to give; he has little or no awareness of others as people but only as stereotypes and consequently has little capacity to empathize with them; he shows a minimal respect for reality and is always ready to substitute magical manipulation for realistic reaction and interaction. The combination of infantile dependency, manipulativeness, exploitation, shallowness, insensibility to give anything of himself, and the very extraverted approach to reality renders the manic-depressive unfit for the complex tasks of parenthood and puts his children at risk for some form of depression at all stages of their development. (P. 314)

During the course of normal development within an average predictable environment, the self-esteem of the child varies within normal limits, along with his self-confidence. The esteem that he has for his parents, as well as his confidence in them, also remains within normal limits. As Winnicott [39] pointed out, this disillusionment and disappointment with regard to the parents increases gradually over time and is constantly counterbalanced by the idealizing tendency in the child. The parents need to further the sense of reality by helping the child to see them more realistically, although they should also be able to accept graciously the "glory" thrust upon them by the child and not frustrate him or her with unbecoming "unempathic modesty." When the developmental environment contains abnormal amounts of narcissism and omnipotence generated by a parent figure, the regulation of self-esteem may become precarious. Here is a good illustration of this seen from the child's point of view [4].

When she has little attacks, it's not so bad. She would be talking big, and we go into the stores and buy things and order all sorts of clothes, and I'd feel like a princess. She made me feel like a princess. She'd say: "You don't have to think small." I'd sometimes go to school feeling grand and pretending I was some sort of princess and that all the children would know about it and stare at me and think that I was great. Sometimes I began to feel so great that I got on everybody's nerves, and the kids soon started to tease me for putting on airs. I hate myself now when I think of it. But when mother was like that, she'd dress me up and do my hair. We'd sit for hours in front of the mirror, and she'd say that we were both beauties and that you couldn't find a pair like us in all the world. You know, I really believed it, and I began to think that I might become a film star or go on the stage. She always said: "You've got to think big because you are big." When she talked and talked and talked, I also talked and talked and talked, and my friends at school thought I talked too much, and that I was too bossy, and that I wanted everything my way. If it weren't for the kids, I think that I would have believed everything my mother told me. She made me feel special, and they just made me feel ordinary. (Pp. 293–294)

Because of the disorder of affective functioning, the parents with this type of illness are quite unable to help their children with their affects. In the following example, the father is relatively normal and is therefore able to assess the deviant behavior of his manic-depressive wife more accurately [4].

When she acted inappropriately toward the children, he often felt that it was not because she did not know what to do in the circumstance but because she was so preoccupied with her own thoughts that she could not think about the situation. He cited a recent example in which the household pet, a kitten, had been run over. The children had been extremely upset. Without a word of explanation, she had bundled them all up in her car and had taken them to a fun fair and encouraged them to take as many rides as possible. This was the way her own mother had dealt with family crises during her childhood, and she was repeating the same pattern. Both children had vomited, and the baby also had been sick. When they had arrived home, they all looked very ill and depressed. He said his own parents would have allowed him to have a good cry and thus work the sadness out of his system. He thought that getting the children excited was not the way to deal with their grief. (Pp. 301–302)

In the above example, the woman in question was not without insight regarding her parenting capacities. She realized that she was not a good mother and that her husband was a much better mother than she; even as a man, he seemed to know better what to do when the children were upset. When the babies screamed at her, she first became afraid of them and then wanted to scream back at them and attack them. She had been a bad daughter to her mother and now she was a bad mother to her children. These kind of parents create extremely vulnerable children. The son of this woman said that the way he felt at school on any particular day depended on how his mother was feeling at home: If she was sad it got him down and he had sort of dark feelings inside him with images of her sitting in a chair at home with her head bowed down. He always expected things to turn out bad for him, and then added, "I don't suppose I'll live very long." When asked to qualify this, he said that he just thought that he would get some kind of sickness [4]. "I think I've got an open door to my body — any germ that wants to get in just has to walk in" (p. 304). This sense of vulnerability haunted many of the children in this series, and the feeling of "skinlessness" (as Virginia Woolf referred to it) was heightened by a similar phenomenon in the parents and their total lack of resourcefulness in coping with it. Defeated and dilapidated egos typified the family setting. Despite the bad and damaging acts perpetrated by these parents on their children, when observed at close quarters in their homes, one could only conclude with Freud that in life there were no villains, only victims — a dismal covey of hapless victims.

In many instances, the children treat the gross parental aberration by disavowing or repudiating the parental tie. In one family of six children where the father suffered from paranoid schizophrenia, all the children called him by his first name. When the eldest child was asked about this she simply said: "He doesn't seem like a father." She added that he also did not appear to recognize the fact that they were children and would often play very roughly with them. "Once he had me in one hand up above his head and said he was going to let me drop and I was scared because I felt it was something he could do and would do. I just don't like him fighting with my mother. I'll kill him if he hurts her. I used to have nightmares about this. It always started with them hugging and kissing like any ordinary couple and then he would be beating on her, jumping on her and trying to throttle her. When I asked my mother why she did not move away from him, she would say that he couldn't help some of this and that she still wanted them to respect him no matter what." These responses from the children remind us, once again, that the parental lines of behavior are conterminous with the general run of human urges but gradually overstep the edges of normality or conventional expectation. This is true for both aggressive and sexual drives. Incest is a constant theme running through family life, sometimes as a delusional idea or accusation and sometimes as an actuality. Psychotic mothers are often changed by the illness, becoming less attractive and occasionally quite repulsive. There would be an understandable turning away of the spouse, and at this point, the delusion would take the form of infidelity or incest. In a few of our cases, what was originally ascribed to delusion later was revealed as truth. As with aggressive play, affectionate play between parent and child gradually gave way to sexual activities. The unpredictability and the lack of continuity in the psychotic parent is what saps the very foundation of the child's security.

The parent's hold on reality is crucial for parental functioning. There is a down-to-earth quality needed in the care of small children, and without this pregenital competence, neglect becomes inevitable. For example, Mrs. D's earliest memory was of her mother going crazy and jumping naked into the river. Later her stepmother would warn her that unless she pulled herself together, she would go crazy like her mother. "I heard this so often that after a while I came to believe that it was going to happen and I didn't care any longer." She married at 15 to get away from a terrible home. She became immediately and totally dependent on her husband and looked to him to care for all her wants. Almost compulsively, she began to have child after child, and with each new birth, the other children were pushed further out of her consciousness. "I could not care for one child and I had six of them around me asking for things and it would send me crazy. I let them do whatever they liked provided they looked after themselves." She recalled a dream in which she had only two options open to her: the choice of falling off a cliff or being attacked by a wild beast. "All my life seems to be like that dream. I really have no place to go." She did not toilet train her children, did not discipline them, did not get meals for them, did not help them with their homework, and had no idea what they did when out of her sight. She was quite unable to differentiate one from another except for one daughter who seemed "just like me." (This child has since had a schizophrenic breakdown.) Mrs. D complained that life was not real, people were not real, and that she herself did not feel like a person. "I have nothing in me except my bones." Even at this rock bottom level of functioning, she was capable of surprising altruism. "I don't want my children mixed up in my sickness. I don't want anyone to know that they have a sick mother, and I don't want them to get involved with me. The best thing I can do for them is to keep away from them." She remembered how hard it was for her to grow up with a sick mother in the house. She knew that she should never have had any children, but since they were there, she did not want to make them sick like herself. She recalled the children teasing her about "being cracked" like her mother. "If someone adopted my children, it would be the best thing for them. When I see other mothers, I know they are something. I am just nothing, and you can't be nothing and be a mother at the same time."

It is clear, from the content of these examples of children of psychotic parents that fantasy and experience feed constantly on each other, leading frequently to an escalation into terror. Television images and dreams add their quota of fear. In the following example, a 9-year-old boy is coping with his father's active psychosis.

Sometimes I think and then I get nervous and I start to cry and I get my cat and go to bed. But if I sleep, I dream things about my dad that is very scary. I watch TV and see monsters and then I see monsters when I go to bed. I think they are real in my dreams and I put the cover over my head and I throw up. Sometimes I become the monster in the nightmare and Dad shoots at me with a gun and I die, or the monster dies and I wake up. I am sometimes scared all the time like somebody is going to be killed. (At this point in the interview, he became acutely nervous and said: "I am nervous now and I feel the room is moving and tilting over. I am getting dizzy." He began to sway.) My mom feels I would be better if I could yell at my dad but I don't feel any better if I do. It's hard for me to yell. Sometimes my mother yells things about my dad when he gets nervous and she gets a headache just like I do. She gets so nervous she has to lie down just like I do. Then everything gets worried in my body and I have to throw up. Sometimes if I can play with my mother's fingers, I feel better. When my dad is sick, he gets mean and I think he can hurt my mom. I feel sad because he says he's getting old and he's bad and getting sick, and I feel sorry for him. I feel bad when my cat has teeth and claws and I get mad because she bites me and it hurts. I'll step on her tail. When I do that, I feel sad and I'm mad and then I feel sad. If I could stop dreaming I would feel much better, I think. The monsters wouldn't be there, and I wouldn't become a monster and get killed. In some dreams, I get sick and the sickness spreads all over my body very fast, and I think I am going to die.

Below is an excerpt from a teenage girl with a chaotically schizophrenic mother. This example also demonstrates how fantasy and experience constantly feed on each other.

Last night I had a dream in which I was in Egypt on the site of a dig and we uncovered a mummy in its tomb and one of the archeologists (who looked like my dad) took a knife and put it into the eyes of the mummy ripping off the cornea and leaving the iris and the pupil bulging out. The stomach of the mummy would also open and you could see all the stuff inside. The archeologist began to laugh but then dropped dead and I knew it was a curse. (This reminded her of an incident when she was 5 years old and had walked out of her home alone and was telling the neighbors that there was a murderer in the house and that he was killing someone. No one believed her. She began, in a somewhat strange way, to laugh at the idea of the mummy being disemboweled.) It makes me think about my Mom. She is crazy enough, but just think of her with her stomach all open and her eyes popping out. A thousand years from now, when people dig her up, they would know that she was crazy, and they would wonder if someone killed her because she was crazy.

Conclusions

Eugen Bleuler [7], the father of schizophrenia, did not take sides in the nature-nurture controversy rampant at the time, possibly because of the influence of Freud and his concept of the "complemental series." From the turn of the century onward, Freud pursued the "etiological equation," focusing on the interlocking between inheritance and experience, in which the diminishing influence of one factor was balanced by the increasing influence of the other. He felt that the influences could be grouped into preconditions that were indispensable for producing a disturbance, but were so general in their effect that any one of a large number of disorders could ensue. Concurrent causes, on the other hand, were equally general but not indispensable. It was the specific group of causes that were not only indispensable but led to the emergence of particular disorders. Psychotic parenting brings in factors of preconditioned, concurrent influences that are harmful and specific effects that influence the thinking, feeling, and behaving of the child from the very beginning of life. Bleuler [7], who had a wry sense of humor, said that "of all the blessings and misfortunes it is our fate to meet with in life, those connected with our choice of parents are the most important; nothing in the world can be matched with them for significance." He went on to add that parents cultivated the givens in the child. They nurtured his "heart" so that he could feel properly; his mind, so that he could think of ways to deal with his predicament; and his body, so that he would be fit enough to adjust better. "Anyone, therefore, who wishes to be happy must seek out for himself the right parents, or forever afterwards, he cannot do much to alter things."

All evidence goes to indicate that the influence of psychotic parenting is as variable as any noxious factors impinging on the child. It is not only the intensity and the duration of the psychosis in the parent that matters, but also its vicious selection of the child as victim. Many psychotic parents avoid their children, who feel a sense of loss and abandonment; they may also affect the children indirectly by behaving in ways that are highly embarrassing. There are also parents who become psychotically abusive. In his *Memoirs,* [15] Schreber uses the phrase "soul murder," which has been understood to describe the cruel child-rearing concepts and practices of Schreber's father. Shengold [34] adapted the term to involve the experience of traumata "imposed from the world outside the mind that is so overwhelming that the mental apparatus is flooded with feeling. . . . The terrifying 'too muchness' requires massive and mind-distorting defensive operations in order for the child to continue to think and feel. The child's sense of identity (that is, the maintenance of the self-representations) is threatened" (p. 538). Shengold assumes that *actual* overwhelming experiences of sexual and aggressive assaults during the course of development have a different, and he thinks, more destructive and pathogenic effect than do the fantasies of being aggressively and sexually attacked. The problem for the child is a paradoxical one: he or she can only deal with the terrifying experience by conjuring up the image of a good parent, and yet it is the good parent that is behaving so badly toward him or her. As Shengold puts it, the child, out of desperate need, is compelled to register the parent *delusionally* as good, which is a mind-splitting or mind-fragmenting operation. "In order to survive, these children must keep in some compartment of their minds the delusion of good parents and the delusive promise that all the terror and pain and hate will be transformed into love" (p. 539).

Shengold compares this to the Orwellian "doublethink" of 1984. Yet he goes on to state that "human beings are mysteriously resourceful, and some do survive such childhoods, with their sexuality and with their souls not unscarred or unwarped but at least in some part intact. Others are crushed, predominantly or completely—body and soul, sexuality and soul. Despite the vulnerability of children and the prevalence of bad parents, a completely successful soul murderer is probably rare. Why this should be so *is* mysterious: part of the explanation is innate and endowment. What was it that enabled one of my patients with two psychotic parents to become, from age 4 on, the real parent in the family—a sane, caring person who was able to help her siblings and even take care of her psychotic parents?" (p. 549). He suggests that sometimes the soul-saving force is the presence of another loving person in the child's environment. My patient's experience of psychotic parenting has led me to similar conclusions. However, even those children who seem to be thriving manifestly make use of a false-self defense organization [38] as a means of survival and frequently resort to transitional phenomena of various kinds when they have experienced a set back. Many of these children are also haunted by the fear of breakdown. Not only have they seen their omnipotent parents break down, but during this phase of "environmental failure" during the earliest phase of dependency, the ego is often so disrupted that primitive anxieties erupt and lead to what Winnicott refers to as "an unthinkable state of affairs" [38]. The early trauma seems to be experienced over and over again. It is an unquiet state and no sense of continuity of being is achieved. It is very difficult to put one's clinical finger on these ineffable but ineluctable details that lie in the background of psychotic parenting.

References

1. Anthony, E. J. "It Hurts Me More Than It Hurts You": An Approach to Discipline as a Two-Way Process. In R. Ekstein and R. Motto (Eds.), *From Learning for Love to Love of Learning.* New York: Brunner/Mazel, 1969.
2. Anthony, E. J. The Influence of Maternal Psychosis on Children—Folie à Deux. In *Parenthood: Its Psychology and Psychopathology.* Boston: Little, Brown, 1970.

2a. Anthony, E. J. Mourning and Psychic Loss of the Parent. In E. J. Anthony, and C. Koupernik (Eds.), *The Child in His Family: The Impact of Disease and Death.* New York: Wiley, 1973.

3. Anthony, E. J. Naturalistic Studies of Disturbed Families. In *Explorations in Child Psychiatry.* New York: Plenum, 1975.

4. Anthony, E. J., and Benedek, T. Influence of a Manic-depressive Environment on the Child. In *Depression and Human Existence.* Boston: Little, Brown, 1975.

5. Anthony, E. J. The Family and the Psychoanalytic Process in Children. In *The Psychoanalytic Study of the Child.* New Haven: Yale University Press, 1980, Vol. 35.

6. Anthony, E. J. Psychoanalysis and Environment. In Pollock, G., and Greenspan, S (Eds.), *The Course of Life:* U. S. Government Printing Office, 1981, Vol. 3.

7. Bleuler, E. *Unconscious Ill Turns.* Munich: Reinhardt, 1906, Vol. 4.

8. Bleuler, M. *The Schizophrenic Disorders.* Translated by S. M. Clemens. New Haven: Yale University Press, 1978.

9. Burlingham, D., Goldberger, A., and Lussier, A. Simultaneous analysis of mother and child. *Psychoanal. Study Child* 10:165, 1955.

10. Deutsch, H. *The Psychology of Women: Motherhood.* New York: Grune & Stratton, 1945, Vol. 2.

11. Douglas, G. Puerperal depression and excessive compliance with the mother. *Br. J. Med. Psychol.* 36:271, 1963.

12. Erikson, E. H. *Identity: Youth and Crisis.* New York: Norton, 1968.

13. Frazer, J. *The Golden Bough* (1916). New York: Macmillan, 1927.

14. Freud, A. *The Writings of Anna Freud.* New York: International Universities Press, 1971, Vol. 6.

15. Freud, S. The Case of Schreber. *The Standard Edition.* London: Hogarth Press, 1958, Vol. 12.

16. Freud, S. On narcissism (1914). In J. Strachey (Ed.), *The Standard Edition of the Complete Psychological Works of Sigmund Freud.* London: Hogarth Press, 1957. Vol. 13, pp. 90–91.

17. Gluck, I., and Wrenn, M. Contributions to the understanding of disturbances of mothering. *Br. J. Med. Psychol.* 32:171, 1959.

18. Greenacre, P. The Influence of Infantile Trauma on Genetic Patterns. In S. Furst (Ed.), *Psychic Trauma.* New York: Basic Books, 1967.

19. Grunebaum, H., Weiss, J., Cohler, B., et al. *Mentally Ill Mothers and Their Children.* Chicago: University of Chicago Press, 1975.

20. Hartmann, H. Psychiatrische und Zwilling studien. *J. Psychiat. Neurol.* 50, 1934–1935.

21. Hartmann, H. *Essays on Ego Psychology.* New York: International Universities Press, 1964.

22. Hurry, A., and Sandler, J. Coping with reality: The child's defense against the external world. *Br. J. Med. Psychol.* 44:379, 1971.

23. Kardiner, A. *The Individual and His Society.* New York: Columbia University Press, 1939.
24. Khan, M. The Concept of Cumulative Trauma. In *The Privacy of the Self.* New York: International Universities Press, 1974. Pp. 42–58.
25. Kris, E. Notes on the development and on some current problems of psychoanalytic child psychology. In *The Psychoanalytic Study of the Chila.* London: Hogarth Press, 1950, Vol. 5.
26. Lidz, T., Fleck, S., and Cornelison, A. *Schizophrenia and The Family.* New York: International Universities Press, 1965.
27. Lomas, P. Puerperal breakdown. *Br. J. Med. Psychol.* 33:105, 1960.
28. Main, T. F. Mothers with children in a psychiatric hospital. *Lancet* 11:845, 1958.
29. Miller, A. *Prisoners of Childhood.* New York: Basic Books, 1981.
30. Sandler, J. The background of safety. *Int. J. Psychoanal.* 41:352, 1960.
31. Sandler, J., and Rosenblatt, B. The concept of the representational world. *Psychoanal. Study Child* 17:128, 1962.
32. Searles, H. The effort to drive the other person crazy. *Br. J. Med. Psychol.* 32:1, 1959.
33. Shengold, L. The parent as sphinx. *J. Am. Psychoanal. Assoc.* 11:725, 1963.
34. Shengold, L. Child abuse and deprivation. *J. Am. Psychoanal. Assoc.* 27:533, 1979.
35. Spitz, R. Psychogenic Diseases in Infancy. In *The Psychoanalytic Study of the Child,* Vol 6. New York: International Universities Press, 1951.
36. Turnbull, C. *The Mountain People.* New York: Simon & Schuster, 1972.
37. Tetlow, C. Pyschosis of childbearing. *J. Ment. Sci.* 101:629, 1955.
38. Winnicott, E. W. *The Maturational Processes and The Facilitating Environment.* London: Hogarth Press, 1965.
39. Winnicott, D. W. The effect of psychosis on family life. The effect of psychotic parents on the emotional development of the child. In *The Family and Individual Development.* London: Tavistock Publications, 1968.
40. Zilboorg, G. The dynamics of schizophrenic reaction to pregnancy and childbirth. *Am. J. Psychiatry* 8:733, 1929.
41. Zilboorg, G. Depressive reactions to parenthood. *Am. J. Psychiatry* 10:927, 1931.

9

Changes in parent-child relationships during and after divorce

Judith S. Wallerstein

The collapse of the family structure draws attention to the network of relationships within the family. Relationships between parents and children that are taken for granted within the intact family (unless they deviate widely from acceptable norms) are cast into bold relief during marital rupture and its often extended aftermath. Under the shadow of the marital breakdown, these relationships are newly perceived by the child as significantly more fragile, less permanent, and less reliable. As the child within the divorcing family sees all too clearly, the social context, which provided meaning, and the external structure, which assured continuity, nurturance, and protection, have been badly shaken. In effect, each parent-child relationship has been freed from some of the more powerful psychological and social moorings that had held it in place.

One immediate consequence of marital rupture, therefore, is the eruption of an intense anxiety in the child and the setting into motion of an anxiety-driven tracking of each parent-child relationship. The child of divorce is much more likely than his or her peers within the intact family to maintain an apprehensive watch over each parent's attitude and behavior, as well as over relationships between the parents, with each sibling, and among siblings. This intense, sometimes hyperalert monitoring of relationships is likely to continue over many years following the parents' divorce and into their possible remarriages as well [5].

In his or her worried attentiveness to the state of the relationship with each parent, the child of divorce is fully in accord with our more systematic observations regarding the extraordinary susceptibility of these relationships to change at this time [9]. Like their children, parents, at the time of the escalating marital distress and during the marital breakup and

Although the editors have chosen to place this chapter in the section entitled "The Abandoning Parent," current studies show unequivocally that most parents do not abandon their children following divorce. In my own research, ten years after the marital rupture less than 10 percent of the children had no contact with their fathers. It is important to distinguish the child's *fear of abandonment* from the reality and to recognize this fear as only one of many themes in the child's experience.

317

its aftermath, are also likely to perceive their children in ways that differ from the perceptions of the same child during the previous intact period of the marriage. All of these relationships, including the routine interactions of daily life, may become modified by the new feelings, attitudes, and behaviors that emerge during this critical period. Even more broadly, the particular psychological or symbolic significance of the child to the parent may undergo profound changes as the family structure changes. Sometimes these changes are only temporary during the height of the divorce crisis, but often they endure throughout the child's subsequent growing-up years.

It is, of course, not surprising that the ways in which parents and children relate to each other are altered under the impact of such a crisis. Important in this context, we have observed that parent-child relationships within the intact marriage have often been able to withstand the pressure of the conflict between the adults or the unhappiness of one or both adults and can, under certain circumstances, even remain relatively conflict-free. We have, for example, reported earlier our own findings that over one-quarter of the 131 children whom we followed in the California Children of Divorce Study, beginning with the marital breakup and through the first 5 years of the postdivorce family, had enjoyed warm and nurturant relationships with *both* parents even during the time of the failing marriage. An even larger number had enjoyed a loving and nurturant relationship with one of the two parents [9]. However, this relative immunity of a substantial number of the parent-child relationships to the conflict and unhappiness between the parents seems not to hold in the face of the divorce crisis. Rather, the chain of multiple reactions — social, economic, and psychological — set off by the divorce, which often last for several years before reaching a new postdivorce equilibrium, is likely to sharply affect the perceptions of the children by their parents and the perceptions of the parents by their children and to cast each into a range of new and unfamiliar roles, which, whether temporary or long-lasting, may be at wide variance with the earlier relationships within the same family prior to the breakup.

Overall, what is so striking in all this is that the entire patterning of conscious and unconscious psychological needs, wishes, and expectations that parents and children bring to each other is often profoundly altered under the impact of the divorce and its multiple ripple effects. Psychoanalytic theory has not prepared us for this. It has led us to expect relative continuity in the relationships between parents and children within the vicissitudes and impact of changing developmental stages in child and adult. Family systems theory has called attention to the complex multiple effects of change within the family system. Nevertheless, it too has provided little psychological undergirding for understanding the ways in which the crisis of divorce can transform the usual interactions between parent and child. Some of the changes that we observe following the breakup reflect a new intimacy and affection occurring only after the divorce and with no visible roots in the predivorce relationship. Conversely, other changes reflect a sudden cooling or even severance of relationships that may have been consistently close and loving during the marriage. Certain kinds of relationships are newly created and are specific to the postdivorce family. These include the visiting relationship in single-custody homes and the special parent-child relationships that evolve under joint-custody arrangements. Others appear as divorce-specific changes. These include peerlike relationships between parents and their children, as well as role reversal in which the child assumes important aspects of the parental role. Still other relationships that are not altogether new have no real counterpart within the intact family. These include alliances and alignments between parent and children whose purpose is to harass and punish the parent who is seeking the divorce.

My overall purpose is first to delineate the expectable divorce-specific general changes across a wide spectrum of divorcing families and, second, to call particular attention to some of the psychopathological relationships that characteristically emerge at the marital rupture and tend to represent the more extreme manifestations of the general expectable trends. These changes in role, in tenor, in the context of the relationship, in mutual perception, and in psychological and symbolic meaning to each other can be examined for the light that they can shed on the impact of marital rupture on the network of parent-child relationships within the family. More broadly, the examination of these relationships during and after the critical divorce period provides access to the potential arc of change within each evolving parent-child relationship. The ways in which these relationships can stretch to accommodate the altered needs and requirements of adults and children illustrate the potential elasticity of the parent-child relationship and show its capacity to survive through accommodation to even severely deforming pressures. And importantly, such changes may be to the benefit or to the serious detriment of one or both participants.

It may well be that some of the attitudes, impulses, and feelings that thus emerge so powerfully during the divorce crisis are present within the intact family as well, where they have been carefully hidden or constrained by the mutual need to maintain the intactness of the family. The enlightened or unenlightened self-interest of the family members in maintaining the family system may have muted feelings that surface at the time of the marital rupture. The relationship of each parent and child within the ongoing intact family is likely to be buffered and constrained by the presence of the other parent, as well as by the entire network of family relationships. If so, in accord with what Anna Freud has described as "the profitable nature of negative experience," the close examination of stable and of altering parent-child relationships during breakdown may shed significant light on the hidden seams in parent-child relationships within the intact family [1].

We discern two decisive and contrapuntal themes in parent-child relationships that can emerge characteristically during the marital rupture and its extended aftermath. The first of these reflects the parents' conscious or unconscious negative view of the children as economic, social, and psychological burdens, as well as unwelcome and sometimes persistently irritating reminders of the marital failure. The anxiety that the children experience at the time of the marital rupture may reflect, in part, their sense of the profound resentment that they evoke in their parents at this time and the awareness that they may be standing in the way of their parents' powerful, albeit conflicted, wish not only to dissolve the present marriage but to wipe out its prior existence and history as well.

Running directly counter to the parental wish to be rid of the child can be a passionate attachment to the child. At the time of divorce crisis, parents are likely to need the child with new intensity during the difficult transition period. They are liable to lean on the child and to turn to the child for help as confidant, advisor, mentor, sibling, parent, caretaker, lover, concubine, ally within the marital conflict, an extended conscience or ego control, a pivotal supportive presence in staving off depression, or even to protect against ego disintegration and suicide. Sometimes it is the parent's conscious intent to seek the child's help only during the height of the crisis or the transition. Not all parents, however, regard the child's new role as temporary, and some of the pressures that arise in response to the parent's neediness may last for many years.

The overall impact of the divorce on the parent-child relationship as proposed here is thus paradoxical. The marital rupture serves to separate parent and child and to drive a wedge between them across which each regards the other anxiously, fearing and expecting decreased availability and even abandonment. Yet, at the same time, the impact of the divorce may bring parent and child closer together—so close that the generally necessary and protective generational differences and distance may be in jeopardy.

The Divorcing Process

Perhaps it is important to set the stage realistically at the outset by noting that the divorcing process is significantly more difficult, more distressing, and considerably longer than many people realize. The decision to divorce ushers in expected and unexpected changes whose complexity and scope exceed the usual expectations of the participants. We have elsewhere noted that there has been insufficient recognition of the disabling impact of divorce itself on the psychological functioning of the adult, particularly on the capacity of the adult to carry on his or her expected roles and responsibilities in the domains of work and family life during the marital rupture and during the months, and sometimes years, that follow [9]. In the great majority of households we have studied, we have described feelings of bitterness and scenes of conflict that increase sharply with the actual separation. We have also noted the high incidence of depression and regression among divorcing adults [9]. And, as I have suggested elsewhere [6], it may well be that the structure of the intact marriage, whether happy or unhappy, often serves as an extended ego control that holds in check a host of primitive angers and sexual impulses, which can erupt when the marital structure topples [5].

This period of disequilibrium in the lives of the family is likely to last several years. Our finding was that the average time that the newly divorced, white, middle-class woman in the California study required in order to reestablish a sense of continuity and stability in her life was between 3 and 3½ years following the marital rupture. The men required an average of 2 to 2½ years before they reestablished a sense of stability in their lives. The divorce remained a live emotional issue at the 5-year mark for at least half of the adults and for most of the children and adolescents [9].

STAGES OF DIVORCE

I have earlier conceptualized several successive stages in the divorcing process that, despite overlap, are significantly distinguishable one from the other [5]. The first stage, which may be considered the acute phase, is precipitated by the decision to divorce, by the decisive separation of the married couple, and by one parent's departure from the household. This phase is characterized by a stressful, often very chaotic ambience. Parents may behave in ways that differ markedly from their customary conduct, and children may be confronted with unfamiliar and frightening behaviors in one or both parents including moderate to severe depression, heightened overt conflict, verbal accusations, threats, rage, and even physical violence. The duration of this acute phase characteristically ranges from several months to over a year or two following the separation.

The second, or transitional phase, which characteristically follows, spans a period of several years. During this period adults and children embark on unfamiliar roles and relationships within the new family structure. They often face unanticipated changes in all domains of family life during these years — changes that are likely to occur at a very different tempo than anticipated at the time of the decision to divorce and that require unexpectedly complex and painful adaptations from parents and children. The transitional stage ends as the postdivorce family is reestablished as a new, stable, functioning unit. Remarriage is a frequent occurrence during and following the transitional phase and, once again, major changes that require complex and sometimes painful adaptation from adults and children are introduced into family life.

Thus, divorce may be understood as a multistaged process of rapidly and radically changing family relationships, which begins with the marital rupture and its immediate aftermath, continues over several years of disequilibrium during the transitional period, and finally comes to rest with the restabilization of the new postdivorce family unit [5]. The parent-child relationships we will describe are primarily associated with the acute phase and the early period of transition.

Diminished Capacity to Parent
Parents experience a diminished capacity to parent their children during the acute phase of the divorcing process. This phenomenon is widespread and should be considered an expectable, general divorce-specific change in parent-child relationships. This diminished parenting is reflected at its simplest level in a wide range of observable attitudes and behaviors that include less physical care of the children, less time spent with the children, less play and discussion with the children, and a greater inconsistency, even disorganization, in physical care and household routines. Hetherington and coworkers [3] recorded disorganization, deterioration of discipline, diminished level of parental expectations, rising angers, and diminished care in divorcing families, all in significant contrast to a comparison group of intact families, and noted that parenting had specifically declined during the divorcing process and its aftermath. Our own observations are remarkably congruent with those of Hetherington and coworkers despite the wide differences in demography between the two populations studied [9].

Additionally, and as importantly, the diminished parenting includes a decline in emotional support and emotional nurturance for the children, a significant decrease in pleasure in the relationships, a marked decrease in attentiveness and sensitivity to the children's needs, and a steep escalation in inappropriate expressions of anger. The grave difficulty that parents often experience in discussing the decision to divorce with their children reflects in part the conflicts that beset their relationships with their children at this time. The characteristic resolution of such conflicts appears to be to withdraw from the children at a time of the children's heightened need for emotional support and explanation from their parents. Since the children are also likely to have become anxious and angry in response to the domestic crisis and more likely to be cranky, unruly, and less gratifying at this time to their parents, the resulting household ambience is one of rising conflict and anxiety accompanying the decreased physical and emotional availability of the parent to the child [7].

There are, of course, many individual determinants that are relevant to each parent-child configuration within each family. The parent's capacity to parent at the time of the divorce, as at other times, is influenced by a wide range of factors. Thus, each parent's emotional and physical availability to the child may be influenced by the parent's need to find a job, to return to school, and to reestablish a social life. Availability may also be influenced by the parent's physiological and psychological response to the divorce; the presence or absence of relief; a sense of new freedom, depression, agitation, or conflict; excitement with a new love affair; and jealous preoccupation with the marital partner's lover. Whatever the dominant mood or salient tasks, one expectable effect of divorce is a temporarily diminished capacity to provide emotional support for children and to maintain the organization of the household and the supervision of the physical and psychological care of the child in ways that are appropriate to his or her needs at this time.

Increased Vulnerability of the Child

One direct consequence of diminished parenting is the terrified sense of many youngsters that *both* parents are withdrawing emotionally at a decisively critical time. Divorce is a very lonely time for children. Unlike the social network that rallies for the ceremonies of death and the support of the bereaved, when divorce occurs the usual supports are likely to drop away. Friends of the family, neighbors, and teachers feel awkward and uneasy about what their roles should be with the children. In our study only one-quarter of the youngsters had grandparents or members of the extended family who helped them during the time of the marital rupture, and a mere 10 percent of the children were comforted by family, friends, or other adults they knew [9].

Thus, the impact of the diminished parenting on the parent-child relationship is magnified many times not only by the marital rupture but also by the relative absence of other supports. As a result, the period of the marital rupture represents an intense stress for the child in the midst of failing support from both the family and the wider surrounding community. And most ironically, the parents, who are generally charged with responsibility for the child's protection and well-being, are the very agents of this stress and failure to support.

One immediate effect of the diminished parenting combined with the loneliness of this critical period is in the child's greater sense of his or her vulnerability and relative helplessness to influence the major conditions of his or her life. The sense of powerlessness that burdens so many children at this time represents, in this view, a correct reading of their temporarily diminished place in the parental scheme of things. There are many potential sequelae to this changed balance of power in family relationships that a child perceives. One result, which may have far-reaching consequences for child and parent, is that the child, especially the younger child, is more likely to bend to the parent's wishes, threats, or blandishments. Conversely, older children or adolescents who are old enough to direct their own activities may be propelled into a position of far greater power and responsibility vis-à-vis the parent or may use the parental emotional withdrawal as the spur toward earlier spurious or real independence or precocious pseudo- or real adolescence. These new directions are likely to have lasting effects on the psychological development of the young person.

The Wish to Abandon the Child

One not uncommon, more extreme component of the parent-child relationship can be the adult's conscious or unconscious wish to abandon the child coincident with the breakup of the marriage. Although parents who litigate over visitation or custody have captured the attention of the community, the litigating group represents approximately only 10 percent of the divorcing population. Our own work reflects a larger population of divorcing families in which neither parent (perhaps only temporarily) wants the child. As we have noted, many parents perceive their children as economic burdens at a time of economic stress, as social burdens at a time of experimentation with new social relationships, and as unwelcome reminders of the marital failure and the years wasted in the wrong marriage. The abandonment fantasy can be acted out and expressed in various guises. Sometimes the directness of the parents' behavior is startling.

John was 2 years and 2 months when his mother decided to file for divorce. She had been devoted to him during the marriage and had invested in the child her wish for the intimacy and companionship that the marriage had failed to provide. When she reached her thirtieth birthday, she filed for divorce, abruptly weaned the child and placed him in full day care, and sought full-time employment. This extraordinary confluence of weaning, school placement out of the home, mother at full-time work, and the breakup of the marriage had a severe impact. When we saw John, who had earlier been described as a healthy, well-developed child, he was acutely anxious, disorganized, and wildly aggressive. His fantasy was that he was a dangerous child who had destroyed the family and had driven both parents away.

One not uncommon fantasy is the wish to hold on to only one of several children and to abandon the others. Some parents express this openly. Mrs. S told us tartly, "If I had my way, I'd pick up my youngest child and keep on walking and never look back at the others." Several mothers complained bitterly saying, "Who will ever want a woman with two children?" A significant number of women turned against their sons remarking angrily and sometimes bizarrely on their resemblance to their fathers. One young mother remarked about her 3-year-old: "He always reminds me of his father. Sometimes he'll get a jar from the refrigerator, and he'll throw it on the floor. If I punish him, he looks at me as if he doesn't understand me. That's just like his father." Sometimes parents split their ambivalence by marking off one child in the family as "his" and another as "hers." Children could be treated well or poorly in accord with this arbitrary assignment of loyalty, which is usually unrelated to the child's own preferences. The chosen child is treated well, and the rejected child may be rejected with a startling cruelty. Time and again we are surprised to observe how little anxiety divorcing parents experienced in openly rejecting one child, who is obviously grieving at this rejection by a parent he or she loves dearly.

Nor is it unusual at the time of the marital rupture for us to observe parents seeking a return to their own adolescence or young adulthood when they were unencumbered by children. We have witnessed an increasing number of families in which the marital rupture occurred coincident with one parent's wish to pursue interests or activities of earlier years. One such mother of three children aged 9, 6, and 4, who had been at home as a housewife and mother during the marriage, coolly informed her children that she now had little time for them because of her interest in sports. She spent several nights weekly with new associates at meetings and every weekend on the ski slopes, leaving the children with young and inexperienced baby-sitters. Another parent decided to pursue an operatic career and was planning a trip to Italy to study voice, expecting to take his young adolescent children with him. Although he had been a considerate and thoughtful father during the marriage, he had given no consideration to the children's resistance to leaving their school and neighborhood, or to their unfamiliarity with the new country or language. One mother of teenage youngsters abandoned her household to move in with her new lover. She came home once weekly bringing a sackful of groceries. When the children berated her, she screamed at them. The presence of an 11-, 14-, and 15-year-old supervised by a 21-year-old seemed to cause her relatively little concern, although throughout the prior marriage she had been a devoted mother.

One especially worrisome behavior among children may be related in part to a child's conscious or unconscious perception of the parent's emotional withdrawal. A significant subgroup of children appear to exercise less care on their own behalf immediately following the family breakup. The increase in accidents requiring medical intervention that we have observed is striking. These injuries appear in part to reflect poor parental supervision of children previously accustomed to good care. Thus, according to our observations, following the marital separation children were involved in hazardous play that would not have been permitted had the parents been functioning at their usual level of parenting. A significant number of children who sustained accidents were preoccupied at the time with fantasies of sinking into quicksand, being hit by a car, or exposing themselves to dangers by standing in the street. While these fantasies and the associated behaviors undoubtedly reflect the depression of the children, they have their counterpart in the diminished parenting and in the fantasies of the adults and their often powerful unconscious or conscious wishes to erase the marriage and its products.

This diminished parenting in divorcing parents and the response in the heightened anxiety of the children are widespread. In most families this dip in parenting is time-limited, and the parenting of the custodial parent resumes its earlier level of care within 2 years following the marital breakup. When the parents are more profoundly troubled, the diminution in parenting and its counterpart in the anxiety and depression of the children may endure for many years.

The Child as Battle Ally

The struggle for and through the children embodies the intense conflicts that often accompany the failing marriage. Although competition for a child's affection may occur in the intact, even well-functioning family, disruption of the family system brings the parents' natural competitiveness into sharpened focus. The angers of the disruption reinforce this parental competition for the children. Moreover, hostility is no longer constrained by mutual need. It is not uncommon for angry, sometimes distraught parents to cast their children into a great many roles in these marital battles. These roles can range from that of audience, whose presence appears sometimes as a necessary backdrop to the parental fighting, to that of committed, fully positioned battle allies. The children range in their participation from astonished, frightened observers to a denunciatory Greek chorus and ultimately, in some instances, to a full alignment with one parent against the other. Many of the anger-driven parent-child relationships that emerge at the time of the marital breakup are very new and diverge greatly from the prior pattern within the unbroken marriage.

When a child willingly played an active role in the battle between the parents, he or she customarily sided with the parent who opposed the divorce. Children saw themselves as fighting to restore the family unity, to redress the presumed injustice, or to diminish the suffering that the divorce had inflicted on one parent. By and large, the active participation of the children had its origin in strong parental disagreement regarding the decision to divorce. The children's conscious behavior was powered by loyalty to the disrupted marriage or by the quixotic impulse to defend or rescue the parent who was identified by the child (sometimes mistakenly so) as the victim [8].

It is not unusual for a child to take the part of the parent who is not present and to represent his or her interests. The child's sense of him- or herself is often that of guardian of the family honor, a gallant Horatio standing at the bridge. For example, waking up at 3:00 A.M. soon after the marital separation, Karla saw a man's car parked outside her home. She cried and sobbed the next morning, saying to her mother, "It's too soon. It's too soon. He's not my dad." She began to stay up until morning to keep an eye on her mother and her boyfriend and to prevent them from going to bed together.

Additionally contributing to the child's active participation in the marital battle is the rise in physical violence between the parents that often occurred at the time of the marital rupture among parents who had not fought physically with each other during the marriage. Over half of the children in the California Children of Divorce Study saw physical violence between their parents at the time of the marital rupture [9]. Most of these youngsters were badly shaken and frightened by the spectacle. Often they tried heroically to intervene to protect the one parent, usually the mother, and to control the violence.

Some children were co-opted by the demands and threats of the angry parent to engage in activities that they themselves did not condone but felt that they had no choice but to take on the role of the parent's ally. Others believed the paranoid accusations by disturbed parents. But most children, especially older-latency children and young adolescents, joined the alliance willingly. Approximately one-fifth of the 131 children within the California Children of Divorce Study entered the fray actively at the time of the marital breakup on behalf of one parent [8]. For example, Mary, who was 11 years old when her parents separated, was enraged to learn of her father's new girlfriend. Siding with her very angry mother, Mary regularly listened in on the telephone arguments between her parents. She took the initiative in calling her father frequently to shout accusations at him telling him that he was immoral and that he was letting his children starve. Mary loudly denounced her father to neighbors, friends, and teachers at school, telling them all, "I hate my father!"

The Child as Spy
Some parents encourage their children, or sometimes only one child, to provide information about the other parent's activities. Usually, a parent is in search of details regarding the divorcing partner's social or sexual liaisons, although sometimes the interest is in the economic circumstances or life-style of the other parent. Children are requested or ordered to open bureau drawers in the other parent's house, to open closets, to search for the presence of women's lingerie (in their fathers' homes), to report who is present during the visit, and to provide a wide range of information that has no practical usefulness whatsoever for the pressuring parent and that often only burdens the child. Children who are pressed into these espionage services are enjoined from telling the other parent about the information sought and are routinely interrogated and debriefed after each visit.

The cooperation of children with these requests is fairly widespread. Our own findings suggest that over half of the 8- to 12-year-old youngsters in our study rendered such reports to one parent regularly during the first year or more following the marital rupture [9]. The motivation underlying the children's cooperation in assuming the role of spy has its roots in pity for the suffering parent, in fear of punishment if the request is denied, in a wish to keep the peace, in a need to placate the parent, in the child's sense of his or her vulnerability and powerlessness to reject the request, and sometimes in the excitement of the spying role. The complex dynamics that guide the children in their cooperation or refusal is especially evident in families where siblings meet to develop a united stance to withstand the parental pressure and where, as often happens, one child breaks ranks, complies with the adult's request, and is then dubbed a "traitor" by the siblings.

Mrs. A always greeted her four children at the door when they returned from their weekly visit to their father with a torrent of questions about the father's girlfriend, how she looked, what she wore, what the degree of intimacy was between father and the woman, and so on. The older children, led by the 16-year-old boy, met together and decided to lie to their mother and to conceal the presence of the girlfriend during their visit. To their great chagrin, the 8-year-old boy, whom they labeled as a "traitor," always provided the mother with the information that she sought. A few years later when the child was 11 he explained his behavior as follows: "I always felt in the middle and disloyal to both parents, but Mom seemed to me the most hurt and angry. I couldn't stand to see her unhappy so I stuck by her side."

The Child as Messenger
One task that children generally find painful, burdensome, and humiliating is that of carrying messages back and forth between the feuding parents. Although the message itself is usually innocuous, the child feels caught in an awkward role, burdened with being the bearer of an unwelcome request. These children suffer out of all proportion to the significance of the communication. They fear that the message might anger the receiver or that they might incur the wrath of the sender if they forget to deliver the message. Either way, they feel they can only lose. They are especially humiliated in being asked to remind a tardy parent to pay a bill for expenses incurred on their behalf. The child's utter misery in asking a parent to pay for trousers or dental work is usually ignored by both parents.

Richard, at age 10, wrote a school composition entitled "What I Wish For the Most." He wrote, "I wish that my mom and dad would get back together so we could be a happy family. Or if they don't do this, I wish that they wouldn't fight about buying me clothes, like 'you get his pants' and 'you get his shirt.' I hate that!"

Parent-Child Alignments

Sometimes parents and children join in a somewhat strange, close, and enduring divorce-specific alliance to do battle together against the other parent. These powerful alliances or alignments occur most often between the preadolescent child and the parent who angrily opposed the divorce. The adult's participation is almost always rooted in a sense of moral outrage combined with seemingly boundless anger at having been betrayed and cruelly exploited for so many years. Thus, women who had worked to support their husbands' professional education only to find themselves rejected for a younger woman are likely to turn to their children as allies. Or men who feel rejected by their wives' interest in another man seek the help of their children to inflict punishment. The avowed agenda of these alignments is likely to be the restoration of the failing marriage; the unspoken agenda is almost always revenge.

It is always difficult to discuss such involvement with the participants. The adults are likely to deny their participation and to insist that the children are acting on their own. For example, one mother, in response to our futile efforts to diminish her pressure on her son in his numerous efforts to involve the father in serious legal difficulties (the boy was reporting regularly to the mother's attorney regarding the father's drug intake), denied her own role in this mischief. She told us, "I'm a good Christian woman. I never get angry. But my son," she added ominously, "will never forgive nor forget." It is equally difficult to discuss this relationship with the children since they are likely to respond as spokespeople for the adults in a language that is often stilted, moralistic, and unchildlike. The extreme identification of these youngsters with the parent and their views of themselves as representing that parent not only make it almost impossible to talk to them, but often lead the older youngsters to exercise a strict censorship to keep their younger siblings from talking candidly as well.

These anger-driven alliances and mutual identifications serve a range of psychological purposes for both parent and child. The loneliness of the divorce period for parent and child is reduced significantly by the new partnership. The child's fear of being abandoned is alleviated by establishing him- or herself as a trusty companion. The direction of the anger outward against the opposite parent serves as a powerful antidote to the intolerably painful feelings of rejection and helplessness that both child and parent experience. Nor is it accidental that many children join cause with a parent with whom their relationship during the marriage had been tenuous or emotionally impoverished and take up an angry campaign against the parent who earlier had been cherished and loved.

Additionally, for the child, the parent-child alignment provides the opportunity for a splitting of the ambivalence in the relationship with the parents and the creation of a convenient, clear repository of virtue and villainy. This anger at one parent is often sanctioned and openly encouraged by the remaining parent and even supported by a moral stance befitting a religious war.

Not surprisingly, our findings indicate that children and adults who join in these endeavors are less psychologically stable than siblings who refuse to do so and adults who refrain from encouraging their children to act out the angers of the divorce. Youngsters who participate are more likely to be distressed and frightened at the time of the separation, to feel their position to be especially tenuous, and to be vulnerable, as we have noted earlier, to parental blandishments. Additionally, children who are emotionally hungry from many years of parental neglect find the one parent's attention dazzling and irresistible. There is, thus, little question that many of these children enjoy the role into which they are newly cast. They are loyal, resourceful, and valuable in their capacity to act out the parent's strategy. They are also able to inflict considerable psychological suffering on the parent whom they attack.

Although we have too little information regarding how long such alliances endure, our evidence is that they do not last past the youngster's adolescence. An example from our own longitudinal study reflects the shame that youngsters experience in later years regarding their behavior at the time of the breakup when they had attacked a parent they had previously loved dearly.

Mrs. J, a mother of four children, filed for divorce after many years of marital unhappiness marked by her husband's frequent absences, drug taking, alcoholism, and occasional agitated, depressive episodes. She had been a devoted mother who had provided economic and emotional support for her children at great personal sacrifice. The relationship between the children and their mother had been tender and loving during the marriage.

When Mrs. J filed for divorce, Mr. J did not object until he heard that his divorcing wife was involved in a relationship with a man. At that time he became enraged and successfully courted his children, enlisting them in an all-out assault on their mother, which continued for almost a year. Under their father's continued coaching, the children, ages 12, 11, 9, and 8, turned on their mother with great anger, calling her "a whore, acting like a teenager, wearing her skirts too short." The children angrily proclaimed, "She has fallen. She's a hippie. She doesn't care at all about her children." The children insisted further that they wished to remain in their father's custody and that they would not have anything to do with their mother. Needless to say the woman was astonished and heartsick. Eventually she was awarded custody of the children largely because the father lacked the emotional and financial resources to sustain his claim in court. At that time the children protested bitterly, stating that they would not live with their mother and that she represented a corrupt influence on their lives.

Five years later we interviewed Ruth, age 16. Looking back over those years she expressed her profound appreciation for her mother's devotion and her recognition that her mother had raised the children single-handedly after many years of struggle amidst poverty. Ruth recalled vividly her own alignment with her father. She said, "I don't want to make my dad sound rotten, but he was very persuasive. I'm really ashamed to tell you how my father brainwashed us. We were terrible to my mom. I'm still surprised that she was so willing to keep us after all that we said and did to her."

Medea: Vengeance Through the Children

The use of the children as the instrument of revenge is given its most savage expression in the myth of Medea, which represents the destruction of the children by their mother within the context of the husband's adultery and departure from the marriage. The particular confluence of historic factors and feelings that led Medea to the destruction of her children is worth noting. Whenever similar experiences and feelings converge within the divorcing family, the children and the children's relationship with the opposite parent are psychologically at very high risk.

We may recall that Medea was the princess who employed her witchcraft to betray her father and her own country in order to aid the Greek hero Jason to obtain the golden fleece, which was the quest that had brought him to her land. Following his victory, Jason took Medea with him to his home across the sea where they married. After Medea had borne him two children, Jason tired of her and turned his affection to a younger woman. Recognizing that Jason no longer desired her, Medea concluded, perhaps accurately, that since he no longer needed her she was being cast aside. She concluded further that Jason had exploited her shamelessly as a stepping stone to his success and that her suicide might provide him with a welcome removal of herself as an obstacle to his new marriage. In an uncontrollable, probably psychotic, rage and profound despair she murdered her children. In so doing she achieved the horrible revenge that she sought. She succeeded in wounding Jason in the cruelest way available to her. In the same act she symbolically destroyed the marriage in its entirety, including its history, by erasing the only products of their union. Finally, she triumphed in overcoming her sense of having been helplessly trapped by recapturing her earlier power (and perhaps her earlier magic) in the symbolic murder of her husband and herself via the destruction of the children. Her own punishment is also implicit in her terrible revenge since there are several implications in the story that she was a loving parent and that her children trusted her.

The central components in Medea's experience and macabre behavior are not unique to Medea or to women. The sense of moral outrage, of having been cruelly exploited, and of having been rendered helpless within the context of betrayal and sexual jealousy give rise to intolerable feelings and set off a towering rage that has an extraordinary destructive power. Women or men, despairing of any other course, have been driven to seek revenge; threats of murder of oneself and one's spouse together with the children occur often enough and are periodically enacted in contemporary society. More often, men and women alike have sought to destroy not the children but the other partner's relationship with the children by depriving him or her of access to them.

A significant portion of the cases that are repeatedly brought to litigation, which exhaust the family resources and impoverish adults and children, have their psychological roots in these dynamics. Similarly, the psychological motivation of those who perpetrate child snatching, in which one parent steals the child from the legal custody of the other and escapes into a foreign country or goes into hiding (variously estimated at 100,000 children a year), is often akin to that of Medea in the despair, helpless rage, and the wish for revenge that the perpetrator experiences. Our findings are that the intense angers rooted in Medea-like psychodynamics have an extraordinary capacity to remain undimmed by the passage of time. Such consuming angers, because they are long lasting even when not acted out, may indeed psychologically, although not physically, consume the children by terrifying them over many years.

The Child as Peer and as Helper
Many marriages that are failing in some important regard have nonetheless successfully contributed to the economic, social, or psychological well-being of the marital partners. Even a conflicted marriage may have provided a modicum of security, a stable household, and a sense of shared responsibility and protection. Or, perhaps, even more profoundly, the

unhappy marriage may still have provided for a mutual dependency, a shared identity, and most of all, from the perspective of the child, a coparenting relationship that enabled each parent to complement and buffer the other in the many complex full-time tasks that parenting demands.

The falling away of customary supports within the marriage, combined with the humiliation of the narcissistic injury inflicted by the divorce and the painful persistence of attachment to the divorcing partner [11], is likely to result in severe ego regressions in adults whose customary functioning separately or together may have been adequate or even very good. Feeling suddenly alone and in need of help, many parents turn to their children for sympathetic understanding and support at this critical time. And many children respond to their parent's need with sensitivity and profound caring and come directly and forthrightly to their parent's aid. The emotional dependence of the adult on the child, the turning toward the child as to a peer, and the counterresponse of the child to the adult (also as to a peer) is an expectable divorce-specific change in parent-child relationships.

At the simplest level, the custodial parent relies heavily on the competent child, especially the older child and the adolescent, to participate actively in the household and in the decision making of daily living; young people work hard and long, and their contributions are substantial. As parents and children join to deal with the problems and routines of life, they are brought together in new ways that directly help the parent and also promote emotional, psychological, and intellectual growth in the child. One of the more moving aspects of the divorce experience is the fact that as parents turn to their children for advice, solace, friendship, and nurturant care, boys and girls move into the breach in a variety of unaccustomed ways to support and maintain the parent, to allay anxiety, and to take care of the parent. Often the child's response has a far-reaching effect on the parent. The child who provides comfort and real aid to a distressed parent is able to speed the recovery process within the entire family. Many youngsters are proud of their new competence and independence and take their new role in the family very seriously. As one 14-year-old noted gravely, "I have to be very careful in what I do. I want to help my mother, and I also have to set a very good example for my younger sisters."

Perhaps the empathic response that is catalyzed by the custodial parent's crisis is most striking in its appearance among young girls who are just approaching adolescence. Dejected mothers are cared for tenderly by children who are able to follow their moods with great sensitivity and to respond with maturity and tact well beyond their years. These young-sters are helpful in stabilizing parent's moods and in anchoring them to the here and now. They intuitively seem to be aware of the parent's depression and to attempt within the limits of their understanding not to overtax the parent or even to protect that parent from pressure. Women have told us many years after a divorce, "I would not have made it except for this child." We have earlier described the development of empathy in status nascendi in the remarks of Ann, age 10, who with unusual insight described her capacity to identify with her mother [9]. She said, "I know that my mother wasn't really ready for the divorce because I put myself in her place. I can think just like my mother thinks." Ann's mother, in turn, told us that Ann was wonderful in her wordless response to the mother's changing moods. "She knows inside when I'm lonely," said her mother [9].

It should be noted, however, that a significant group of adolescents, as we learned at our study's 10-year follow-up, were resentful of having to take on so much responsibility at the time of the breakup and during the years that followed. Regarding the divorce as a voluntary decision of the parents, these youngsters felt that they had been forced to bear the brunt of their parents' mistaken marriage and that they were unjustly required to take responsibility at home for disturbed or incompetent parents or for parents who themselves enjoyed an active social and sexual life. A signifi-cant number of these young people expressed anger at their parents because they, the children, had had to give up so much of their own childhood and adolescence, including irreplaceable playtime and school-time, in order to care for their parents and younger children and to assure the continuity of the household. Others deplored the lack of supervision and support from parents, especially during crucial adolescent years. Mary, age 16, told us, "My house was always empty. That's how I got into all that trouble with sex and hash." By and large, these resentments, which surfaced years later, were not expressed easily or openly at the height of the divorce crisis [6].

In the most adaptive situations, the relationship that developed be-tween parent and child at the time of the marital rupture and during its aftermath reflected a peerlike quality in its mutual decision making and in its sharing of concern and the responsibilities of daily living. The more visible emotional strands are those of friendship and compassion for the parent and the pride that the young people take in the independence conferred by their new role within the family. The underside of these relationships is the young person's resentment and longing for the bene-fits that they associate, sometimes unrealistically, with the intact family.

All of these complex feelings and conflicts join with, reinforce, and intensify the phase-specific interactions of child and parent as these unfold within the divorced family over the years.

Role Reversal and the Overburdened Child

A major hazard that divorce poses to the psychic integrity of the child is the multifaceted dependency of the severely distressed, regressed parent. In some of these intense relationships, which characteristically grow at the time of the marital rupture, the adult requirements on the child extend far beyond the customary parameters of the normal parent-child relationship. Often there are compelling, anxiety-driven needs that are not met just by the willing and generous enhanced participation of the child in household chores or decision making or by the new kindness and gentleness of the concerned empathic child.

It is not uncommon in these singular relationships for the distressed and lonely parent to turn inappropriately to the child to meet a wide range of urgent psychological and social needs during the acute phase of the divorcing process. Often the adult utterly fails to recognize the unreality of these expectations. Nor does the adult who may have a history of reasonably adequate or even sensitive parenting prior to the divorce seem able at this juncture to perceive the emotional burdening of his or her child, which occurs within these coercive relationships, or to connect the symptoms that the child soon develops as expectable responses to the parental pressures. While it is striking and poignantly moving to note the amazing capacity of young children to respond, at least verbally, to the parental need for help, to resonate to the parent's moods, and to feel responsible for the care of the parent, it should be noted that these relationships are also likely to be seriously detrimental to the children's well-being and further development and are often associated with the appearance of moderate to severe depression in children.

The expectation that the young child who never before took responsibility for his or her own physical care should not only take responsibility for him- or herself but, in addition, should provide some measure of support for the distressed parent is sufficiently widespread to be considered a divorce-specific response. It may well be, of course, that children within intact families are more supportive of their parents than we have recognized and provide more emotional nurturance to parents at critical times than we usually have been willing to perceive. Nevertheless, it remains startling to learn that Sammy, at age 4, comforted his grieving mother whose lover had just left saying, "He should not quit in the middle. That's not right." Or to learn from Mrs. B that she discussed all of her problems with her 6-year-old child because "he understands everything. He told me I should not marry now." Or to hear from Dr. C that his 6-year-old is "psychic" and "understands everything with the sensitivity of an adult."

The needs that are thrust on young children at this time with force and urgency have their roots in the complex interactions of the marriage, which, despite its failure, had been successful in meeting at least some of the parent's ongoing needs or in alleviating at least some of the myriad of anxieties that arise in the course of daily living. These needs are suddenly uncovered as the marital relationship ruptures, and the associated anxiety that then erupts is often overwhelming. Thus, although lacking in love and fidelity, a significant number of marital relationships provide one or both partners with an external structure that helps to govern their lives. This external structure is not only relevant to the ongoing routines of daily life but has significant ramifications and implications within the intrapsychic functioning of the adult as well and may provide a major support for the adult's sense of his or her adulthood. Indeed, following the marital breakup it becomes common for the divorcing adult to be preoccupied with issues of identity and with anxious questions regarding who he or she is separate from the other and separate from the marital structure. Those with greater strength and emotional resources seek redefinition successfully and reestablish themselves with a sense of renewal and perhaps an enhanced sense of self. For others, the separation may be experienced as an amputation and may pose a threat to their overall psychic integrity.

Furthermore, the presence of another adult, however unloving or unloved, can still serve significantly to protect against the real dangers of living alone and the fantasy dangers of being alone, whether alone in the house or alone in the world. This presence of the other disappears with the dissolution of the marriage. Newly divorced men and women alike report intensified fears of being alone. Many adults master these anxieties successfully. For a certain number, however, these anxieties, which were in abeyance during the marriage, are now overwhelming and threaten the adult at every turn.

All of these needs and many others in the absence of the marital partner or an available adult relationship are likely to be brought to the child. The particular demands on the child vary with the psychological condition of the individual parent, the degree of regression and deterioration of functioning, the specific emotional toll of the divorce, and the availability of other adult sources of support. The very presence of the child has the power to stave off the dangers of loneliness and aloneness and to reduce the terrors of abandonment. Similarly, the child's presence has the power to reinforce the reality of the external world and to mute suicidal preoccupations, which are not uncommon at this time, by providing an external presence that gives structure, emphasis, and continuity to the day.

One common expression of the reliance of the parent on the child is evident in the number of parents who seem unable to separate from their children, especially at night. Young children are kept home from school during the days that the parent needs their presence. They stay up late frequently to watch television with a lonely parent. They are regularly brought into the parent's bed at night. However, when the parent decides to spend the night with a lover, the child is requested to sleep in his or her own bed. Young children accompany their parents to adult parties and to adult social events. They are taken into their parents' full confidence. The child who is cast into this role is often young, far too young to understand the complexities of the issues that the parent sets before him or her. It is not unusual for such a relationship to occur primarily with an only child. Perhaps the young child and the only child are singularly able to provide the uncritical love, the uncritical approval, the unconditional acceptance, and the unconditional overall set of confirming responses that the adult requires at this time. Perhaps it is also the young child who is most vulnerable and helpless and unable to seek other options and is thus most malleable in the face of a parent's need. And perhaps finally, in the parental regression, it may be the very young child to whom the parent can most readily relate as a coequal during the crisis.

THE CHILD AS CONCUBINE. The dependence of the child on the parent and the many acute needs of the parent sometimes lead to a parent-child configuration in which the child is perceived almost entirely by the parent as present to minister to the parent's needs, howsoever these may arise. In many regards the role of the child in these relationships is that of concubine, although there is no necessary sexual component to these relationships. Nevertheless, the central core is the child's total subservience in catering to the parent's needs and whims.

Mrs. M divorced her husband of 10 years after several years of drinking and drug taking by both parents. The marriage followed an exciting love affair that lasted several years before being brought to an abrupt end. The only child of the marriage was Gail, who was 8 years old at the time of separation. At the time of the divorce Mrs. M was drinking heavily and was depressed. Following the marital separation, Mrs. M began to take her daughter Gail to adult parties and other adult social activities. Commenting on this, the mother noted in a stilted manner, "I want to make my daughter happy by taking her to be with better people and to find our way and our enjoyment together." The pattern of relationship that emerged was that Gail was kept home from school when her mother needed companionship; she was kept up late, as well, when her mother wanted her present; she shared her mother's bed when her mother wished her to do so; she was the victim of her mother's violence and was occasionally beaten with a stick when the mother became angry; at times she was her mother's drinking companion and occasionally suffered with hangovers. Gail, in turn, advised her mother when to go out and whom to date and whether or not the mother should make love. The mother withheld Gail from seeing her father whenever the mother felt so inclined although the child had no other stable relationship and yearned intensely to visit with her father.

In our assessment, Gail presented herself as a child who smiled a lot, pretended to be silly, liked to clown, and entered into a variety of different roles with relative ease. She emphatically denied any unhappiness. Gradually she emerged as a very frightened, depressed youngster, preoccupied with fears of abandonment and suffering with many disabling symptoms including severe night terrors, chronic constipation, social isolation, and poor learning.

During the failing marriage, the relationships within this family were different from their course following the separation. The relationship between the two adults had served to buffer Gail and to deflect the mother's needs from falling entirely on the child. Subsequent to the divorce, the isolation of the mother and her deterioration led to the extraordinary burdening of this young child and to the serious deterioration in Gail's psychological health and development.

Thus, as is demonstrated with the preceding example, the need for the child is greatly intensified as the child acquires new psychological meaning within the context of the far-ranging and devastating impact of the divorce itself. The adult who is rejected by the marital partner feels unloved and needs desperately to be reassured that he or she is lovable. The child, perhaps, especially the young child, is able to provide this assurance. The adult who has been displaced by a lover feels humiliated and needs to be highly valued; the child is able to repair the parent's damaged self-esteem. The adult who has left the marriage to pursue another lover or a career feels guilty of having betrayed the marriage, the child, or the values by which he or she was raised and needs to be assured that he or she acted virtuously or out of necessity. For reasons that are not completely self-evident, the child has an extraordinary capacity to grant indulgences, to forgive, and to help the parent feel like a good person. The parent who has left or is leaving the marriage feels unneeded. There are few relationships as responsive to the wish to feel needed as that provided by the young child. Extended fights over custody are often rooted in this intense need by each parent for the child's presence.

The characteristics of the parent in these relationships is that he or she is likely to be highly stressed by a divorce that he or she did not expect or desire and to be regressed, socially isolated, depressed, anxious, and angry. Sometimes the parent may organize around a core of anger at the opposite parent in order to stave off the threatened regression. Sometimes the parent is deteriorated or agitated. A common denominator in the psychological functioning of these parents appears to be an impaired reality testing, especially as reflected in the adult's capacity to judge the behavior of the marital partner or to judge the child realistically or appropriately. It is almost as if the breakup in the marital relationship affects the nature of the object relationships that the very distressed parent can maintain, so that the former spouse and child take on new faces and distorted meanings that derive sometimes almost entirely from the intensified inner needs of the regressed parent. At its most extreme, ego boundaries between parent and child can be eroded, and the parent becomes unable to distinguish him- or herself from the child.

THE CHILD AS ADULT. In some instances the impairment in the parent's reality testing regarding the child emerges with startling clarity. For example, Jay is 3½ years old, and his father (who sought the divorce) is a competent and successful young businessman. Jay's father assured us that he talks to the boy "eye to eye and man to man. I explain everything to him. He is very important to me, more important than anyone else in the world. He takes 99 percent of my love and attention." Typically father and son spend their three-day weekends together in a busy round of adult activities that include drinking parties, adult sports events, and a range of activities with the father's adult friends. Father and son sleep together in the same bed. The father makes extraordinary demands on the child, not only for participating in the full-scale adult schedule, but for behaving appropriately and responding to the father's long, dramatic conversations with him about the present and future.

In our assessment, Jay appeared a very troubled, intensely anxious, almost phobic child. His social and emotional development was below an age-appropriate level. His play was dominated with fantasies of death and of being run over by a truck. One prominent fantasy was that of a little boy and a father, both of whom were dying. During his play the child excitedly placed a nude father doll in bed with a little boy doll.

THE CHILD AS MENTOR. Sometimes the young child appears able to take a directive role in relation to the needy parent and to instruct the parent regarding his or her behavior. For example, Helen, age 8, gently admonished her mother, who was apathetic and depressed following the marital separation. "Mom," said the child, "you know when a baby is born he can't even talk. All a baby can say is baby talk like ga-ga- or goo-goo. Well," said the child, "you understand very well what the word *no* means, and you can talk, but you're not used to saying no, and you can't use it." Or Jimmy, at age 6, was distressed because following his parents' separation his father took him to the movies constantly during their visits together. Jimmy asked us to tell his father that the movies were poorly selected. He added that he is worried about his father. Jimmy thinks his father takes him to the movies because he, the father, is unable to talk about the sad events in the family.

In a true sense the adulthood that is a prerequisite for competent parenthood is shaken in a significant number of adults by the impact of the divorce and the destruction of the marriage. In these families, the regression in the adult's capacity to parent reaches far beyond the temporary diminution that we have described. Instead the child is perceived and responded to primarily in terms of the urgency of the adult's need as the replacement for the departed parent and as a needed self-object. In effect, for a significant group of parents, the capacity to maintain a true object relationship with the child is diminished at this time, and during this crisis the child serves as the kind of powerful self-object that the distressed parent at least temporarily requires. It may well be that the distinctness of the normal parent-child relationship has a greater vulnerability to the vicissitudes of the parent's capacity to maintain his or her separate adulthood at the time of the divorce crisis. Moreover, it appears that psychic separateness between parent and child may give way more easily than in other relationships.

The periods in which parents utilize young children in such ways are likely to be of relatively short duration and occur primarily during the acute phase of the divorce (during the year or two following the marital breakup). They tend to terminate when the parent has successfully been able to establish a significant tie with another adult. Sometimes, at that time, they terminate abruptly. The child may then feel cast away and suddenly ejected from the central position that he or she has held in the parent's emotional orbit. In this sense the plight of the child is not necessarily eased when the singular needy relationship comes to an end.

Nevertheless, the primary function of these relationships is not at all related to the child's needs but provides emergency assistance to the adult and is developed to facilitate the transition from the loss of the marital relationship and the marital structure to another adult relationship. When the adult experiences difficulty in making this transition, as many do, or when the new relationship also fails, the reliance on the child for the maintenance of emotional integrity may continue for several years, and the intensity of this close dyadic relationship may also continue during this extended period.

For their part, children involved in these relationships are characteristically sober, usually mature for their age, verbal, and sensitive. When there has been a selection, children are likely to be selected for this role because of their sensitivity, their vulnerability, and their love and pity for, as well as their fear of the adult. These relationships, of course, place children at high risk. The children that we have observed in them have been wretched and frightened. They are depleted and threatened by the many changes in their own lives and by the drastically changed face of the caretaking adult. They feel that they have no independence and that they must share the feelings of the adult as they shoulder the responsibility placed on them to maintain the parent's functioning, to restore the parent, and sometimes to restore the marriage. They are likely to show a range of severe symptoms that, not surprisingly, include grave developmental difficulties in learning and in adjusting to friends. Our clinical experience also suggests that distressing somatic symptoms are not unusual in this group.

The Visiting Relationship
Perhaps the most difficult and challenging psychological task for parent and child within the postdivorce family is to transplant the parent-child relationship that developed within the rich soil of family life into the strange, relatively impoverished, and very limited ground that the visit provides. It is no surprise that a great many parent-child relationships fail to survive the shock of the move and fail additionally to take root outside the family. What is surprising is that many parent-child relationships that were failing within the structure of the marriage take on new life and growth within the narrow constraints of the visit [10].

The visiting relationship is a new relationship that is created at the time of the marital rupture and has no true counterpart within the intact family. The processes by which this new relationship is established and maintained are complex, and the many difficulties that attach to this relationship have been insufficiently acknowledged by clinicians, as well as by the divorcing families themselves. Yet, our findings point very strongly to the fact that the mastery of the part-time parent–part-time child relationship is critical to the continued psychological development and self-esteem of both child and parent [4].

At the time of the marital rupture and for many years thereafter, children and adolescents are preoccupied with the many dimensions of the visit. The questions that concern the children are myriad. Will the visiting parent arrive? Will he or she arrive on time as promised? Will the custodial parent allow the child to go freely and to enjoy the visit? Will there be other people present at the noncustodial parent's home, and if so, who will they be and what will their relationship be to the parents? Where will the child sleep? Will the parent be attentive or distracted, fresh or fatigued, interested or bored, pleasant or angry? Will the visit be interesting or boring? Will it be too short or too long? Additionally, for girls, especially young adolescents, anxieties associated with erotic fantasies because of the "datelike" nature of the visits are ubiquitous. All of these questions represent the most common concerns that loom very large in the child's mind, often preempting the child's thoughts during the intervals between the visits.

Similarly, parents are preoccupied with obstacles that also loom large because of their very heavy emotional loading. The visit usually requires a return of the departed parent to the family residence, a brief meeting between the adults, and some modicum of verbal interchange and cooperation around the logistics of the visit. Often such brief meetings at the threshold during the visit lead the adult to reexperience intensely the hopes and dreams of the marriage combined with the angers, the disappointments, and the sorrows of the divorce. For many people such meetings engender intolerable distress. Additionally, the visit, at its minimum, demands that both adults accommodate to the other's needs and wishes, as well as to the needs and wishes of the child, and often to the needs and wishes of more than one child. The arrangements that are the routine, although sometimes complex, adjustments of life within the intact family pose seemingly insurmountable obstacles for the divorcing family in which the expectation of continuity, cooperation, and accommodation to the other person has been profoundly disrupted. Not surprisingly, the visit can be a major source of conflict.

As a result, many children regard the visit with terror — a crossing of a no man's or no child's land. They wait anxiously and restlessly at the window for the visiting parent to arrive, and they return with a mixture of relief and anxiety wondering about the reception that they will encounter. Nevertheless, children cling to these visits with great devotion and often regard the visit as the high point of their week, month, or year. From the child's perspective, contact with the visiting parent is a central strand in his or her self-concept. With the exception of a few children who reject their parents either by themselves or in alignment with the one parent, children not only prize the visits but feel rejected and abandoned when the visiting parent does not appear. The sense of profound loss, the feelings of being rejected, and the implications for being unlovable that the rejection conveys to the child are not likely, in our observation, to be mastered during the child's growing up years, except perhaps in prolonged psychotherapy.

The tensions that are stirred by the visit are likely to diminish over time in most families. What remains, however, for parent and child is the formidable task of building a meaningful relationship within the narrow constraints of the visiting contact. For many adults this represents a task that is very difficult to achieve, and they soon become discouraged and yield to the impulse to stay away. Many adults, especially those who have been rejected by the marital partner, become depressed not only at returning to the family residence but at each successive separation from the children. Eventually they restrict their visiting or give it up altogether. Others, feeling guilty at having left, find that each visit with the children renews and sharpens their guilt, especially if the children have been left in the care of a distressed or inept parent. Still others, men who remarry women with children or have new children within the remarriage, find that they have difficulty in maintaining an emotional commitment to both sets of children. As time goes by they turn increasingly to the children with whom they reside and relinquish their emotional investment in the children from the earlier marriage [9].

A recent survey of a national sample of children between the ages of 11 and 16 in divorced families reported that close to one-half of the children had no contact with their outside parent (customarily the father) during the preceding 5 years [2]. In our own work where we have made a brief, concerted effort to help fathers maintain their visits to children and have addressed practical issues, as well as the father's depression or anger, only 10 percent had no contact with their children at the 5-year mark, and almost all had some contact with their children during the preceding 5 years [9]; over one-third of the fathers and children were able to create and maintain an emotionally nurturant relationship that held firm during the 5 years following the divorce and represented a continuing strong influence in their lives.

The pattern and form of the visiting relationship vary widely. Many visiting relationships enhance the child's development; some may reinforce an infantile attachment. One of the grave hazards is the propensity of the visiting relationship to remain fixated at the developmental level of the child at the time of the separation and to resist change in response to the child's growth. For example, one 8-year-old child continued to sit on her father's lap at dinner as she had done at the time when the marriage broke up when she was 4 years old. Only her stepmother recognized the extraordinary inappropriateness of this behavior for both father and child. Youngsters often have difficulty communicating their changing needs and wishes, and adults may be reluctant to acknowledge the passage of time. Other hazards include the intense, unrealistic idealization of the visiting parent or the eroticization of the visiting relationship so that it becomes a rendezvous that father and child look forward to with rising excitement as the peak activity in their schedule. One deplorable visiting pattern is the exploitation of the child by the visiting parent where the child is required to undertake tedious, time-consuming chores throughout the entire visit. Such children essentially work hard to earn the child support that is their due.

The parent-child relationship that successfully transplants to the confines of the visitation does not reflect continuity with relationships within the earlier intact family. There is, in fact, no correlation between the visiting pattern postdivorce and the father-child relationship within the marriage [10]. Moreover, the relationship between the parents and the amount of conflict between the parents, although powerful influences at the outset, have little impact on the visiting patterns that evolve over time. Success and failure rest primarily on the commitment of the visiting parent and the children to each other and their capacity to reinforce this commitment with gratifications within the relationship that outweigh the inherent difficulties and frustrations.

There is no other family relationship that depends so heavily on voluntary part-time association; that needs to adapt so flexibly to the changing developing needs, aspirations, and goals of the child and the parent; and that needs to withstand the impact and the inevitable frustrations and resentments that arise in the course of the youngster's growing up years. Therefore, when the visiting relationship works out happily and successfully for child and parent, it takes on special significance for both.

Conclusion

The long-standing issues of dependence and independence, love and hate, and separation and individuation that are woven into the continuing fabric of all parent-child relationships are importantly redefined by marital rupture. In calling attention to the major currents and crosscurrents set off by the marital rupture, I have suggested that divorce separates parents and children, that parents experience a diminished capacity to parent at this critical time, and that this diminished capacity not infrequently hides an impulse to abandon the child. These behaviors and feelings in the parent find their counterpart in the child's steeply rising anxiety and sense of powerlessness, which render the child more vulnerable to the parent's conscious and unconscious demands. I have suggested further that parents and children also come much closer together at this time in new mutually dependent ways as peers, sympathetic friends, comrades, and sometimes allies in the battle against the other parent, and that parents turn to their children for the help that they need at this critical time in their lives, fully expecting the child to stand temporarily in the needed role. Sometimes, like Medea of ancient history, they even use their children as instruments of revenge.

I have suggested that parents and children develop singular relationships at this time in which the hapless child is expected by the regressed adult to assume the role of parent, mentor, confidant, lover, or concubine — as the "other" whose very presence deters loneliness, depression, and ultimately prevents ego disintegration. Moreover, it appears that these overburdened young children attempt bravely, if pathetically, to move into the expected roles. And, finally, I have delineated the visiting role as an entirely new undertaking that has no counterpart within the intact family and that challenges both parent and child to create and maintain a meaningful parent-child relationship outside of the family structure.

Unlike the disturbed parent-child relationships of child abuse or incest, many of the divorce-induced changes that I have described do not represent a minority or a deviant group, but rather an expectable response that can be considered a general, divorce-specific response to the disorganizing crisis of the marital rupture and its aftermath. In most families the lapses in parenting are time-limited, and the adult will recover his or her earlier capacity to parent when the acute stage of the divorce comes to an end, usually within 2 years of the marital rupture. When the parents are more profoundly troubled and the stress level remains high, the singular parent-child relationships that arise at the time of the marital crisis may endure for many years.

It may be, as we have suggested, that the feelings and behaviors that emerge at this time are part and parcel of parent-child relationships within the intact family where, carefully constrained by the presence of the other parent and by the network of family relationships, they remain hidden from view. What clearly emerges is the extraordinary potential of the parent-child relationship to take a great many forms and to stretch to accommodate to the acute psychological needs and requirements of the adults as well as to the anxiety and genuine concern of the children, as these are modified under the powerful impact of radical family change.

Acknowledgment

This work has been supported by a grant from the San Francisco Foundation and the Zellerbach Family Fund.

References

1. Freud, A. *Difficulties in the Path of Psychoanalysis.* New York: International Universities Press, 1969.
2. Furstenberg, F. F., Jr. Parenting Apart: Patterns of Child Rearing After Divorce. Paper presented at the American Sociological Association, San Francisco, 1982.
3. Hetherington, E. M., Cox, M., and Cox, R. The Aftermath of Divorce. In J. H. Stevens, Jr. and M. Mathews (Eds.), *Mother-Child Relations.* Washington, D.C.: National Association for the Education of Young Children, 1978.
4. Kelly, J. B., and Wallerstein, J. S. Part-time parent, part-time child: Visiting after divorce. *J. Clin. Child. Psychol.* 6:51, 1977.
5. Wallerstein, J. S. Children of Divorce: Stress and Developmental Tasks. In N. Garmezy and M. Rutter (Eds.), *Stress, Coping and Development in Children.* New York: McGraw-Hill, 1983.
6. Wallerstein, J. S. Children of divorce: Preliminary report from a 10-year follow-up. *J. Am. Acad. Child Psychiatry,* in press.
7. Wallerstein, J. S., and Kelly, J. B. The effects of parental divorce: Experiences of the preschool child. *J. Am. Acad. Child Psychiatry* 14:600, 1975.
8. Wallerstein, J. S., and Kelly, J. B. The effects of parental divorce: Experiences of the child in later latency. *Am. J. Orthopsychiatry* 46:600, 1976.
9. Wallerstein, J. S., and Kelly, J. B. *Surviving the Breakup: How Children and Parents Cope With Divorce.* New York: Basic Books, 1980.
10. Wallerstein, J. S., and Kelly, J. B. Effects of divorce on the father-child relationship. *Am. J. Psychiatry* 137:1534, 1980.
11. Weiss, R. S. *Marital Separation.* New York: Basic Books, 1975.

10

Abandoning parents and abusing caretakers

George H. Pollock

The dread of abandonment, particularly intense in childhood, is an almost basic universal fear. Although its form and shape may change during the life course, the fundamental elements remain quite constant. Initially the focus is on external presence or absence of the protective, familiar, loving parent—especially the mother. This, too, remains a presence throughout the life course, becoming especially intense in old age when one is helpless, relatively out of control, and very dependent on others for nourishment, safety, companionship, and reality testing. When one is physically or emotionally ill, we may again see the emergence of this dread of abandonment. The familiar takes on reassuring significance that one may take for granted under other circumstances.

When an actual abandonment has occurred, the dread has become an actuality and many traumatic and pathogenic consequences can occur. To be certain, there are many variables that contribute to either the muting or accentuation of the reactions, but reactions do occur even without obvious pathogenic consequences. In my analytic work with adults who were adopted at birth, some of the most painful affect revivals center around the confrontation of "Why did my real mother give me up?" The actual abandonment, even though adoptive parents are loving, kind, and benevolent, still raises questions in the mind of the adopted individual. In another type of situation, an individual who miraculously survived Nazi concentration camp horrors told of the total abandonment he felt—by his country of origin (not Germany), by his family (although they all perished in the Holocaust), by his co-religionists, by his God, and by humanity. A sense of total aloneness and isolation, so traumatic in the reality sense, did revive abandonment fears from his earlier childhood and adolescent years.

A distinction should be made at the outset that abandonment is not the same as, though related to, the loss of love, loss of esteem, or the loss of reality pleasures. In similar fashion, it is also to be distinguished from, although intimately related to, separation anxiety, which can occur in

This work was, in part, supported by the Anne Pollock Lederer Research Fund of the Chicago Institute for Psychoanalysis.

349

many forms and situations, and loss of support. Finally, one should differentiate those situations where actual abandonment or desertion did occur from fears and anxieties about abandonment where the desertion did not occur in reality. Clinically, one sees the latter situation in instances of the depressed mother and/or father where the child constantly fears the parent will leave or commit suicide. The former situation is found in those tragedies where suicide actually did occur and the child feels betrayed, abandoned, and deserted. This situation, with which many clinicians have had contact, is related to but different from the reactions of children and adolescents where there has been the loss of a parent through death other than suicide.

The reactions of children whose parents have divorced evokes fantasies of parental abandonment, which indeed does occur, although reality says otherwise. The reactions of adults whose parents divorced when they were children is closer to the situation described above where actual and complete desertion did not take place. Finally, we have at times worked with adults whose parents were absent for long periods during their childhood because of institutionalization for illness, incarceration for legal transgressions, or because of military or civilian duty overseas. Again, we find similarities in all of these situations; however, the critical differences are crucial in understanding the pivotal effects of what the child feels is desertion and abandonment. When other family members (e.g., a parent, siblings, grandparents) are able to maintain some semblance of integrity, support may help in the alleviation of the trauma. In some clinical instances, I have found that the traumatic effects of the abandonment are still present in the adult, but they are less contributory to the pathogenic process than when no other family member is available to provide support.

Anna Freud [12] observed during wartime that young children preferred remaining with their mothers in London, even though there was a great deal of external danger and tension, to going to the country where things were peaceful, but without their mothers. I believe that this "abandonment anxiety" is more precise than the use of the term "separation," which covers many situations. And in the movie "John, 17 Months" by Robertson [27], we see very movingly the impact of a sudden, temporary abandonment of this child and the progressive deterioration in his psychological and social adaptation as a result of this situation. In a most vivid scene at the end of the film account where the child and mother come together, one can see the fear, rage, and disappointment that the child has toward the mother.

We must closely examine the actual meanings of terms such as "separation anxiety," "loss of love," "abandonment," and "desertion" if they are to be of ongoing value. Parenthood has many dimensions — a child and his or her parent or parents may feel unloving on different occasions, but the basic feeling of trust, confidence, and deep affection allows this affective-traumatic state to pass without serious consequence. Actual desertion, physical and emotional abuse, and abandonment have different consequences, especially if they are long lasting, permanent, and persistent. The child's fear of abandonment is no longer a fantasy when accompanied by the reality, but it is an actuality — a basic rejection allied to the most primitive concerns: death through total rejection.

Liebert [20], in his recent psychoanalytic study of Michelangelo, pays particular attention to the role of abandonment in this artist's psychological development and later life reactions.

Otto Rank [26] has written about the myth of the birth of heroes where there was parental abandonment and, in some instances, the wish on the part of the parents (especially the father) that the child be killed or left to die. Noteworthy is the fact that the "heroes" mentioned by Rank are male children and of course are rescued by animals or simple people who have compassion for helpless babies. Among the many myths and biographies Rank mentions that fit this theme, I wish to note only a few special ones. Oedipus was abandoned three days after birth and, at the time of his abandonment, his ankles were pierced to ensure his helplessness; the name itself means "swollen foot." Others that are noteworthy include Moses, Paris, Perseus, Tristan, Romulus and Remus, Jesus, and Siegfried. The formula in the myths seems similar: banishment or death sentence of the baby, abandonment, discovery, adoption, and a heroic adult life. In the early days of man, filicide, especially of female children, was not uncommon. It may well have been an accepted means of limiting population size. In some parts of the world, this practice, including abortion before birth, still exists today. Therefore, the deeper anxieties of children may parallel that which was and still may be in existence today.

In literature one can find occasional references to the theme of the abandoned child. Emily Brontë's mother died when she was 3 years old. In her own prose creation, *Wuthering Heights* [4], published a year before her own death at age 30 of tuberculosis, Brontë's angry, disappointed hero Heathcliff, we learn, was an abandoned young child. He was wandering around Liverpool when he was found and "adopted" by the Earnshaws, who gave him the name of Heathcliff after their son who died in childhood.

Franz Kafka has a moving episode in his novel *America (Amerika)* [15], in which a young woman describes her plight to the hero, Kurt Rossmann. She was an illegitimate child whose father sent for her and her mother to join him in the United States. Shortly after their arrival in New York, he abandoned them without explanation or further contact. The young child and her mother were lost beyond discovery among the eastside tenements of New York City. When Therese, the informant, was about 5 years of age, her mother was looking for some shelter for the night. There was a snowstorm and the mother's hands, numbed by the cold, let go of the child, not realizing what had happened to her. Hanging onto the mother's skirts, the child stumbled and fell, but her mother desperately kept moving ahead. The mother, without work, without food, without shelter, carried bundles of useless odds and ends — in some ways reminiscent of the "shopping bag ladies" of today. The mother coughed up a great deal of blood, but still found no place where she and her child might rest and be warmed. From night until 5:00 A.M., the desperate pair continued to wander about aimlessly but without any respite. The child was bewildered and her only explanation was that her mother wanted to run away from her. For safety's sake, the child clutched more tightly to her mother's skirts, while sobbing intermittently. She was fearful of being left in the unfriendly corridors and streets on which they walked.

In the morning, mother and little daughter were leaning against a house wall in an exhausted state. The child had lost her bundle in the night's frenzied activity and her mother beat her for this, although she felt no blows. They reached a building where mother thought there might be some work. The child waited for mother while mother began to climb a ladder, reaching a level where bricklayers were involved in construction work. Mother walked on until she fell over the wall, with bricks and a heavy plank following her fall to the ground below. The child's last memory of her mother was seeing her lying there on the ground, her legs askew, covered by the plank, with people shouting angrily. This moving account of a child's witnessing her mother's dramatic death and all of the pain, fear, and actual deprivation she felt before the mother's demise is one of the most vivid descriptions of the phenomena that clinicians, on occasion, hear about from their patients who, as children, witnessed the suicide or the discovery of the body of their recently deceased parent. The anguish, confusion, bewilderment, pain, and powerlessness inflicts a deep wound on the child's psyche, in addition to the loss of the parent and the subsequent consequences.

In later adult years, regressions to these early traumatic states can occur when reality imposes conditions on the individual that allow for the emergence of this deeply repressed material. Parental loss through death, divorce, desertion, and prolonged institutionalization have many features in common, but there are also significant differences that should not be overlooked in our quest for simple universal formulations. Family disruptions, dislocations, and extreme psychic and physical upsets in surviving caretakers further complicate the situation and obviously increase risk vulnerability in later adult years.

Before leaving this section, I wish to note that fairy tales, myths, and religious stories have also addressed the theme of abandonment and desertion. Bettelheim [1] has recently written about the meaning and importance of fairy tales in the lives of children. He notes that "many fairy stories begin with the death of a mother or father; in these tales the death of the parent creates the most agonizing problems, as it (or the fear of it) does in real life" (p. 8). However, one might see this in an allied fashion (i.e., the fear is that of abandonment of the child at a time when he or she cannot care for him- or herself and so is in danger of dying). Thus the deeper inner concern is about survival of the self, which, of course, is related to and also displaced outward onto the parent's survival. This, too, Bettelheim affirms when he notes that "the child is subject to desperate feelings of loneliness and isolation, and he often experiences mortal anxiety. More often than not, he is unable to express these feelings in words, or he can do so only by indirection: fear of the dark, of some animal, anxiety about his body" (p. 10). One way of dealing with the mastery of such concerns is through fairy tales that can be enlightening about the world, its dangers, its safety measures, and its conflicts. But again, as Bettelheim states, "The fairy tale's deepest meaning will be different for each person, and different for the same person at various moments in his life" (p. 12). Thus, "which story is most important to a particular child at a particular age depends entirely on his psychological stage of development and the problems which are most pressing to him at the moment" (p. 15); I would add to this list the family structure and situation in which the child finds him- or herself.

The fear of abandonment may not be restricted to a particular period of development, but the fear and actual abandonment when it occurs does have developmental specificity. Thus a child who was abandoned at age 3 may react differently, taking into account the other variables, than a child who was deserted at 8. The earlier fears or actual events get registered, may be repressed, and may give rise to a vulnerable individual in later life, but later abandonments without such an earlier experience may get registered in a different way without repression and even without increasing later risk of abandonment.

In an ongoing study, I am investigating writers of children's stories, including fairy tales. An aspect of the life of James Barrie [24] suggests that the meaning of writing for a particular age group is a crucial aspect of the process that is one-sided if it concentrates solely on the reader or the listener. Thus far my research indicates that every production has within it autobiographical facts. The theme, content, form, style, plot, characters, and dialogue all come from what is meaningful to the writer and what the writer thinks will be of interest to the reader or listener. In similar fashion, biographers select the subjects of their writing for personal autobiographical reasons. I have also found that in autobiographies, diaries, journals, memoirs, notebooks, and the like a certain amount of fictive narrative is present. Thus, autobiography has in it fiction, and fiction or stories have autobiographical facts in them. Narrative memory with its subjectivity is fascinating to many adult readers — perhaps this is why there are so many autobiographies and biographies that are published and read. Like fairy tales for children, folklore narratives for primitive societies, and Bibles for religious groups, biographies and autobiographies allow adults to study the meaningfulness of other lives in comparison to their own.

The Case of Rudyard Kipling

It is my purpose now to describe a critical period in the early life of Rudyard Kipling and indicate how he retroactively handled a traumatic episode through literary creativity and how we need to reexamine concepts of neurosogenesis and trauma. Unlike my earlier studies, the "object loss" of young Kipling was not due to death, but to a sudden, prolonged, unexpected separation from his parents that extended over a period of years, during which time he was brutally assaulted regularly and systematically both emotionally and physically. That this period of abuse affected him is without question. That it permanently impaired him is doubtful. The temporary abandonment during critical years, even though the child is later reunited with his or her parents, does have an impact on later development, but perhaps in a different manner than situations where there is permanent desertion.

My data are derived from biographies of Kipling, his own autobiographical account of this chronic crisis written years after it occurred, his sister's memories of him, and especially from his story "Baa Baa, Black Sheep" [16]. In this story, although the names have been changed, the details are close to what he believed actually occurred, and we can assume that it is an accurate depiction of what he felt about his early traumatic situation as viewed from a later perspective. This creative production, which is only thinly disguised autobiographical fantasy and/or reality, seemingly had cathartic significance for Kipling and may have constituted the end result of his mourning-liberation process from this extremely trying period of his life. Kipling, in the first chapter of his story "The Light that Failed," includes elements derived from this earlier life experience, but the content is more removed from the events of his early life than is so vividly depicted in "Baa Baa, Black Sheep."

Before beginning with some biographical detail, let me digress briefly into a literary sidestreet. In 1978, the "long-suppressed biography" of Kipling by Lord Birkenhead was published in the United States. His son, Robin Birkenhead, in the introduction to the volume, indicates that near the end of the Second World War his father was commissioned to write the official biography of Kipling by Mrs. George (Elsie) Bambridge, Kipling's only surviving child. The family agreed to make unpublished documents available to Lord Birkenhead, but the daughter also stipulated that there would be close supervision of the writing. The biography had already been attempted and abandoned twice by two other writers who presumably found the supervision too exacting.

Lord Birkenhead entered into a contract with Mrs. Bambridge that was quite unfavorable to him in terms of copyright and finances. Mrs. Bambridge retained complete control of the book at all stages — even to the extent of removing any passages from it that she disliked; she could stop its publication completely if she wished. However, the Bambridges were most cordial and cooperative. Captain Bambridge died while the book was being written, but his wife, Kipling's daughter, continued her contacts with Lord Birkenhead in a most friendly fashion. The biography was completed in 1948 and there was every anticipation that it would be published. Mrs. Bambridge's unexpected response was shattering — an immediate and complete ban on its publication. Despite inquiries as to whether any particular passages or interpretations were objectionable, there was a firm and uncompromising refusal on the part of Mrs. Bambridge and she could not be swayed from her decision; the efforts of eminent literary figures to mediate were of no avail. Financial negotiations resulted in an agreement to pay the author £4,500 on condition that he not publish any biography of Kipling. Since Mrs. Bambridge had no heirs, it was expected that the work would appear after her death. In 1951, Mrs. Bambridge found another biographer, Charles E. Carrington, whose authorized biography of Kipling appeared in 1955. Presumably only Carrington and Lord Birkenhead had access to the Kipling archives and papers.

Mrs. Bambridge told Carrington that the Birkenhead biography was full of amateur psychoanalysis and that the writer hated Kipling and his works. I have found little to buttress this assessment. I have not found the Birkenhead biography filled with amateur psychoanalytic interpretations: Freud or psychoanalysis do not even appear as entries in the index to the volume!

Lord Birkenhead continued his research on Kipling, including visits to India and South Africa, and revised his biography in the 1960s. Lord Birkenhead died in 1975 and Mrs. Bambridge died in 1976. It then became possible to publish Birkenhead's book, over 30 years after the original draft was first suppressed. The third Carrington edition was published in 1978, as was Angus Wilson's biography and the Birkenhead biography — all after Kipling's daughter's death! I will comment on the 1978 Carrington biography later in this essay.

In my research I have relied on the biographies of Birkenhead [3], Angus Wilson [37], and Carrington [6], concentrating on the period of the parents' abandonment of Kipling and his sister during their childhood. The "Baa Baa, Black Sheep" story and Kipling's autobiographical description are consonant with the views put forth by Birkenhead. Much literary and psychological research remains to be done on the biographical controversy, but I shall return to the main road of my thesis now.

BIOGRAPHICAL FACTS

Rudyard Kipling's parents were married on March 18, 1865 and left for India immediately. Lockwood Kipling, the author's father, had been appointed Professor of Architectural Sculpture in the School of Art at Bombay. Lockwood and Alice Macdonald Kipling landed in India in May and on December 30, 1865, Joseph Rudyard Kipling was born in Bombay. Alice Kipling had six days of an agonizing, dangerous, and protracted labor. Rudyard's infancy was passed in the teeming city of Bombay. He was a difficult child to control but his mother was able to soothe him and, during a serious bout of whooping cough, it is noted that she could do so by reading to him.

Because Rudyard's birth almost killed Alice, when she became pregnant again in 1868, the doctors sent her to England for the delivery. Rudyard accompanied his mother and they arrived at Bewdley, where her parents lived. Rudyard was an active child and was fascinated with his grandparents' home. Alice again had a dangerous confinement in June. The newborn daughter was apparently stillborn and remained so until the doctor revived her. When the baby was 5 months old, Alice returned to India with her two children. On April 15, 1871, Rudyard (Ruddy) now 5½, and Alice (Trix), his 2½-year-old sister, left for England with their parents. Mrs. Kipling had lost a baby at birth the year before. The Kiplings, answering an advertisement, had decided to take their children to England and board them out with two strangers at Southsea: The Holloways cared for children whose parents were in India. The Kiplings did not know the Holloways and they were not personally recommended to them. Relations on both sides of the family had offered the children homes, but for reasons not exactly known, these offers were refused. The children were not prepared in any way for the separation and as Trix said in her later published memories of her brother, "It was like a double death, or rather, like an avalanche that had swept away everything happy and familiar" [10].

The home Rudyard and Trix lived in for the next 5 years was known to them as the "House of Desolation" or "Forlorn Lodge." The parting from their parents and from India was sudden. Rudyard was told that he must learn quickly to read and write so that he could read the letters and books sent by his parents from India. Trix indicated later that the horrible little house they were sent to was far from the sea and the common; it had a very small garden. Mrs. Holloway ("Aunty Rosa"), a tense woman, her husband ("Uncle Harry"), a retired naval captain, and their son, Harry, lived there. Mrs. Holloway had a "false voice," and Harry, who was several years older than Rudyard, had "crafty eyes." Mrs. Holloway, who had always wanted a daughter but had none, shared her bedroom with Trix and made her the "favorite." Rudyard shared a bedroom with Harry. Mrs. Holloway was a harsh evangelical disciplinarian and Rudyard became the target of her rigidity. The demands were strict, the punishments severe, and except for the protection of Uncle Harry and the support of Trix, Rudyard was severely reprimanded for the slightest deviation. For example, he was put into solitary confinement in a dark basement room in which mildew grew for two to three days without fire or heat. Separation from his sister and banishment to the basement room for 24 hours were imposed for spilling a drop of gravy at dinner, crying when the letters from Bombay were read, or when the slate was not properly put away. Discipline was one of "The Woman's" (as Rudyard Kipling called Mrs. Holloway) favorite words and she applied it liberally.

Humiliations were many, and Harry (referred to by Rudyard as "the Devil-Boy"), was an even more painful cause of suffering — mentally and physically. Rudyard shared an attic room with him, sleeping on a hard iron bed. When Harry trapped the children, he would report their inconsistencies and minor transgressions to his mother. After the death of Uncle Harry in 1874 (the one seemingly kind figure in the household), the cruelty increased. Rudyard would be beaten or sent to bed without supper if he offended Harry or committed a trivial offense. Trix tried to help Rudyard, as did the overworked and frightened maid, Jane. Birkenhead notes that the children never ceased to speculate as to why they had been deserted and why they had been sent to this House of Desolation. Mrs. Holloway told them it was because they had been naughty and that she had taken them out of pity, but her husband told them kindly that this was only "Aunty's joke," and that India was too hot for them. They did not believe him because they recalled that they had once been to the hills for the hot weather season in India without any problems. Harry told them they were workhouse brats who had to be taken in out of charity and that their toys did not belong to them. It is possible they thought they were adopted and might never see their parents again.

Trix felt that "Aunty" did her best to weaken the affection between brother and sister. She said Trix was always right and Rudyard was wrong. The children did not communicate their unhappiness to their parents because their letters were often dictated by Mrs. Holloway and always strictly censored. The constancy of accusation, detection, homily, and punishment did not wear Rudyard down. "He was too busy struggling to adjust himself to these crazy and inexplicable conditions, and to keep his head above water" (p. 20) [3].

Mrs. Holloway taught the children to read together. Trix was praised and Rudyard was criticized. Trix learned to read before her brother, but when he did read, he read everything he could find. Although Ruddy spent a month each year at Christmas time with his real aunt and uncle, he never confided his misery to them at these times. He seemed to be a stout, cheerful boy who was active, showed no signs of ill treatment, and made no complaints about his Southsea life. He had a very active imagination; the stories teeming in his head he could recite with great fluency. His creative talent was already in evidence. He was, however, frightened of the dark and especially of what might be under his bed. His family had no idea of what went on at the House of Desolation. After his holidays, he would return and cry himself to sleep for the next two or three nights until he once again became absorbed in the grinding routine. He seemed to be stoically resigned to his fate.

Sometime in March 1877, Rudyard was shut away from Trix for two days because he was a "moral leper." Trix heard "Aunty" storming at Rudyard in the hall. After some time she saw her brother going down the garden path, wearing a cardboard placard on which the Devil-Boy had printed: "Kipling the Liar." Trix ran out and tried to tear it off, but could not. Instead she took Ruddy's pocketknife and cut each stitch until it was off. Ruddy crept to school very shaken. Aunty Rosa caught Trix and brandished the cane she had never used on the child. Trix screamed, "You are a wicked woman." She threatened to tell everybody how cruel she was to children and that they hated her. Aunty threatened Trix with the cane, but Trix said, "That's right; thrash me as if I was Ruddy — you know how I bruise and when I'm black I'll go to the police and show them, and have you punished" (p. 26) [3].

In March 1877, Mrs. Kipling left India for England and came to the house at Southsea without notifying the children. Trix had no recollection of her mother until the reunion with her in 1877; she was 9 years old then. Trix apparently had forgotten her mother and was taken with the gentleness of her voice, the softness of her face pressed against hers, and the blueness of her eyes. Rudyard said he knew his mother immediately. "When she went into his bedroom to kiss him goodnight he flung up an arm to ward of the blow he had learned to expect" (p. 27) [3]. Soon Mrs. Kipling took the children from the House of Desolation.

Birkenhead asserts that Kipling undoubtedly remembered vividly and bitterly his privations, but he and his sister never talked of the Southsea days. Forty-three years later, when he was in Southsea to inspect the submarines, his wife noted in her diary: "Rud takes me to see Lorne Lodge . . . where he was so misused and forlorn and desperately unhappy as a child, and talks of it all with horror" (p. 27) [3].

That Rudyard probably gave Mrs. Holloway a difficult time is most possible — at least initially. She may have felt it was her duty to correct his "boorish tendencies," which she did with a heavy hand. Nonetheless, the traumatic aspect of this "treatment" and the sudden abandonment by his parents cannot be ignored [31].

Eleven years after Kipling left the House of Desolation (to which his sister later returned), he wrote his moving story "Baa Baa, Black Sheep." It was one of the few stories that he did not send to his family either in manuscript or in proof. Birkenhead notes that when Lockwood Kipling read the painful savage outpourings in cold print he was so upset that he and his wife tried to make Trix say it was all exaggerated and untrue, but she could not pretend that they were happy there [10, 11].

Even though he had later difficulties, which may or may not relate to the period in the House of Desolation, Kipling had formidable powers of recuperation. Afterward he had "an endless reserve of vitality, resilience and bumptiousness" (p. 28) [3]. His daughter, Elsie Bambridge, told Lord Birkenhead, "I think the bitter experiences and injustices of life in 'Lorne Lodge' were the making of much that was best in Rudyard's character; they supplied the discipline that was lacking" (p. 28) [3]. Interestingly, Rudyard Kipling remained to the end of his life a believer in corporal punishment and in discipline. He told his daughter that he had often been beaten and that he richly deserved it [3]. What remained from his Southsea days was Kipling's "morbid reticence in which he was to shroud every secret corner of his mind from external scrutiny — in a constant, almost animal wariness and timidity, and an undying instinct for self-protection" (p. 28) [3] — in some ways similar to what one may see in concentration camp survivors.

Kipling had many encounters with death throughout his life. His brother, John, born in April 1870, immediately died at birth. One year later Rudyard left India, was left by his parents, and entered the House of Desolation. While there, his only friend, "Uncle Harry," died leaving him to the additional persecution by Mrs. Holloway and her son. Much later, following the sudden death of his dear friend, Wolcott Balestier, he married his friend's sister, Carrie, in 1892. His son, John, was killed in action in World War I in 1915. Earlier, in 1899, his beloved eldest daughter, Josephine, died at age 7. He himself suffered from undiagnosed stomach distress for many years, developing a cancer phobia. Ultimately, he died from a perforated duodenal-gastric ulcer on January 18, 1936 at age 71. Despite his internal grief, he rarely expressed his emotions. Periods of grief and depression have been described, but with stoical resignation, he seemingly kept his feelings to himself — a souvenir of his means of mastering the tensions he endured in the house at Southsea?

KIPLING'S AUTOBIOGRAPHY

At age 70, Kipling published his autobiography, *Something of Myself — For My Friends Known and Unknown* [17]. The first chapter, entitled "A Very Young Person," begins with the following quotation: "Give me the first six years of a child's life and you can have the rest." Did Kipling mean that the good years in Bombay before the House of Desolation protected him from the terror he experienced later? He describes the pleasant early years in India with his ayah (nurse) and his mother who sang beautiful songs at the piano, the smells, and the greenery. When a chicken attacked him, he recalls his father drawing a picture of the tragedy for him with a rhyme beneath:

There was a small boy in Bombay
Who once from a hen ran away.
When they said: "You're a baby,"
He replied: "Well, I may be:
But I don't like those hens of Bombay."

This consoled Kipling and he thought well of hens evermore. It may be that this early experience with poetry played a role in his later career as a children's writer and poet.

Kipling describes the evangelical nature of the Southsea house, the beatings and starvation, the constant bullying and torture, and how he was sorry when the old captain died because he had been the only one there who threw Kipling a kind word. He notes that the lies he found it necessary to tell may have played a role in his later inventive literary efforts. When he read with eagerness and enjoyment, he was subjected to a new deprivation — no reading; so he read more earnestly and stealthily. He never refers to Mrs. Holloway by name, instead calling her "The Woman." He refers to her son, as mentioned previously, as "the Devil-Boy."

Kipling's fantasies and play were his salvation activities from the constant cross-examinations, punishments, and humiliations. Later when his aunt asked him why he never told anyone how he was treated, he wrote [17], "Children tell little more than animals, for what comes to them they accept as eternally established. Also badly-treated children have a clear notion of what they are likely to get if they betray the secrets of a prison-house before they are clear of it" (p. 17).

Kipling then describes how his eyes became weakened, perhaps as a result of reading so much in bad light. His schoolwork suffered, and as a result, he received a bad report that he feared showing "The Woman." When the bad schoolwork became known, he was beaten and sent to school through the streets of Southsea with the placard "Liar" between his shoulders. He had a "sort of nervous breakdown" when he imagined he saw shadows and things that were not there. His aunt heard of this, had him examined, and he was found to be half-blind. He was accused of "showing off" and, as a punishment, was isolated from his sister. Very soon after the eye examination, his mother suddenly appeared and rescued him from the House of Desolation. He was encouraged not to think of his past. At the end of the first chapter in his autobiography Kipling describes his apparent pleasure, after being removed from the House of Desolation, at being able to read as much as he liked, that he could ask as many questions as he liked, and that he could write what he thought without being accused of "showing off" by doing so. He also learned that his mother had written verses and that his father also "wrote things."

From this autobiography, his sister's remembrances of him, and the countless unpublished letters, diaries, and conversations with his biographers — official and unofficial — one can construct a picture of Kipling. But when one goes to his stories, notably "Baa Baa, Black Sheep," the reader has the opportunity to see how the transformation of remembered reality into a creative product has taken place. However, the very moving account of Kipling's years in the House of Desolation is somewhat changed. He and his sister Trix are called Punch and Judy, the puppets. Mrs. Holloway, Uncle Harry, and Devil-Boy are identical to what we know of them. Ruddy becomes the Black Sheep. The closing description of the reunion with mother is particularly touching. The story closes when Judy tells Punch that everything is different now that mother is back and it is as if she never had been gone. The closing paragraph, however, says [16]:

Not altogether . . . , for when young lips have drunk deep of the bitter waters of Hate, Suspicion, and Despair, all the Love in the world will not wholly take away that knowledge; though it may turn darkened eyes for a while to the light, and teach Faith where no Faith was. (P. 274)

BIOGRAPHIES OF KIPLING
The biography of Kipling written by Angus Wilson [37] before or about the same time as the publication of the Birkenhead volume should be mentioned because it suggests some answers to significant questions and illuminates areas of Kipling's life that deserve special note.

Wilson [37] wrote that Kipling "was a man who, throughout his life, worshipped and respected (a rare combination) children and their imaginings. He took part in children's games, . . . not, as so many adults do, in order to impose his own shapes, but to follow and learn as well as to contribute. He would very happily leave adult company to play with children even in his sixties" (p. 1). His intense absorption could transform a small space into a whole world — much like a child does. And in similar fashion, Wilson suggests, Kipling could convert a child's smallest journey into a wondrous exploration. These two abilities come to fruition in many of Kipling's best stories. Yet Kipling's children are "so real, so unselfconsciously revealed in their play, that he quite avoids that decadent feeling of self-indulgent empathy with children's ways that so often nauseates" (pp. 5–6) [37]. Wilson suggests, and I agree, that Kipling "never fell out of love with the small happy boy he had been in India" (p. 6). And so, his children's masterpieces, including the *Just So Stories*, the *Jungle Books* stories, Puck's tales, and *Kim*, still delight young and old.

Wilson calls attention to the importance of parents, especially of mothers as they are frequently seen in Kipling's poetry and stories. Kipling's feelings about his mother undoubtedly form the basis for this emphasis. Rudyard's mother came from an interesting background. She was the oldest daughter of a large family of minister's children, all of whom were lively and talented. She played an instrument, sang, and composed songs and verses. Some of her stories may have been published before she married and went to India. Her engagement to Kipling's father was long—it was over four years before marriage occurred and the ostensible reason for this was lack of money. Kipling's father went to India because it was there that he could get a job. He was one of three subordinate teachers appointed to teach utilitarian crafts. The pay was poor and private work was needed to supplement the family's income. The difficult financial circumstance may have been the reason that Alice Kipling went to England along with Rudyard, but without her husband, to have her second child. Alice ran the household, wrote for magazines and newspapers, and used her exceptional social skills to help her husband's advancement. When asked some years later why Rudyard and Trix had been left to board in England at early ages, Alice gave her need and wish to be with her husband and help him with his work as the reason.

Kipling's father was known for his detailed knowledge. His mother had a volatile nature with a nervous, hypochondriacal undertow. These were melded together in Rudyard, who was a careful craftsman but also one with quick and impressionistic insight.

The decision to board the children with the Holloways was made so that the children would not be separated in England, which might be necessary if they lived with relatives there, and possibly because of other family complications. Because the payment to the Holloways was a heavy burden on the meager salary of Kipling's father, Alice could not afford to return to England to see her children in the six years they were at Southsea. She also may have felt that the futures of the children would be better served if she could give all of her efforts and great talents in helping her husband's career. We can, if Wilson is correct, understand the motivations of Kipling's parents in placing the children with the Holloways, but an unanswered question remains: Why did they not check on the boarding family before entrusting two very young children to their care? There is indication that Alice's three sisters and her mother did visit the Holloways and felt "Aunty Rosa" was fond of the children and seemed to be a very nice woman [37]. How then do we explain the difference in the accounts of Rudyard and his sister from their relatives' impressions? Is it possible that there were two different behaviors (i.e., public and private) and each could be valid? Or should we consider the possibility that the Southsea experience was a combination of reality, fantasy, and a frightened, angry reaction of an abandoned, deserted child?

Rudyard was a masterful, aggressive, interesting, inquisitive, and overindulged child. Mrs. Holloway was concerned about her finances, especially after her husband's death when his pension ceased or was markedly reduced. Those years were as bad for "Aunty Rosa" as they were for Rudyard. She may have felt that she had to tame the arrogant and boisterous little boy who had no religious identification. Rudyard's parents were not religious people although he was baptised in the Church of England and the families on both sides were Wesleyan-Methodists. The Holloways—especially Mrs. Holloway and her son—were very religious and "Aunty Rosa" had vigorous evangelical beliefs. Kipling noted that before Southsea he had never heard of Hell, so he was introduced to it in all of its terrors. Mrs. Holloway was a Calvinist Evangelical of the Church of England and her efforts seem to have been in the direction of saving the wicked Rudyard without sparing the rod or other punishments. The strain of bullying, ostracism, and fright did not "save" Rudyard, however; but, as Wilson [37] suggests, it left him "forever exceptionally reticent except to children and his very few intimates. More immediately it aggravated an eyesight defect so that his vision was seriously affected" (p. 32).

Rudyard's aunt (Alice's sister) wrote Alice that all was not well with Rudyard, and she immediately came to save her children. Wilson [37] sees the Southsea experience as "the conflict of two eras, a conflict between the idea of childhood liberated, and a precious source of creation that was taking root in the mid-Victorian middle-class world, and an earlier, fast disappearing idea of sinful childhood to be repressed and chastened, as Aunty Rosa believed was her Christian duty" (p. 32).

After leaving Southsea, Trix returned to spend several periods at the House of Desolation and, in 1880, Rudyard himself paid a visit there when he came to fetch his sister for a holiday at their uncle's home. So we have another query that needs answering: Why did Rudyard allow Trix to return to the House of Desolation without informing his parents about Mrs. Holloway's behavior?

Although there is no evidence of Kipling's hate, Wilson [37] points out that a feature of Kipling's work consists of "the deliberate cruelty of the goodies to the baddies in order to teach them a lesson, or simply as a necessary expression of mastery" (p. 49). Might this be a manifestation of Kipling's identification with the aggressor and/or a means of handling his own hostile impulses? Wilson observes that Kipling was a fierce man and a very gentle one. Despite the latter, there was somewhere within him a pleasure when exposed to the pain of others.

C. S. Lewis [19], citing G. K. Chesterton, finds two essential features of Kipling: (1) Kipling discovered or rediscovered the poetry of common things, perceiving "the significance and philosophy of steam and of slang" (p. 234), and (2) Kipling was "the poet of discipline" (p. 234). His emphasis on discipline of every shape included military discipline. For example, "there is nothing Kipling describes with more relish than the process whereby the trade-spirit licks some raw cub into shape. That is the whole theme of one of his few full length novels, *Captains Courageous*" (p. 238) [19]. It is also to be found in all of his army stories and sea stories. Lewis notes further that what is even more antipathetic is Kipling's presentation of the "breaking" and "raw hiding" process (p. 239). Those who have hated Kipling for this emphasis dismiss him as a fascist with "public school" brutality, and yet, as Orwell [22] notes, Kipling was no fascist, although he might be thought of as prefascist or sadistic. The sadomasochistic core may well be traced back to his experiences at the House of Desolation. It may be that this experience, as well as the "Baa Baa, Black Sheep" story, is a defensive cover memory hiding an earlier series of traumas, but there is no evidence to confirm or refute this possibility.

Lewis [19] suggests that "the very same methods which he [Kipling] prescribes for licking the cub into shape, 'making a man of him' in the interests of the community, would also, if his masters were bad men, be an admirable method of keeping the cub quiet while he was exploited and enslaved for their private benefit" (p. 240). This is consonant with his behavior at Lorne Lodge and his later emphasis on work, discipline, and bullying, especially of those in lower positions. Kipling, notes Lewis [19], is "eminently a moralist; in almost every story we are invited, nay forced, to admire and condemn. Many of the poems are versified homilies" (p. 244) — shades of Mrs. Holloway! Kipling had been badly hurt as a child and at times there are "moments of an almost quivering tenderness" (p. 249) [19] when he writes of children or for them.

As already mentioned, George Orwell [22] did not believe Kipling was a fascist, although he perceived a definite sadism and brutality in his writings, which went along with his imperialistic orientation. Pritchett [25], reviewing Angus Wilson's biography of Kipling, emphasizes Kipling's "moving about" — from India to England, then back to India and to England again, with sojourns to the United States, South Africa, and his later wintering in France. It is true that in his first few years of life he did make several trips to England, with the last one being the "abandonment"; perhaps his later "rides" to various parts of the world were attempts to deal with his losses of land as well as family. He spoke Hindi before he spoke English and later he became a multilinguist who could talk to soldiers, engineers, workmen, farmers, and literary and political figures. He had a child's ear for language — perhaps again a derivative of his necessity to observe and pay close attention to sounds lest he get into trouble at the House of Desolation.

Pritchett [25] suggests another possible motive for sending Rudyard and Trix to England: it was a sign of social status and economic success to be able to do this. As we will shortly see, Rudyard's mother may have had significant unresolved sibling problems that make this explanation plausible. Aside from the Holloway experience, Pritchett [25] calls attention to the later influence of Kipling's schooling at Westward Ho. "Once again, the parents made a choice that looked good and was within their means. . . . The place flourished as an anomaly: intended to train boys for empire-building and the military life, it was run by a progressive crank and intellectual who shared the artistic tastes of the Pre-Raphaelites" (p. 35).

Kipling was badly bullied his first year at Westward Ho, but the perceptive headmaster gave him free rein of his excellent library. Kipling soon spoke and read French and even some Russian. "As for the bullying, we know from Stalky & Co., he soon had his own elite gang or tribe, who were clever at running the traditional school boy secret society, out maneuvering the bullies and inventing the schoolboy guerilla practice of cunning and crude practical jokes" (pp. 35 – 36) [25]. Kipling did not go to the university; he was a born watcher and listener, an imagemaker but not a thinker. Here again, one might speculate on the possible adaptive assistance of watching and listening that was so necessary to keep his balance at Southsea.

INTERPRETATIONS

Using data from biographers who examined unpublished documents and who had personal interviews and contacts with Kipling's family, Kipling's own autobiography, remembrances of his sister, and his pertinent published stories (especially "Baa Baa, Black Sheep"), I have attempted to reconstruct what may have occurred and what Kipling constructed and reacted to during a crucial period in his later childhood (age 5½ – 11). In an attempt to understand, I have speculated about the various aspects of the Kipling situation so that a more comprehensive formulation might be presented. I do not believe that Kipling's great talents can be explained by the traumas he endured or the identifications he made, which guided and directed his creativity. Viewed retrospectively some conclusions can, however, be presented.

Let me first explore the situation of Kipling's parents. His mother, Alice Macdonald, was the second child and first daughter of a large surviving family of seven children. Her oldest sibling, a brother Henry, was born in 1835. Two years later, Alice, the author's mother, was born (1837). Georgiana, a sister who married the famous artist Burne-Jones, was born in 1840. A brother, Frederick, the friend of Kipling's father and the one who introduced Alice to John Lockwood Kipling, was born in 1842. In 1843, Agnes was born. She, too, married a famous artist — Poynter. Louisa, born in 1845, married Baldwin, the head of a railroad and the father of the later Prime Minister, Stanley Baldwin. The last sibling, Edith, was born in 1848.

As already noted, Alice married late and very likely was destined to remain unmarried until John Lockwood Kipling appeared. Alice was slightly older than her husband. She was described as a lively young woman who was flirtatious. Angus Wilson [37] notes that she had been engaged once or twice before her marriage. Alice was impetuous, witty, and sharp-tongued. There was a legend that in a fit of anger she threw a treasured relic, a lock of John Wesley's hair, into the fire [37]. She played, sang, composed songs, and wrote poetry. Carrington [5] describes her as a little woman with a very lively and witty tongue, whose power of speech was unsurpassed and whose insight was swift and accurate. Her sisters, too, had great charm and married very well.

John Lockwood Kipling is described by Carrington [5] as a man of wide reading and close observation. He had a zest for technical arts and crafts and "an almost feminine sensibility to textures and tones and scents" (p. 3). He was also an artist, using pen, brush, and modelling clay. Small in stature, he was always good humored and liked by all. Incidentally, he met his wife-to-be in the spring of 1863 at a picnic party at Lake Rudyard in England. In celebration of this momentous occasion, the first child was called Rudyard, although the author's first name was Joseph (the same name as that of the author's paternal uncle).

What do these observations, and some made by Angus Wilson and others, suggest? I believe that Alice was probably the dominant figure in the Kipling nuclear family of origin. It may be that Alice assumed a more aggressive, masculine identification, either based on an ascending sibling rivalry with her older brother or descending sibling rivalry with her younger sisters. Her marriage, at a late date for those times, provided her with the chance to help her more "feminine" husband who was not as successful as the spouses of her sisters. She was a proud person who had great needs for the success of her partner and particularly her children, whom she bore at great risk to herself and to them. Her husband obtained his post through the intervention of her sister's husband, Burne-Jones, who was a famous artist. John Lockwood Kipling also was immersed in art. In India, he could have more status than he could attain in England where he would be in competition or at least in comparison with his wife's famous, later knighted, brothers-in-law and her wealthy nonartist brother-in-law. This could have been a possible motive for Alice's need and wish to remain in India to help her husband's career and for giving the impression that she could afford to send her children to England for schooling.

Angus Wilson [37] suggests that financial circumstances were not the best during Rudyard's first five or six years; nonetheless, the Indian servants and the dedicated parents gave the children much support, love, and encouragement. Because the family had pride and a wish not to be dependent on their more economically well-off English relatives, I suspect they elected to place their children with the Holloways at Lorne Lodge in Southsea. In all probability the cost was moderate and the parents, fearing that the children might become sick and die, rather quickly arranged for the placement. This argument may be strengthened by the fact that Alice's third child, a son John, died shortly after birth and about a year before the fateful trip to the House of Desolation.

One additional factor, again noted by Angus Wilson [37], should be kept in mind. Alice had a "volatile nature with its nervous, hypochondriacal undertow" (p. 17). This was similar to her own mother's "nervous disposition," which was manifested by fatigue, psychosomatic ailments, and periods of alternating gaiety, depressions, and sudden despairs (p. 10). These tension states were also seen in Alice's oldest brother, Henry, in Alice's younger sister, Georgiana Burne-Jones, who had alternating moods of wit and gloom, and in Kipling's sister Trix, who had years of "serious hysteric disorder" (p. 10) [37]. Angus Wilson, following Rudyard Kipling's famous cousin's (Angela Thirkell) lead, suggests that Kipling may well have "attributed his own black moods, his habitual insomnia, the periodic exhaustions of his vitality, his restlessness" (p. 10) to personality characteristics inherited from his mother and her family. Kipling did express anxiety about the inheritance of cancer from his family — anxiety closely related to his later severe abdominal pains, which remained undiagnosed for a long time. I am not suggesting the inheritance of a manic-depressive predisposition in Kipling, but this cannot be excluded.

Angus Wilson suggests that Kipling's fear of inherited cancer overlaid a greater fear of mental breakdown. "He was a gentle-violent man, a man of depressions and hilarity, holding his despairs in with an almost superhuman stoicism. Manic-depressive does no more than repeat this in big words" (p. 342) [37]. Kipling persistently avoided introspection and questioning of the source of despair, anxiety, guilt, and other feelings that so many of the characters in his best stories feel. This defense against insight might well have been used in the adaptive service of keeping the repressed repressed, thus avoiding further anguish for himself.

From a psychological point of view, the possible identification of Kipling with his mother, her talents, and her vulnerabilities and the possible maternal fixation that extended to his wife Carrie, a woman also described as assertive and in some ways similar to his mother, must be considered. Like Alice, who was introduced to John Lockwood Kipling by her brother, Rudyard was introduced to his wife Carrie by Carrie's brother. The marriage to Carrie occurred shortly after the sudden death of her brother. I ask: Did Rudyard feel some survivor guilt from the death of his own brother when he, Rudyard, was 5? And was the marriage to Carrie connected with his own early family of origin and his apparent temporary abandonment by that family? Did he fear that brother John's fate or Carrie's brother's fate might be his if he succumbed?

Carrie was described as a depressed and melancholic woman, again having some similarities to Alice. Edmund Wilson [38], citing Viscount Castlerosse, notes that Carrie was more than a wife to Rudyard: "She was a mistress in the literal sense, a governess and a matron" (p. 47). In some ways Edmund Wilson's reference suggests that Carrie was Rudyard's nurse. "Kipling handed himself over bodily, financially and spiritually to his spouse. He had no banking account. All the money which he earned was handed over to her, and she would dole him out so much pocket money. He could not call his time or even his stomach his own" (p. 47).

When Carrie was with him he would become quiet and submissive and yield to her command that it was time for him to go to bed when she so determined. Apparently there were no "signs of murmuring or even incipient mutiny" (p. 48) [38] in response to these controls, although Kipling did develop a duodenal ulcer. Could it be that Sarah Holloway — "Aunty Rosa," "The Woman" — represented an aspect of mother that Kipling could only deal with in a displaced sense?

Edel [8] has described the intense relationship between Charles Wolcott Balestier (Carrie's brother) and Rudyard Kipling. Balestier's sudden death evoked a profound grief in Kipling — perhaps harkening back to Kipling's grief at the time of his own infant brother's death, which was followed by his suddenly leaving India and his parents and his period in the Southsea House of Desolation. Kipling collaborated with Balestier on the novel, *The Naulahka,* a combined American Western and Anglo-Indian tale. Balestier died suddenly in Dresden of typhoid fever. Kipling received word of Balestier's death in India. His grief was "long and profound" (p. 333) [8]. Kipling resolved to marry Balestier's sister, despite his mother's opposition to the match. Edel suggests Carrie was a replacement for her dead brother in Kipling's life. Five weeks after Balestier's burial, Kipling married Carrie Balestier. I am inclined to see Carrie as more of a maternal figure for Rudyard than a substitute for her brother; however, both components might have existed.

Pritchett [25] felt that Carrie "once more" was a stern mother figure to Kipling. "She managed his financial affairs, his contracts, his correspondence. She is said to have opened all his letters and to have dictated the replies. Her daughter said she cut her husband off from stimulating intellectual company and indeed she was out of her depth in it. But she fiercely protected his privacy and stood between him and the plague of visitors who descend like vultures on famous men" (p. 41). Kipling apparently was very content with Carrie's rule, especially since he had an excessive reliance on his parents, even in middle life. Kipling found a tough wife; his mother had been a tough wife and mother.

We are told by Carrington and others that, as an adult, Kipling shunned publicity, was an elusive and retiring figure, and that few knew him well because he was a very private person. Green [13] suggests that as a child and later Kipling showed evidences of behavior derived from both parents — "his mother's nimbleness of mind and wit, her skill in words, her vision and her inaccuracy as to detail, with his father's amazing memory and insatiable curiosity and breadth of interests" (p. 19).

I will now return to the apparent changes in Kipling that occurred after the Lorne Lodge experience. Green [13] proposes that the biggest mistake the Kipling parents made was in not preparing the children for the coming separation and explaining the reasons for it. Since Rudyard was a precocious child with "a mind bubbling over with imagination and curiosity," he could easily have understood and accepted the reasons for his "exile" (p. 30). This I doubt, but an acknowledgment might have allowed him to express his feelings openly. Earlier he was described by his maternal grandparents and other relatives as a talkative, inquisitive child who was forward and more self-assertive than most Victorian children (p. 9) [5]. The later changes that occurred in him may have originated in or been emphasized by the circumstances of "a childhood in exile from the family" (p. 4) [28]. After this experience, he emerged physically damaged; afterward he always wore glasses. And he had an inward-driven sensitiveness and need for self-protection. Edmund Wilson [38] observes that in parallel fashion to his life, some of Kipling's most authentic early stories deal with children forsaken by their parents, as he felt he was, and the most poignant of his later stories deal with parents bereaved over their children's deaths, as was also true with his family. "The theme of the abandoned parent seems to reflect in reversal the theme of the abandoned child" (p. 68) [38].

And yet, Carrington writes that Mrs. Holloway was a good woman and a devoted housewife, not as tyrannical or cruel a foster mother as one would conclude from Kipling's writings and his sister's reports. In fact, Carrington goes on to say that after Kipling left Lorne Lodge there was no breach of the two families, and Trix returned and remained with Mrs. Holloway for several years. He [5] suggests that Rudyard was a "restless, clumsy boy, very little used to genteel discipline. He sprawled over the sofas, he talked continually, he asked the most searching questions, he knew more than little boys were expected to know and paraded his knowledge in the company of elders, he had Anglo-Indian notions of nursery etiquette, he was unresponsive to demonstrations of sentiment. . . . It was disgraceful, 'Aunty Rosa' must have thought, that at nearly six years old, he had not yet begun to write. . . . If he had been spoiled by indulgent parents in Bombay, 'Aunty Rosa' was determined to do her duty by him in Southsea, to correct his manners and cure him of 'showing off' " (p. 12). This she did. The long years at Southsea affected his character and his personality to some extent, but the child abuse that was inflicted upon him did not impair his later creativity and his love of children, and did not result in the serious psychopathology one might have expected. Shengold [31], in a very scholarly essay, has suggested some possible reasons as to why Kipling was spared and why his capacity for love was not destroyed. Other considerations that may also be valid are suggested here.

Carrington, in the preface to the 1978 revision of his official biography of Rudyard Kipling, points out that Kipling's memory was faulty when he wrote his autobiography, *Something of Myself*, so that some doubts about the validity of his recollections in old age must be seriously addressed. This autobiography [17], completed a few days before his death, was never checked over or revised. Carrington, gaining access to new data after Kipling's daughter's death in 1976, presents some of the new data in several appendices to the 1978 edition of his biography. The new work ends with an epilogue—a memoir by Mrs. George Bambridge, Kipling's daughter.

In Appendix 1 [6], Carrington describes the biographies and biographers of Kipling that preceded him (i.e., Hector Bolitho, T. Corling, Eric Linklater, and Lord Birkenhead). Most of these authors gave up writing the official biography because of the stringent supervision imposed on them by Mrs. Bambridge. Elsie Bambridge, Carrington reports, disliked Birkenhead. She felt he was a "bright young thing" (p. 609) and unlike her father, herself, and Carrington, who were creatures of the prewar age [6]. But Elsie's real objection was that the Birkenhead biography "was riddled with the amateur psychoanalysis that had become fashionable in the 1930's" (p. 610). She felt Birkenhead's interpretations were wrong. She consulted T. S. Eliot who agreed with her although he later told Carrington that the word he used was "insufficient." Carrington believes Lord Birkenhead was most honorable in his behavior of keeping silent about the entire matter.

Carrington does raise questions about the authenticity of portions of "Baa Baa, Black Sheep." He notes that Alice left Trix alone with Mrs. Holloway for three years after Rudyard left the House of Desolation. One can raise questions of accuracy, reality, or fantasy. But even if the latter played a role in the story and Kipling's later life, it cannot be ignored or dismissed as having no significance.

Gilbert Ryle [29] has noted that:

There often arise quarrels between theories, or, more generally, between lines of thought, which are not rival solutions of the same problem, but rather solutions or would-be solutions of different problems, and which, nonetheless, seem to be irreconcilable with one another. A thinker who adopts one of them seems to be logically committed to rejecting the other, despite the fact that the inquiries from which the theories issued had, from the beginning, widely divergent goals. In disputes of this kind, we often find one and the same thinker—very likely oneself—strongly inclined to champion both sides and yet, at the very same time, strongly inclined entirely to repudiate one of them just because he is strongly inclined to support the other. He is both well satisfied with the logical credentials of each of the two points of view, and sure that one of them must be totally wrong if the other is even largely right. The internal administration of each seems to be impeccable but their diplomatic relations with one another seem to be internecine. (P. 1)

We do not have the answer to Kipling's creativity. We can, using the methods of the historian and archeologist, attempt to reconstruct a life from bits and pieces — from various episodes that can form some sort of pattern. Kipling had the capacity for hard work, an abundant supply of energy, great sensitivity, and the ability to see the world through the eyes of a child. This he put to use in his creative writing, despite his traumas, losses, and anxieties.

Kipling's poem "If" reveals how he managed to survive the difficult years that evidence indicates were upsetting in one way or another. It gives us insight into this great poet's life.

If you can keep your head when all about you
Are losing theirs and blaming it on you,
If you can trust yourself when all men doubt you,
But make allowance for their doubting too;
If you can wait and not be tired by waiting,
Or being lied about, don't deal in lies,
Or being hated, don't give way to hating,
And yet don't look too good, nor talk too wise:

. . . Yours is the Earth and everything that's in it,
And—which is more—you'll be a Man, my son!

The Case of Saki (H. H. Munro)

While investigating the role and effects of abandonment in the life of Kipling, I began to wonder about other writers who were, like Kipling, born in an outpost of the British empire but were removed from their birthplace at an early age for various reasons and sent to England. It is my intention to study these individuals further, especially since geographic dislocation can have symbolic meaning that can be deep and far-reaching. Usually the land of birth is referred to as the "mother country" or "fatherland." Rarely, if ever, does one hear of the brother- or sister-land. Among the writers I have studied, I now wish to turn my attention to H. H. Munro, who took as his pen name Saki.

As Graham Greene [14] observed, "There are certain writers . . . who never shake off the burden of their childhood. . . . All later experience seems to have been related to those months or years of unhappiness" (p. vii). Dickens, Kipling, and others were surprised by their defenselessness in the face of overwhelming traumas. There are great similarities in the early life of Kipling and Saki and, as Greene observes, Saki's reaction to misery was similar to that of Kipling. Kipling, as noted previously, was born in India; Munro was born in Burma. Family life for such "colonial" children is always broken and, again, as Greene notes, the miseries recorded by both Kipling and Munro probably were experienced by many children born to civil servants or colonial officers in the East. Though there are similarities between Kipling and Munro, there were also differences. The best stories of Munro are about childhood — its humor, its anarchy, its cruelty, and its unhappiness.

Langguth's recently published biography [18] of Munro, based on the writer's papers and notes, is the first such account of the writer's life, excluding the earlier biography written by his sister, Ethel M. Munro. Ethel Munro's account of her brother's life obviously is subjective, and there are indications she avoided certain areas of her famous brother's life narrative that she felt would present him in an unfavorable light. In some ways there is an analogous circumstance to Kipling's daughter's "censorship" of the biographies of her father. We also know that many of Kipling's letters are unavailable because Kipling, like so many others, scrupulously burned incoming mail and copies of his responses when he had finished with them. Nonetheless, some to whom he wrote (e.g., H. Rider Haggard) did save the original letters of Kipling and these are useful in reconstructing patterns and responses of the past.

I am grateful to Langguth for his biography of Saki. He does state the facts as he gathered them. The interpretations and speculations are my responsibility. Also, Ethel Munro's biography [21] is of great value, not only for what she does state so vividly — what she omits from commenting on is of interest.

BIOGRAPHICAL FACTS

In 1872, Mary Frances Munro, who had borne three children in less than three years, was pregnant again. Each of the earlier births took place in northwest Burma, where her husband was stationed as an officer of the British military police. Although the births had been uneventful, Munro's husband decided that the fourth delivery might be less hazardous if it occurred in his family's home in Devonshire, England. There in "safe" western England, on a quiet country lane, a runaway cow charged at Mary Munro. The shock resulted in a miscarriage. The fetus died, as did the mother, leaving three young children suddenly motherless. They were far from their home in Burma and their entire family life was disrupted. Ethel Mary was 4 years old, Charles Arthur was 15 months younger, and Hector Hugh Munro—who later took the pen name of Saki—was 2 years of age.

The father, who had to return to his post in Burma, realized he could not care for his three young children and decided to entrust them to his own widowed mother and his two spinster sisters. Aside from "an unyielding strictness in observing the Sabbath . . . the children's grandmother was gentle with them" (p. 8) [18], but her two daughters were "turbulent" (a description used by Ethel after their deaths). Morley [21], in his introduction to the short stories of Saki, notes that "probably more than any writer who ever lived he has made a study of aunts and nephews. His sister's biographical sketch, which tells with moderation of the appalling auntly regime of their childhood gives us a clue to this. Aunts and werewolves were two of his specialties. Of what other writer can it be said that his Life could not be written until his aunts had died" (p. vii). Ethel Munro notes that Hector was a delicate child, and a trusted doctor declared that all three of the children "would never live to grow up" (p. 637) [21]. Ethel writes little of her parents or of Burma, but of the "up bringing" by her aunts that was quite "wrong" she notes [21]: "the house was too dark, verandas kept much of the sunlight out, the flower and vegetable gardens were surrounded by high walls and a hedge, and on rainy days we were kept indoors" (p. 637). "Fresh air was feared, especially in winter; we slept in rooms with windows shut and shuttered, with only the door open on the landing to admit stale air. All hygienic ideas were to Aunt Augusta, the Autocrat, 'choc rot,' a word of her own invention" (pp. 637–638). "The grandmother, a gentle and dignified old lady, was entirely overruled by her turbulent daughters, who hated each other with a ferocity and intensity worthy of a bigger cause" (p. 639). Ethel once asked a friend of the family what had started the antagonism. "Jealousy," she said, "when your Aunt Tom, who was fifteen years older than Augusta, returned from a long visit to Scotland, where she had been much admired, and spoilt, and found her little sister growing up, also pretty and admired, she became intensely jealous of her—from that time they have always quarreled" (p. 639). This household to which the three young abandoned orphans were brought sounds familiarly like Kipling's House of Desolation, except that there were two "Aunty Rosas."

Aunt Tom (she was never called Charlotte), the elder sister, is described by Ethel as a reincarnation of Catherine the Great. "What she meant to know to do, that she did. She had no scruples, never saw when she was hurting people's feelings, was possessed of boundless energy and had not a day's real illness until she was seventy-six" (p. 639) [21]. "Whatever she did was dramatic, and whatever story she repeated, she 'embroidered'" (p. 640). Without any sense of humor, Ethel nonetheless was an extremely funny storyteller (shades of the later Saki?).

The children had a life of their own to which they only admitted animals and a favorite uncle, Wellesley, who came to visit once a year. Other children scarcely came into their lives. They went to a children's party once a year at Christmas, but were not allowed to eat the attractive, exciting-looking food "for fear of consequences" (p. 638) [21].

The other aunt, Augusta, depicted by Saki in one of his stories, "was the autocrat of Broodgate [Broodgate Villa was the house Munro took for the family after his wife died and before leaving for Asia] — a woman of ungovernable temper, of fierce likes and dislikes, imperious, a moral coward, possessing no brains worth speaking of, and a primitive disposition. Naturally the last person who should have been in charge of children" (p. 640) [21]. The punishments were sadistic in their own way — debarring the children from invented pleasures, which they would have had, had they not misbehaved, and "fearsome silences" — "nothing could be said" (p. 640).

When the aunts fought with each other, it was like a pitched battle with yelling on each side. When Augusta had to go to bed for an entire day, it was almost a holiday for the children; they became more venturesome and daring. Augusta's religion was not elastic and definite. "Neither aunt permitted her religion to come between her and her ruling passion, which was to outwit the other" (p. 641) [21]. This could give rise to a tremendous fight, but they never swore. "One good effect the quarreling certainly had on us — it looked so ugly, we never copied them — never in our lives have we three had a row" (p. 641). Aunt Tom was busy with her gardening; making yards of useless embroidery had a soothing influence on Aunt Augusta.

One can see why Ethel might not have dared to write about her aunts while they were still alive! Langguth [18] notes that "writers may remember the good times of their childhood but they make use of the bad. Few grandmothers figure in Hector's work; instead, his stories abound with aunts, whose emotions range from unfeeling to diabolic" (pp. 8–9).

To return to Ethel's account, she continues [21]: "We had early learnt to hide our feelings — to show enthusiasm or emotion were sure to bring an amused smile to Aunt Augusta's face. It was a hateful smile, and I cannot imagine why it hurt, but it did; among ourselves we called it 'the meaning smile'. . . . With an autocrat like herself, the most unexpected little things would upset her. Both aunts were guilty of mental cruelty; we often longed for revenge" (p. 642). "Charlie really came off worst — Aunt Augusta never liked him, and positively used to enjoy whipping him. Hector and I escaped whipping, being considered too delicate" (p. 643). The children were fond of their grandmother, who was kind and gentle, but never on Sunday. She was strict on that day: "No toys, no books except Sunday books, Dr. Watt's ghastly catechism, a collect and piece of a hymn to be learnt and repeated to her, stories read to us from 'Peep of Day,' and church, of course, in the morning" (p. 643).

"Once in four years my father came home on leave (he was then a major in the Bengal Staff Corps, and Inspector-General of the Burma Police), and for six weeks we had a glorious time" (p. 647) [21]. At these times, the children did not fear Aunt Augusta. At other times, again like Kipling's Aunty Rosa, the children felt mesmerized by their aunt: "The look in her dark eyes, added to the fury in her voice, and the uncertainty as to the punishment, used to make me shiver. She had the strange characteristic of being unable to be just annoyed at anything, she had to be so angry that she would work herself into a passion" (p. 647) [21]. Ethel notes that the children seldom visited her mother's family in Kent and regrets this, as her maternal grandfather and his daughters were full of fun and life.

I shall not continue with Ethel's biography except to note that the parallels between Kipling and Munro are many — both returned to the lands of their birth, both traveled extensively, both were very taken with the East. Hector chose his pen name Saki from the cupbearer in Omar Khayyam's poem "Rubaiyat." Both Kipling and Munro understood children from their own personal perspective — their own childhood was still within them and could be expressed in their writings. Their writings were disguised and not-so-disguised autobiographical accounts of their personal beliefs and value systems. Both had suffered abandonments and severe trauma afterward, yet both were creative and relatively free of overt serious psychopathology. Saki, to the best of my knowledge, never married — nor did the other Munro children. Saki volunteered for the British Army in 1914 and was killed by a sniper's bullet in a trench in France. Never once in his biography does Ethel mention their mother or the effects of losing her and their father, but she does emphasize the evils of their aunts in their care of her and her brothers. The Munro children had their own Lorne Lodge.

INTERPRETATIONS

To return to Langguth's life story of Munro, he suggests, as did Angus Wilson about Aunty Rosa's treatment of Kipling, that a characteristic of the Victorian age that had come from the Queen herself was her dislike of children, especially toward Edward, her son and successor. The culture seemed to respond to this regal attitude "by encouraging a wholehearted repression of children for their own good, a task to which Aunt Charlotte and Aunt Augusta brought an awesome vigor" (p. 9) [18]. Aunt Tom seemingly was less severe with Hector than Aunt Augusta, who was quite vengeful. As noted above, Ethel did not publish her biography of Hector until her aunts had died. Hector could also revenge himself with gratification through his writings, although he too waited until Augusta was securely buried. Hector learned to humiliate his oppressors in a dozen ingenious ways on the printed page.

As also mentioned previously, Munro took the name of Saki from the "Rubaiyat," of Omar Khayyam. When one reads this poem, one can find suggestive evidence that it relates to Munro's identification with his dead mother and might explain his daring risk-taking ventures in the First World War that did indeed end with his being killed in the trenches. He copied five stanzas of the "Rubaiyat," which Langguth [18] republishes.

Yet ah, that Spring should vanish with the Rose!
That Youth's sweet-scented manuscript should close!

. . . And when like her, oh Saki, you shall pass
Among the guests star-scattered on the grass
And in your joyous errand reach the spot
Where I made One — turn down an empty glass!"

. . . So when that Angel of the Darker Drink
At last shall find you by the river brink,
And, offering his cup, invite your Soul
Forth to your Lips to quaff — you shall not shrink. (Pp. 61 – 62)

Langguth [18] strongly suggests that Munro was a homosexual and he presents persuasive evidence for this. However, this possibility was never mentioned by Ethel in her biography. With the death of his father, who never remarried and who returned to England on his retirement to be with his children, Munro prepared himself to leave journalism and become a full-time writer. This he did quite successfully, although there were periods of despair that stemmed not from unsuccessful work, but from loneliness and isolation — still the abandoned child!

At the age of 43, Saki enlisted in the British Army (August 25, 1914). Again, Langguth [18] suggests that "Munro had chosen to enter the ranks because his inverted tastes would find the pickings easier there" p. 251). It may be, however, that another deeper motive — a death wish to perhaps be like his mother — motivated this action. He was a model soldier, advancing in the ranks. He had offers to remove him from the front lines but he refused. As his friends were wounded or killed, Munro's euphoria about the war slowly leaked away.

In the autumn of 1916, Munro came down with malaria and he was sent back to headquarters, but he got up from bed on November 11, 1916 and reported back to the trenches, even though he should have remained in the hospital. On November 14, 1916, Munro, resting in a crater, saw one of the men light a cigarette. Lance Sergeant Munro knew this was very dangerous. He shouted his last words, "Put that bloody cigarette out" (p. 277). Fighting started, but a sniper had already killed Hector Munro at age 46 [18].

The Case of Eric Blair (George Orwell)

In the churchyard in the village of Sutton Courtenay where Orwell is buried, his grave is marked by a plain grey-brown stone on which has been inscribed:

Here Lies
Eric Arthur Blair
Born June 25th 1903
Died January 21st 1950

The inscription was specified by Orwell himself in the first part of the final sentence of his last will. The will was drawn up on 18 January 1950, three days before his death, in University College Hospital, London, where he had been a patient since the preceding September. Having chosen his epitaph, he went on to conclude the sentence with a request that no memorial service be held for him and no biography of him be written; and then he signed his name, Eric Blair. (Pp. xvii–xviii) [33].

There have been many biographies and biographical memoirs written about Eric Blair and I have attempted to study several of these in preparation for this chapter. Blair died of tuberculosis, despite efforts to use newly discovered drugs that have been used to combat this disease. He did not respond and seemingly waited for death while discussing translation rights for his already published *Animal Farm* and making arrangements for the publication of his last major work, *Nineteen Eighty-Four,* which appeared in London on June 8, 1949 and five days later in New York, only a relatively short time before he died at the age of 46.

We can appreciate Blair's prophetic insights in his literary works, especially in *Animal Farm* and *Nineteen Eighty-Four.* It is not my intention at this time to discuss in depth his most interesting and meaningful creative life from a psychoanalytic perspective. Instead, I hope to focus on some details that seemingly parallel the early significant features of the lives of Kipling and Saki. The writings of all three are disguised and derived from their own lives, especially the early years. One might say the writings are autobiographical even though literary in manifest purpose. Both Munro (Saki) and Blair (Orwell) are better known by their adopted rather than by their assumed names. All three (Kipling, Saki, and Orwell) were self-sacrificial, each in his own way, and each bearing the imprint of his unique painful childhood experiences. All three were "abandoned colonial children" who "lost" their parents in one way or another and who wrote about the overseas lands where they were born. Saki and Orwell both died at an early age. As will be seen, the early school experiences of Orwell have a strong parallel to those of Kipling in the House of Desolation and of Saki in the house where his tyrannical aunt was a constant threat. Orwell's predictions and his writings derived from many sources; the emphasis here deals with the emotional impact of his earlier life experiences, but I am mindful of the other significant variables that contributed to the amalgam from which he sprung, which later shaped and directed his literary and life pursuits.

Although he never legally changed his name, Eric Blair is known throughout the world as George Orwell. He had "tramped" around London and Paris and used the pseudonym of P. S. Burton. When his first book, based on these experiences, was to be published, he wrote to his agent suggesting three other pseudonyms. He himself favored George Orwell and thus his first published book, *Down and Out in Paris and London,* marked the appearance of this nom de plume. "The Orwell is a river in Suffolk, south of his parents' home" (p. 6) [36]. Stansky's and Abrahams' [33, 34] two-volume biography of Orwell, based on personal interviews and careful study of original documents and archives, is a magnificent source for data about *The Unknown Orwell* and *The Transformation* of Blair to Orwell. However, there are many other useful books, some of which I have consulted and read. The "latest" excellent biography is that of Bernard Crick [7]. As in my studies of Kipling, I have been impressed by the importance of comparing biographies and biographers; before dealing with Orwell, a few comments about this literary pursuit seem to be in order.

Obviously, as new facts emerge, later biographers have the advantage of utilizing them in their work. Similarly, as we understand more about the inner life of man, these insights may be useful in "filling in" the inferences to be made when factual details are unavailable. Nonetheless, differences between biographies and even autobiographies written at different times exist. Perhaps the study of biographers can help us understand these varied presentations and interpretations of a life — a follow-up study where outcome is already known. Methodologically this presents the problem of selecting those antecedent events that expectedly relate to outcome. One may not consider alternatives when prediction has already been tested. Nonetheless, if one considers all possible contingencies and variables, the task becomes insurmountable. Crick's [7] biography introduces some of these methodological issues in a most enlightening way. Since much of the work of the biographer, the psychoanalyst, and the historian have similar problems in this domain, I will briefly discuss these issues here.

Orwell's books and essays were more or less written directly from what he observed and experienced. For example, *Burmese Days, Animal Farm,* and *Nineteen Eighty-Four* had clear political purposes and were anti-imperialist or expressed Orwell's concerns and fears where special privilege and bureaucratic manipulation, even for the public good, were the goals. He was a great essayist and a brilliant journalist. Crick points out that he addressed particular themes positively (e.g., love of nature, books, and literature) and others negatively (e.g., mass production, distrust of intellectuals, suspicion of government, contempt for and warnings against totalitarianism [of the right and the left], imperialism, racialism, and censorship). He favored simple language, speech, the good in the past, fraternity, individuality, liberty, equality, and patriotism. As Crick [7] notes, "he was indeed, a 'revolutionary patriot.' For he saw our heritage and the land itself as belonging to the common people, not to the gentry and the upper middle classes" (p. 21). That this philosophy might be related to his preparatory school experiences will be discussed shortly.

Despite his own philosophy, however, Orwell did observe and write about human issues that have had and continue to have universal importance. His observations in *Animal Farm* and in *Nineteen Eighty-Four* and the social science, economic, political, and psychological insights expressed in these novels, though stemming in part from his earlier life experiences and fantasies, have a validity of their own. Unfortunately they also have predictive value in terms of totalitarianism. What he stated so clearly and vividly in his novels could be intuitively applied to the broader political scene, whether right or left in its orientation. Furthermore, *Animal Farm* and *Nineteen Eighty-Four* are significant discussions of elitism and power manipulation, despite their fictive format.

Crick [7] points out that Eric Blair did not suddenly change his character when he called himself "George Orwell" for the publication of his first book. Instead, as we know from psychodynamic developmental theory and observation, the process of transformation was gradual, subtle, and had particular antecedents.

Crick has made a major contribution to biography in his short essay on biography and "character" [7], which is embedded in the "Introduction" to his book. Because of my interest in the methodology of biographical and autobiographical writing as these relate to free association and personal myths, and because of my reading of several key biographical studies dealing with the same individual and finding discrepancies, I feel a brief discussion of Crick's comments are indicated.

As Crick [7] simultaneously read a lot of biography, he began to grapple with the problem of evidence and he grew "skeptical of much of the fine writing, balanced appraisal and psychological insight that is the hallmark of the English tradition of biography. It may be pleasant to read, but readers should realize that often they are being led by the nose, or that the biographer is fooling himself by an affable pretense of being able to enter into another person's mind" (p. 29). Crick notes that "smoothing out or silently resolving contradictions in the evidence and bridging gaps by empathy and intuition" (p. 29) does not remove gaps in evidence or contradictions. "None of us can enter into another person's mind; to believe so is fiction. We can only know actual persons by observing their behavior in a variety of different situations and through different perspectives" (p. 30).

Well-written biographies are like novels, and good novels have embedded in them bits of the author's autobiography, even though it is disguised. One must look for evidence, even though it may point to contradictory conclusions. Biographies that read like fiction are extreme examples of an "empathetic fallacy" (p. 30) [7]. At the opposite pole is the "purely empiricist presentation of the evidence" (p. 30). So one must avoid "seductive short-cuts and pseudocertainties even of 'empathy'" (p. 30), without abandoning the evidence and chronicle of events as they unfold. "Gaps in the evidence are inevitable and should not be disguised either by expanding with surmise what we do not have, or by contracting, for the sake of balanced chapter lengths, what we do have" (p. 31) [7]. Of course one tries to fill gaps or find other sources of evidence, "but when one does have to speculate, when a gap in the evidence seems crucial to the coherence of other parts of the record, one should simply say so clearly" (p. 31).

Crick [7] emphasizes that "the trouble with the empathetic approach to acting . . . was in trying to create the illusion of being someone else, the character is then fixed, frozen, and unchallengeable. The audience loses any critical distance and must accept or reject totally the character as portrayed. But both human freedom and good art demand not a suspension of disbelief, but a critical awareness that an actor is acting [and I would add interpreting] and that the part could be played in other ways. . . . So also with an actual human life and a biography" (p. 32). "We may understand a person better by knowing more about their history and background, but however much we know there is no inevitable inference from these antecedent facts to what someone actually writes" (p. 32). Crick argues against simplistic, formulalistic, and reductionistic explanations — a caution well worth noting. "Freedom, imagination, will and chance are all at play throughout life" (p. 32). This antideterministic caution can be discussed further but will take us far afield from my purpose.

It is possible to see repetitive patterns in the course of a life; evidence can be obtained from "here and now" observations rather than on reconstructions where one can end up with "a kind of speculative teleology" (p. 32) [7]. Careful understanding of creative products over time to ascertain thematic perseverations is a further evidential path that helps us in our task. For example, Crick [7] realized right from the beginning how intricate was the relationship between Orwell's life and his writings. "All of his books except the last two are obviously based upon his own experiences, and it is clear that he deliberately went out to gain experiences in order to write about them" (p. 32). I would suggest that even the last two, *Animal Farm* and *Nineteen Eighty-Four,* were also based on his experiences, which fueled his creative fantasy life, which in turn was translated into his writing.

Only by recognizing the evidence from the "repetition compulsion," albeit repetition in writing, can one give full rein to interpreting the author, the work, and even the audience's response. *Animal Farm* and *Nineteen Eighty-Four* come from Orwell's unconscious, preconscious, conscious, and his creative reality-oriented fantasy life. This will be seen in the discussion of Orwell's "Such, Such Were the Joys," a story of his prep school experiences — how he reacted to them at the time, how he wrote about them many years later, and how these could possibly be related to his classics, *Animal Farm* and *Nineteen Eighty-Four.* Crick [7] calls attention to the problem of retrospective accuracy of memory, especially of earlier events, especially unless supported by external evidence. This same argument can apply to Kipling's "Baa Baa, Black Sheep." However, one cannot ignore parallel experiences, parallel stories, and the awareness that even if facts may be somewhat inaccurate in order to create a literary report, the very "distortions" are also significant and important.

I do not agree with Crick [7] when he writes, "If the domestic privacies are relevant to understanding the writings or the public role of an author, then they must be fully treated and not ignored; but if they are not relevant, they need not be examined and therefore, for the sake of clarity and economy, should not be examined" (pp. 38–39). This ignoring of data is what he himself opposed earlier in his essay. One must state one's orientation and then leave room for alternative or additional interpretations without closing the door on evidentially supported different interpretations. Nonetheless, Crick in his "Prologue" has rendered us a service in opening up issues of biographical writing that are worthy of more extensive thought and discussion.

BIOGRAPHICAL FACTS

Eric Arthur Blair was born in India on June 25, 1903, five years after his sister, Marjorie, was born and five years before his younger sister, Avril, was born. His father, Richard W. Blair, was a civil servant in a department of the Government of India. For nearly 20 years Richard moved to new posts annually; they were not good posts. There were several more extended assignments, the last being one lasting quite long, from a year after Eric's birth until retirement. Life was not a huge success for Richard Blair, an indigent son from an aristocratic background. He had not gone to public school or university because his family could not afford to send him, so his assignment in "the service" was not a favorable or fashionable one. His postings and gradings indicate that he did not get easily or quickly promoted. He retired on a limited pension with very little family inheritance. In 1896, when he was 39, he married Ida Limouzin, who was 21. She was born near London of an English mother and a French father. She had lived most of her life in Burma, where her father had a business. "Ida Blair, eighteen years younger than her husband, was a more lively, unconventional, widely read and in every way a more interesting person" than her husband (p. 47) [7]. She was a realist, much like Kipling's mother, who could adjust to difficult circumstances. Richard Blair was a tolerant and easygoing man, who may not have approved of all of his wife's opinions, but was no martinet or tyrant.

Ida Blair took her two young children back to England in 1904, not in 1907 as other biographers have written. Richard Blair did not see them again until 1907, when he had a three-month leave. Avril, Eric's younger sister, was conceived at that time. Richard returned to India before she was born and did not rejoin the family until 1911, when he retired. Ida Blair did much of the work and child care herself since the family was of limited means. Her 1905 diary notes Eric's episodic ill health, especially of his respiratory system (e.g., bronchitis). He had difficulties with his chest throughout his life, eventually dying of pulmonary tuberculosis. Crick [7] notes that Ida Blair was a benevolent gadabout. "The diary gives the impression of a woman who could be very protective towards her children, but not ever present, perhaps over compensatory when at home" (p. 49).

Eric Blair claimed no memories of life in India and noted in his essay "Why I Write" (1946) that he barely saw his father before he was 8. "For this and other reasons I was somewhat lonely. . . . I think from the very start my literary ambitions were mixed up with the feelings of being isolated and undervalued" (pp. 309) [23]. At 6, he was sexually and socially interested in "the plumber's daughter," but he was separated from her by his mother because she was "common." Orwell notes that when he was 6 he passed through a phase of sexuality. He especially enjoyed "playing at doctors" and got a thrill holding a toy trumpet, which was supposed to be a stethoscope, against a little girl's belly. He also fell "deeply in love" with a 15-year-old girl. One can speculate that growing up in a household with three females — mother and two sisters — without a father in evidence could have stimulated his oedipal longings, including his sexual feelings. Evidence to support this possibility, cited by Crick [7] is an autobiographical fragment that Orwell recalls from age 6.

I am 6 years old, and I am walking along a street in our little town with my mother and a wealthy local brewer, who is also a magistrate [like father?] The tarred fence is covered with chalk drawings, some of which I have made myself. The magistrate stops, points disapprovingly with his stick and says, "We are going to catch the boys who draw on these walls and we are going to order them Six Strokes of the Birch Rod." (It was all in capitals in my mind.) My knees knock together, my tongue cleaves to the roof of my mouth and at the earliest possible moment I sneak away to spread the dreadful intelligence. . . . not till many years later, perhaps 20 years, did it occur to me that my fears had been groundless. No magistrate would have condemned me to Six Strokes of the Birch Rod, even if I had been caught drawing on the wall. Such punishment was reserved for the Lower Orders. (P. 52)

There indeed was a brewer, called Simmons, who was a magistrate and also a friend of his mother's. The doctor game, the distant love of the older girl, the fear of the older man, and the punishment by beating are seemingly related in a classical fashion. Especially important are the fears of punishment. Avril hinted much later that neither she nor Eric, like Simmons, had his close friendship with their mother—especially since their father was off in India.

Fiderer [9] points out the emphasis on whipping and physical punishment in Orwell's writing. For example, in "Such, Such Were the Joys," was a series of whippings; in *Burmese Days,* Orwell's fist book, Orwell indicates the British were in Burma to beat or punish the natives. All of Orwell's hate and guilt about the injustice of colonialism are bound up with images and depictions of physical cruelty. Fiderer [9] also points out that the women "are singled out as the most conspicuous torturers" (p. 4); they instigate the beatings. Fiderer suggests that these horrors of torture, beating, and punishment should be "understood as representing unconscious fantasies" and so are exaggerated. Shengold [30], on the other hand, referring to Orwell's *Nineteen Eighty-Four,* focuses on the hero as tortured by exposure and threatened by starving rats. The torturer is a Stalin-like Big Brother [30]. Orwell was appalled by what he saw in Burma where he, in reality, took a post as policeman. This could be viewed, as was seen in Kipling's life, as a manifestation of his own sadistic impulses. In Orwell's life, however, he was unable to continue on, and so resigned his policeman's post. Nonetheless, Orwell returned to the Indian police, the land of his birth, and probably participated in beatings himself. Furthermore, he was loyal to the British government, volunteered to fight in the Second World War, and actually did fight in the Spanish Civil War.

Fiderer [9] further indicates Orwell's preoccupation with physical torture and beatings in *Animal Farm, Coming Up for Air, A Clergyman's Daughter,* and *Nineteen Eighty-Four.* Although there are unconscious determinants, especially from earlier years, for Orwell's preoccupations, he was prophetic and did accurately describe the real sadistic behavior of the Nazi concentration camps and of the Stalinist tortures and torturers. What these determinants were can only be speculated about. Crick [7], Orwell's most recent biographer, points out arguments and inconsistencies in Orwell's own early life that do not yield a simple explanation. Nonetheless, the textual accounts are there and can be seen in several of Orwell's works. Was it Orwell the sadist, the masochist, the political prophet, or the superb writer who sensed what his readers might "enjoy"? Perhaps it was some of each.

Eric did grow up, until he left for prep school at age 8, entirely among women, having seen his father only for 3 months when he was 4. When he was sent to boarding school at age 8, father returned. However, Eric was sent away to a brutal world, whereas before he was the only male at home. In an isolated passage in a notebook, written in the last year of his life, Orwell recalls overhearing, as a small boy, conversations between his mother, his aunt, his elder sister, and her feminist friends that women did not like men. They were looked upon as large, ugly, smelly animals who maltreated women in every way. He believed, until he was 20, that sexual intercourse gave pleasure only to the man, not to the woman. As explained by Crick [10], the picture in his mind was that of a man chasing a woman, forcing her down, and jumping on top of her as he had often seen a cock do to a hen.

In order to get into the right school, boys of 8 years of age were sent to preparatory schools. Fee-paying, wealthy children, or boys of the landed aristocracy had no difficulty with tuition, room, and board. But children of modest means, whose parents recognized that entry into the Church, the Army, the Civil Service, and the professions depended on one's schooling, especially in view of Richard Blair's experience, had parents who were particularly eager for their sons to get a scholarship to a preparatory school that had a good record of getting its graduates into one of the best public schools. The newer preparatory schools wished to establish and buttress their reputation by selecting for scholarships those boys who would do well and go on to the better public schools (e.g., Eton, Harrow). And so, based on the recommendation of his local convent school, Eric Blair entered St. Cyprian's at age 8 and stayed there until he was 13. Mrs. Blair probably applied in the spring of 1911 and interviews with the headmaster and owner of the school, Mr. Vaughn Wilkes, and the "real power behind the throne," Mrs. Wilkes, took place. Mr. Blair had not yet retired but would do so very soon. His pension and the scholarship Eric was awarded "must have turned 'extraordinarily difficult' into 'just possible'" (p. 59) [7]. The scholarship was kept secret even from Eric, but as he got near his entrance examinations for public school, Mrs. Wilkes told him in order to shame, threaten, and goad him into working harder.

Despite the methodological cautions of Crick and others about the resurrection, reinterpretations, and reconstruction of our past from perspectives of the adult as contrasted with what was experienced as a child, St. Cyprian's was no pleasure for Orwell. In referring to the torments of his childhood, Orwell's posthumously published account of his days at St. Cyprian's is so unhappy and so horrible a picture of institutional despotism that one can see in it the origins of *Nineteen Eighty-Four,* aspects of *Animal Farm,* and a striking similarity to Kipling's "Baa Baa, Black Sheep." Crick [7] agrees that the food was awful and inadequate, as was the heating and sanitation. The code was austere, and the war did not improve conditions. St. Cyprian's was a commercial enterprise and one for which the sheltered, albeit conflicted, Eric Blair was ill prepared. In a seething essay, "Such, Such Were the Joys" (1947), one can detect the rage Orwell [23] still felt after many decades. The school emphasized competition and rankings. Blair's letters to his mother constantly refer to this. St. Cyprian's, in the essay, is described as barbaric and totally unprivate, filled with caning, beatings, cramming, and fear. "Such, Such Were the Joys," which Orwell described as autobiographical, could not be published in Great Britain until after Mrs. Wilkes' death in 1967, when she was 92.

Eric Blair wrote, "By their law I was damned. I had no money, I was weak, I was ugly. I was unpopular, I had a chronic cough, I was cowardly, I smelt" (pp. 65 – 66) [7]. Even with a questioning attitude and suggesting the possibility that some of the horrors described in his essay are embellishments or overstated accounts, Blair's experience at St. Cyprian's was not pleasant, to say the least. Even educationally, the learning was anti-intellectual learning by rote. Favoritism was very much in evidence, especially if one came from wealthy or important families. As Crick notes, the major themes of the essay are cruelty, physical canings, shame, favoritism, snobbing, shame, bad teaching, filth, and bullying. Orwell writes about the enuresis of the hero who, after several nights, is warned that he will be caned if he does not stop. Mrs. Wilkes is the major villain, although her husband does the beating. There is no reason to doubt Eric was beaten for bed-wetting. The beatings were almost public and the picture presented resembles that of Ilse Koch and the Nazi concentration camps. Cruelty was a characteristic of the school, especially in relation to the arbitrariness and uncertainty of the punishment. The beatings could last for five minutes and only increased his sense of desolate loneliness and helplessness.

Mrs. Wilkes was capricious and, if one was in her favor, life was blissful; if out of her favor, it was hell. Eric Blair was generally out of favor. The food for the rich boys was different from that served to the less fortunate children. Wilkes tried to please the well-off and well-connected parents so that the commercial part of the school would be enhanced. When Eric learned that he was a "scholarship" student, it must have made him even more vulnerable. The filth of the dishes, the porridge with hairs and unexplained black things floating about, the slimy water of the plunge bath, the presence of human feces in the unchanged water, the greasy basins, the moldy towels, the dirty and dilapidated lavoratories without locks on the doors, and the evil smells all made it unpleasant for Eric Blair to think of his preparatory school days with any pleasantness.

If Blair felt a fantasied punishment for his earlier oedipal triumphs, he undoubtedly could find his fears actualized in reality. Bullying by the top form, receiving a bloodied mouth, being shoved and laughed at, and the violence of Mrs. Wilkes herself (e.g., pulling boys' hair) brought frequent tears to Eric Blair's face. And yet he did not talk of this to his mother, much as Kipling or Munro could not share their experiences with their parents. Injustice and oppression along with brutality were pivotal features of Orwell's later writings. His experiences at prep school prepared him to reject imperialism, to side with the underdog, and to oppose totalitarianism of the right and the left.

Blair did not reject the First World War or Empire as Kipling did in 1914. As Crick [7] again notes, the War led to his first publication in the *Henley and South Oxfordshire Standard* of a poem titled "Awake Young Men of England" (p. 85). This put him in good favor with Mrs. Wilkes, but only for a short while. His father, aged 60 in 1917, decided to enlist and was commissioned a second lieutenant. A friend commented that she did not believe Eric was fond of his father. He respected and obeyed him but was much closer to his mother and sisters, especially Avril. Avril remembered him as aloof and undemonstrative; others commented on his reserve and self-contained quality as well.

The last two years at St. Cyprian's focused on his hard work to try for a scholarship, especially to Eton. To have a "safety position" he also took the examination for Wellington College, a lesser school, which he successfully passed. Mr. Wilkes, himself, took him to the Eton examination. Eric placed fourteenth, missing Eton by one place, and so went to Wellington, which he did not like. Because of the War, a vacancy occurred at Eton and just before his fourteenth birthday in May 1917, Eric Blair joined Eton College. Eric's chubbiness persisted until his face grew cavernous from two pneumonias. Prep school left Eric Blair an instinctive rationalist, antiromantic, inhibited, and secretive. The hostile world of prep school with its physical violence, emotional blackmail, and favoritism for the fortune may well have left its mark on the sensitive young boy who suddenly was removed from the informality and comfort of his mother's home; also traumatic was that he found his place taken by his father.

"Such, Such Were the Joys" is an unusual account of a young boy's boarding school experience [23]. It opens with: "Soon after I arrived at Crossgates (not immediately, but after a week or two, just when I seemed to be settling into the routine of school life) I began wetting my bed. I was now aged eight, so that this was a reversion to a habit which I must have grown out of at least four years earlier" (p. 1). Mrs. Wilkes becomes Mrs. Simpson, the headmaster's wife, in the story. Orwell describes the beatings by the headmaster, his helplessness, his shame, and the snobbishness of Crossgates with such accuracy that there is little doubt that, even if the account is not fully accurate, it is close and includes his own perceptions, even if they vary in minor detail from the reports of others. The reader is advised to read the essay to catch the full flavor of Orwell's memoir. Let me quote the ending of this long account:

I have never been back to Crossgates. In a way it is only within the last decade that I have really thought over my school days, vividly though their memory has haunted me. Nowadays, I believe, it would make very little impression on me to see the place again, if it still exists. And if I went inside and smelt again the inky, dusty smell of the big schoolroom, the rosiny smell of the chapel, the stagnant smell of the swimming bath and the cold reek of the lavoratories, I think I should only feel what one invariably feels in revisiting any scene of childhood: How small everything has grown, and how terrible is the deterioration in myself! (P. 47)

Even before St. Cyprian's, Eric "was acutely sensitive to dirt and smells; he was repelled by physical ugliness, the paunches, jowls, wrinkles, sagging breasts and stomachs, and flabby thighs and buttocks of adults; he was disgusted by dogs' messes on pavements and horse dung in the street; his nostrils caught the whiff of sweat, bad breath, stale beer, and unwashed armpits; he was offended by mortality, the sense of decay made visible when he came upon the carcass of a frog being eaten by maggots" (p. 37) [33]. Perhaps this correlates with his very sensitive respiratory tract and his subsequent illnesses, but it seems to antedate the fecal, fetid, decaying body of odors associated with St. Cyprian's. That the sudden separations from his home, and earlier from India, were critical events in his life can be assumed, but the reinforcement by Mrs. Wilkes and the ambience of St. Cyprian's further aggravated and may have even induced certain responses that remained throughout Blair-Orwell's relatively short life.

Blair's later life and his transformation into Orwell, the writer, is worthy of fuller discussion, but I shall refrain from doing this now. Orwell wrote very little about Eton, but of the little he did write on the subject, much was critical and deprecatory. Nonetheless, Eric Blair did not rebel or abstain from the Etonian way of life. "Discipline in College — as it took physical form, beating, birching, caning, the Corporal Punishment that Blair called 'disgusting and barbarous' — was in the hands of the boys of Sixth Form (not the Masters, who were not allowed to cane), and much would depend, then, on their intelligence, humaneness, fairness, and emotional balance" (p. 123) [33]. Blair was still being subjected to mass floggings at age 18!

Blair chose not to go to university after Eton, perhaps because he and his family could not afford this further education. His father suggested the Indian Civil Service, and Eric Blair joined the Indian Imperial Police and was trained in Burma. He served there for nearly five years and then in 1927, while home on leave, decided not to return. His resignation was effective on the first day of 1928. As Williams [36] observes, Eric Blair followed the pattern of his family, but he broke with this at age 24. He made a new set of social relationships and assumed a new social identity. This was part of the transformational process of Eric Blair into George Orwell. He rejected imperialism and decided to be the writer he always wanted to be.

After leaving the Imperial Police, Blair took rooms first in London and later in Paris to get to know the poor people. He became ill with pneumonia in Paris and returned to England in 1929. These experiences formed the basis of his early book, *Down and Out in Paris and London*. In late 1932, he assumed the name, never legally changed, of George Orwell. His first novel, *Burmese Days*, deals with imperialism as he observed it. In 1936, he married Eilleen O'Shaughnessy, an Oxford graduate in English. He was married in June, and in July the Spanish Civil War broke out. By the end of autumn, Orwell was preparing to go to Spain to collect material for articles and perhaps fight. He went to Barcelona and went into action in January 1937. His experiences with Soviet-style communism again transformed him into an anticommunist, but he remained a revolutionary socialist. He left Spain in 1937, broke with the orthodox left, and joined the Independent Labour Party. He became ill with tuberculosis in late 1938 and was in the sanitorium. He tried to join the army when the Second World War began, but was rejected as physically unfit. In 1941, he joined the BBC as a producer-commentator of the Indian Service. In 1943, his mother died. He became ill again and left the BBC to become a literary editor. In late 1943, Orwell began to write *Animal Farm*, which he completed in February 1944. It was rejected by several publishers on political grounds, but was published in August 1945, at the end of the War. He and his wife adopted a son in 1944, but in March 1945 his wife died during an operation. His elder sister died in 1946, and his own health began to deteriorate further. During 1947, there was a reappearance of his tuberculosis. He reworked *Nineteen Eighty-Four* but was too ill to write anything else. He went into the hospital in London in September 1949 and in October married Sonia Brownell. He died in January 1950.

INTERPRETATIONS

The emotional, political, social, and economic events of Orwell's life do not explain why he became a writer, even though they played significant roles in what he wrote. As Williams [36] has noted, "The distinction between 'fiction' and 'nonfiction' is not a matter of whether the experience happened to the writer, not a distinction between 'real' and 'imaginary.' The distinction is one of range and consciousness. . . . Orwell began to write literature . . . when he found this nonfictional form capable of realizing his experience directly. Realizing his experience — not only what had happened to him and what he had observed, but what he felt about it and what he thought about it, the self-definition of 'Orwell,' the man inside and outside the experience" (p. 48). The writer organizes and shapes what happened to produce a particular effect. This is based on experience, outer and inner, but the creation is new, even though it comes from these experiences. Williams believes that the process of selection and organization is a literary act. The writer is the external observer, the observer of the inside, the fashioner of the literary creation.

Stansky and Abrahams [33] have written that "the making of a writer is a complex process; and who is to say with any assurance where it begins — with his first book, or his first day at school, the day of his birth, or generations back, lost in a tangle of genealogy?" (p. xv). Becoming George Orwell was part of the process of making himself into a writer and coming to terms with himself and his world. As Stansky and Abrahams observe, "Blair was the man to whom things happened; Orwell the man who wrote about them" (pp. xv–xvi). He did become a writer of extraordinary power. At times Blair and Orwell were one; then the polarities occurred. For seventeen years until his death he wrote and wrote.

In a brief essay, "Why I Write," Orwell [23] states that he knew from an early age, perhaps 5 or 6, that he would be a writer when he grew up. He tried to abandon the idea between ages 17 and 24, but knew he would settle down and write. He describes the childhood shaping forces that were part of the process of becoming a writer. "I had the lonely child's habit of making up stories and holding conversations with imaginary persons, and I think from the very start my literary ambitions were mixed up with the feeling of being isolated and undervalued. I know that I had a facility with words and a power of facing unpleasant facts, and I felt that this created a sort of private world in which I could get my own back for my failure in everyday life. . . . I wrote my first poem at the age of 4 or 5, my mother taking it down to dictation" (p. 309). He goes on to say he gives the ready background material about himself because one needs to assess a writer's motives and this requires knowing something of his early development. "His subject matter will be determined by the age he lives in . . . but before he ever begins to write he will have acquired an emotional attitude from which he will never completely escape . . . if he escapes from his early influences altogether he will have killed his impulse to write" (p. 311). Orwell describes four great motives for writing: sheer egoism, aesthetic enthusiasm, historical impulse, and political purpose. In the concluding section of this short, candid, yet powerful, essay, he asserts that "All writers are vain, selfish and lazy, and at the bottom of their motives there lies a mystery" (p. 316).

Bion's Part of a Life *and White's* Flaws in the Glass

BIOGRAPHICAL FACTS OF WILFRED BION

Francesca Bion tells us in the Foreword of Bion's autobiography [2] that he was born in India in 1897. He came from a long line of individuals who had served in India as missionaries, police, and in the Department of Public Works. At age 8 he was sent to England to attend preparatory school and he never returned to India. Despite this, he retained a strong affection for India and had planned a visit there but died two months prior to the return to the land of his birth.

In a very open fashion, Bion writes of his lonely, unloved childhood in India, of his father whom he feared and did not like, his somewhat cold mother, and his destestable sister who was his only playmate. He cried a great deal, seemed to always be in difficulty, and had a tendency to lie when in trouble. Masturbation, though sinful, was a pleasure. When he entered boarding school in England at age 8, he plunged into a deeper hell of terrors, self-doubts, and guilt. He writes [2] that as he approached Bombay, on the way to England, he saw the railway station, "which even in retrospect can evoke in me nostalgic feelings of great poignancy. I came in time to believe that these feelings were the substitute for what others called 'homesickness.' But I have no home for which I could feel sick—only people and things. Thus, when I found myself alone in the playground of the Preparatory School in England where I kissed my mother a dry-eyed goodbye, I could see, above the hedge which separated me from her and the road which was the boundary of the wide world itself, her hat go bobbing up and down like some curiously wrought millinery cake carried on the wave of green hedge. And then it was gone" (p. 33). Bion was numbed and stupefied. When the "ghastly day ended I was able to get under the bedclothes and sob" (34). And weep he did, silently. "Tears did not cool and refresh—they scalded" (pp. 34–35). He felt secure in bed, where he could weep quietly. Very early he was determined never to reveal his vulnerabilities to others and he was seen as gentle, nonperturbable, and laconic. Despite legitimate triumphs, he always felt he was a fraud who could be unmasked and disgraced. Yet in the First World War he was heroic and won a medal for bravery, which he felt he did not deserve.

INTERPRETATIONS

Bion became a world famous psychoanalytic theoretician and clinician despite the traumas of his childhood and early adolescence. And yet, as noted by his widow, he seemingly loved India even though he did not feel close to his own family. Was his response to the English boarding school a culmination of his despair from India? Did he feel abandoned even before arriving in England? Did the preparatory school provide difficulties of its own for young Bion that allowed him to compensatorily develop ego strengths that helped him in his later life and in his career as a psychoanalyst? One can only conjecture about these queries; however, his response in some ways is similar to the other "colonial" children who were sent to England at an early age to prepare for life. Some made it quite easily, some did not, and some suffered much in their adaptations.

Psychoanalysis brought a new autobiographical mode into being. In the psychoanalytic treatment, both analysand and analyst work together to register, understand, and trace out the significance of earlier life experiences on later life behaviors, feelings, fantasies, and thoughts. Psychoanalysts in one sense are trained and accredited for working with autobiography—in a sense, autobiography becomes the profession. In the psychoanalytic situation, however, a single, consecutive, connected story does not emerge in that form. Partial glimpses, pieces of memory, reactions to the psychoanalyst, dreams, slips, and fantasies all come out as seemingly isolated vignettes. And yet, a mosaic, a series of patterns, emerges that has a logic of its own. Reconstructions, relivings, insights, repetitions, and interactions in and out of the therapeutic situation, all contribute to the process of self-understanding. In a written autobiography things flow as in a story; yet the sequence of unfolding in psychoanalysis may not be as smooth or regular as the autobiographer or the biographer reports. The revelations may be truncated; the resolutions reported as one-sided decisions may be less simple. But to have the psychoanalyst write his own autobiography is a relatively unique event. Others have done so, and I presume someone soon will study the comparative autobiographies of the professional students of biography, the psychoanalysts. The interactions between the observer and the reporter parallel the therapeutic split with which we are familiar in our clinical work. We continually add to our autobiographies, but few if any have a chance to study them and report on them. Bion has done so, and all psychoanalysts train their students and their patients to look as carefully, as objectively as possible, and somewhat skeptically at the autobiographical productions in order to further our insights into ourselves and into our fellow human beings.

BIOGRAPHICAL FACTS OF PATRICK WHITE

In 1973, the Nobel Prize for literature was awarded to Patrick White, who was born in England in 1912 but was taken back to Australia at 6 months of age. Asthmatic, homosexual, and almost 70 when he wrote his autobiography, *Flaws in the Glass* [35], White describes again what by now the reader can recognize as a pattern. His mother determined that she would go one better than any other Australian family by sending her son to an English public school and to an English university as well. Bitterly disappointed with her life, she attempted to vicariously obtain through her son that which she herself had missed. However, her son did not give her grandchildren or a daughter-in-law; instead he was a male child that she labeled a "freak." White did go to King's College in Cambridge after Cheltenham Public School.

When White's mother drove him to Cheltenham Public School at age 13, she exclaimed, "This is the proudest day of my life." White [35] notes that "when the gates of my expensive prison closed I lost confidence in my mother" (p. 12). He never forgave her for the next four miserable years he spent there — his "four-year prison sentence." The school was physically cold, foul-smelling, and afforded him no privacy. The breakfasts were bleak and sparse. White's Australianness made him an outcast. The housemaster's obsession with sex and especially masturbation bordered on the pathological. "He would burst into toshroom or gym hoping to catch us in flagrante. He was the tallest man I had seen. He smashed the light bulbs caning us. He promised to stamp out a 'morbid kink' on discovering my passion for Chekov, Ibsen, and Strindberg, and only stamped it deeper in. Never during my stay in his house did he uncover sex, though he must have disturbed fantasies in his forays through toshroom steam and the stench of sweat-sodden jerseys and mud-caked boots in a more puritanical gym. We were far too frightened" (p. 13) [35]. When his parents and three-year younger sister left him at Cheltenham, White did nothing—he did not cry, although he would have liked to tear off his father's glove and hold his hand to his own cheek. Instead he "throbbed" as his family left on the fast-moving train.

White's mother, unlike his more mild and gentle father, had a violent temper. His mother did the whippings with a formidable riding crop. Mother was relentlessly determined to do everything for his own good, "which included dumping me in a prison of a school on the other side of the world" (p. 9) [35].

INTERPRETATIONS

As we have already seen in the preceding sections, the hostile and aggressive female caretakers were either frightening or directly abusing, and the surrogate caretakers at the boarding school carried on in the tradition of abuse. Nonetheless these young gifted men became creative in ways that were acclaimed by the public.

Postscript

How can I conclude a chapter that in some ways is only a beginning? Although some of the ideas and work had been ongoing for some time, it was only when I was a patient in the intensive care unit that I realized the unifying themes presented above. A diagnosis had not yet been made, this was my first major hospitalization, and the concerns of all who were and are very close to me were in evidence. I, too, was very concerned, felt "my body was abandoning me" and, as a result, I was in jeopardy. My caretakers were and are excellent, but the central ideas I have tried to develop kept returning. Paying close attention to my dreams, I realized that I was "in touch" with aspects of me that existed before conscious memory or willing recollection. Very shortly after my birth, my mother developed a serious septic breast abscess. She and I were separated because it was feared that I, too, might become very ill from contact with her. I was entrusted to unwilling relatives who, in retrospect, were incompetent to deal with and care for a newborn infant. In the hospitalization that I recently had, which culminated in a coronary bypass surgical operation, old archaic feelings unlinked to conscious events appeared. By working at them and the accompanying dreams, I could interpret with great value what these meant to me, where they came from, and how the past was resurrected by the "present" crisis.

The idea of temporary abandonment and noncaring caretakers came together with what I had been trying to put into appropriate perspective. Clinical data from my work with patients, supervisees, and colleagues "fit," and so I pursued the lines of scientific association wherever they led. By using literary figures and biographical data in the public domain, no data about patients has been revealed, although information and levels of understanding derived from my clinical work are abundant throughout. I have shared a fragment of my own autobiography because I believe knowing how something begins (what was in the mind of the conceiver) can be useful in understanding the product that ensues. Reconstructing the history of the psychological lives of creative individuals has and will be the subject of much discussion. Facts alone do not tell us the story. Patterns that are repeated by the individuals themselves and that have similarities in different individuals can open areas for further study. Even with the concerns of methodological issues, there is value in seeing biographies as outcome studies with attempts to identify some contributing antecedents.

Stambolian [32] points out that one is able to recognize various themes, images, and patterns of expression that characterize an author's particular view of reality. Proust calls these phrase-types and asserts that by understanding an artist's unique characteristics and their ongoing similarities enables a reader to further appreciate the writer. But the task of reconstructing involves knowing the special view of reality that is peculiar to a particular writer [32]. This we get from attempting to find evidence about the inner structure of a writer's creative personality and about particular experiences that had shaping significance in the transformation of the writer's experiences in life (external and internal) into a work of art. Stambolian devotes his book to a study of Proust, but his insights can equally be applied to many other creative individuals. Submerged past comes into the present; memory, impressions, reminiscences, and reconstructions occur; and patterns emerge. This allows us to get "new truths," which allow us to move further — have new insights, eliminate gaps in the continuity of our understanding, and explain our own and others' interests, motives, and outcomes. This "psychoanalytic process" can occur in a psychoanalytic treatment setting, in a self-induced psychoanalytic encounter where one feels, experiences, and then observes what is or has emerged, and in the study of other lives. Insight can be the creative outcome.

I wish to close by returning to my central theme: Abandonment as seen from the point of view of the abandoned has many different facets. The impact will depend on various factors (e.g., when the abandonment occurred, the prior emotional organization of the individual, the circumstances of the abandonment, and the "replacements" for the abandoner or abandoners). How can this be handled preventively? Unfortunately, not always easily. There must be preparation, replacement, and continuity of contact with a familiar, which will facilitate a discharge of feelings including fear, rage, and despair; the caretaker must be aware of and recognize this ongoing turmoil.

References

1. Bettelheim, Bruno *The Uses of Enchantment.* New York: Vintage Books Edition, 1977.
2. Bion, W. F. *The Long Week-End: 1897–1919.* Abingdon, England: Fleetwood Press, 1982.
3. Birkenhead, Lord *Rudyard Kipling.* New York: Random House, 1978.
4. Brontë, Emily *Wuthering Heights.* New York: New American Library, 1959.
5. Carrington, Charles E. *The Life of Rudyard Kipling.* New York: Doubleday, 1955.
6. Carrington, Charles E. *Rudyard Kipling: His Life and Work* (3rd ed.). London: Macmillan, 1978.
7. Crick, Bernard *George Orwell: A Life.* New York: Penguin Books, 1982.
8. Edel, Leon *Stuff of Sleep and Dreams.* New York: Harper & Row, 1982.
9. Fiderer, G. Masochism as literary strategy: Orwell's psychological novels. *Literature and Psychology* 20:3, 1970.
10. Fleming, Alice M. Some childhood memories of Rudyard Kipling. *Chamber's Journal* 8:168, 1939.
11. Fleming, Alice M. More childhood memories of Rudyard Kipling. *Chamber's Journal* 9:506, 1939.
12. Freud, Anna Infants Without Families and Reports on the Hampstead Nurseries 1939–1945 (in collaboration with Dorothy Burlingham). In M. Masud-R. Khan (Ed.), *International Psycho-Analytical Library,* No. 96. London: The Hogarth Press and the Institute for Psycho-Analysis, 1974.

13. Green, Roger Lancelyn *Kipling and the Children.* London: Elek Books Ltd., 1965.
14. Greene, Graham *The Best of Saki (H. H. Munro).* New York: The Viking Press, 1972.
15. Kafka, Franz *America (Amerika).* London: Secker & Warburg, 1949.
16. Kipling, Rudyard Baa Baa, Black Sheep (1895). In *Under the Deodars, The Phantom 'Rickshaw, Wee Willie Winkie.* Garden City, New York: Doubleday, 1925. Pp. 240–274.
17. Kipling, Rudyard *Something of Myself – For My Friends Known and Unknown.* Garden City, New York: Doubleday, 1937.
18. Langguth, A. J. *Saki: A Life of Hector Hugh Munro.* New York: Simon & Schuster, 1981.
19. Lewis, C. S. Kipling's World. In *Selected Literary Essays by C. S. Lewis.* Cambridge: Cambridge University Press, 1969.
20. Liebert, Robert S. *Michelangelo: A Psychoanalytic Study of His Life and Images.* New Haven: Yale University Press, 1983.
21. Munro, E. M. *The Short Stories of Saki (H. H. Munro), Including the Biography of Saki.* New York: The Viking Press, 1930.
22. Orwell, George *Dickens, Dali and Others.* New York: Harcourt Brace Jovanovich, 1946.
23. Orwell, George *A Collection of Essays.* New York: Harcourt Brace Jovanovich, 1953.
24. Pollock, George H. On siblings, childhood sibling loss, and creativity. *The Annual of Psychoanalysis* 6 : 443, 1978.
25. Pritchett, V. S. *The Tale Bearers, English and American Writers.* New York: Vintage Books, 1981.
26. Rank, Otto *The Myth and the Birth of the Hero.* New York: Brunner, 1952.
27. Robertson, James *John, 17 Months,* film. London: Tavistock Institute of Human Relations, 1969.
28. Rutherford, Andrew (Ed.) *Kipling's Mind and Art: Selected Critical Essays.* Stanford, California: Stanford University Press, 1964.
29. Ryle, Gilbert *Dilemmas.* Cambridge: Cambridge University Press, 1954.
30. Shengold, Leonard The effects of overstimulation: Rat people. *Int. J. Psychoanal.* 48 : 403, 1967.
31. Shengold, Leonard An attempt at soul murder: Kipling's early life and work. *Psychoanal. Study Child* 30 : 683, 1975.
32. Stambolian, George *Marcel Proust and the Creative Encounter.* Chicago: University of Chicago Press, 1972.
33. Stansky, Peter, and Abrahams, William *The Unknown Orwell.* London: Granada Publishing Co., 1974.
34. Stansky, Peter, and Abrahams, William *Orwell: The Transformation.* New York: Alfred A. Knopf, 1980.
35. White, Patrick *Flaws in the Glass — A Self-Portrait.* New York: Penguin Books, 1983.

36. Williams, Raymond *George Orwell*. New York: Columbia University Press, 1971.
37. Wilson, Angus *The Strange Ride of Rudyard Kipling*. New York: Viking Press, 1978.
38. Wilson, Edmund The Kipling that nobody read. In A. Rutherford (Ed.), *Kipling's Mind and Art: Selected Critical Essays*. Stanford, California: Stanford University Press, 1964.

IV
Specific influences

11

The parents of children with psychosomatic diseases: a critical review of the literature

H. David Sackin

In reviewing the data from a clinical study of children with peptic ulcer, my coinvestigator, Dr. George H. Pollock, and I were impressed by how much the parents of these children resembled each other. The mothers shared certain significant character traits and attitudes: they were all competent, driving, ambitious women who demanded, and usually received, remarkably high levels of performance by the affected child. The fathers were notable for their absence: they were all emotionally uninvolved, physically removed, or both. Since these parents were so much alike in so many ways, we were sure that other investigators had reported findings similar to ours. We also wondered whether the parents of children with other psychosomatic diseases resembled the parents in our sample. Accordingly, I undertook a review of the relevant literature.

This review, then, is based on an extensive survey of the literature on the psychological aspects of psychosomatic diseases in children. Publications were collected for review by means of three separate searches of the literature, examination of numerous bibliographies, and exploration of the cumulative indexes of several psychosomatic journals. All publications ultimately selected for review made some mention of the parents; this was the only criterion for inclusion in the study. References to the parents ran the gamut from a brief comment to a lengthy, detailed account; but in only a very few instances [14, 49, 50, 53, 134, 148] are the parents the primary focus of discussion.

My sources differ in other ways.

1. While several investigators [20, 53, 89, 95, 112, 130, 134, 135, 139, 140, 148] examine and discuss the elements that are common to all psychosomatic processes in children, most authors direct their attention to single disease entities. Judging by the number of papers devoted to each psychosomatic disorder, asthma and anorexia nervosa (and obesity) have commanded the greatest interest; ulcerative colitis has been studied less frequently; and rheumatoid arthritis, hyperthy-

roidism, eczema (and neurodermatitis), essential hypertension, and peptic ulcer have been virtually ignored.[1]

2. The number of cases studied ranges from one to several hundred.
3. Both clinical and experimental approaches of varying degrees of formality and complexity have been used to study patients.
4. Techniques utilized to collect data include psychoanalysis, psychotherapy, supportive casework, counseling, family therapy, diagnostic interview, brief observation in a clinical setting, parental attitude scales, psychological testing, and, in one project [14], clinicians' conceptions of the hypothetical mother of an asthmatic child.
5. The methods used to conceptualize data are predominantly inductive, but in a number of instances the data have been subjected to statistical analysis.
6. The majority of authors have employed a psychoanalytic framework on which to order their observations and to construct their conclusions, but other theoretical models (e.g., family systems, learning theory) are represented.

It is interesting that, despite the wide disparity of sources, there is a remarkable consistency in the descriptions of and inferences about the parents of psychosomatic children. It would appear that almost all investigators, whatever their orientation or approach, have observed similar phenomena and have drawn similar conclusions.[2] Thus, most authors agree, at least in principle, that there is a correlation between the character structure of the parents and the development of a psychosomatic disorder by the child. Several authors [43, 49, 50, 54, 55, 107, 115–117, 147], however, dispute the validity of this correlation. And, even though the dissenters are few in number, their position seems to be typical of a

---

[1] I have chosen to confine my review to this group of psychosomatic disorders, which has been dubbed "The Chicago Seven"; the one addition to this group, anorexia nervosa, was included because of its prominence in the recent literature. My choice was predicated on the fact that, although there is little agreement on how the term "psychosomatic disorder" should be defined, there is *some* agreement that the eight disease entities selected for review are representative of "psychosomatic disorders," however the term may be defined. Therefore, in narrowing the field of inquiry, I have attempted to achieve conceptual focus and clarity while minimizing the risk of oversimplification.

[2] Several authors — Bruch, Pinkerton, and Sperling, in particular — might appear to be overrepresented in this survey. However, the inclusion of what might seem to be a disproportionately large number of publications by each of these authors is simply a reflection of their numerous important contributions to the relevant literature. Furthermore, any possible bias that may result from frequent reference to these authors is at least partially tempered by two factors: these three authors' combined contributions make up a relatively small segment of the total, and one of the three, Pinkerton, disagrees with prevailing opinion.

recent general tendency to dismiss psychosomatic specificity as an outmoded concept. Since these papers appear to represent current opinion, they deserve more than passing mention; I will, therefore, briefly review the segments of each of these papers that assess the influence of parental attitudes on the illness of the child.

Weiner, in a recent review of psychosomatic theory [147], asserts, "Studies of asthmatic families have shown that no single pattern of family relationships exists" (p. 12). However, in support of this contention, the author refers directly to only *one* study of psychosomatic families; he does not mention numerous publications by Minuchin and his coworkers in which they painstakingly elaborate their model of the "psychosomatic family." As additional support for his position, Weiner goes on to say, "Mothers (of asthmatic children) may be: (1) overprotective or oversolicitous; (2) perfectionistic and overambitious for the child; (3) overtly domineering, rejecting, punitive, or cruel; (4) helpful and generatively maternal" (p. 12). As I hope to demonstrate later, this author's first three sets of maternal attitudes are not mutually exclusive; in fact, these patterns tend to coexist in most psychosomatic mothers in a manner that is logically consistent. I cannot understand why the author included the fourth maternal attitudinal pattern — "helpful and generatively maternal": the two sources he cites [88, 115] make no mention of anything resembling these characteristics.

Dubo and associates [43] concluded from their study of 71 children with chronic bonchial asthma and their families that, "No significant relationships of the family situation and the child's asthma are found." However, the variables chosen by these investigators to define "family situation" consist of vague generalities. Thus, for example, under the variable designated "parents' relationship with child," choices are limited to the following categories: "not disturbed," "not and mildly disturbed," "mildly and very disturbed," and "very disturbed." In my opinion, any conclusions based on these kinds of data are suspect.

Fitzelle [49] comments, "The study [his own] has demonstrated that the thesis 'parents of asthmatic children may be set apart from the parents of other sick children' is not one which can be readily substantiated." But this author acknowledges that the method of his study, "psychometric techniques," might be considered "a somewhat superficial approach to the problem" (p. 216).

Rees [115 – 117] asserts, "Studies, including my own, of asthmatic families reveal that no single pattern of family relationship exists" (p. 13) [117]. But he then says, "A group of 170 asthmatic children were compared with a control group of 160 children of similar age, sex, and social status. The asthmatic group had a much higher prevalence of parental attitudes classified as overprotective, perfectionistic, and rejecting, compared with the control group" (p. 13). He continues, "75 percent of maternal overprotective attitudes develop prior to the onset of asthma" (p. 13). Nevertheless, he again insists, "Certain parental attitudes are, therefore, of importance in producing conditions conducive to the precipitation of attacks of asthma, but no one pattern of relationship is necessary or sufficient in the causation of the disorder" (p. 13).

Pinkerton and Weaver [107] state, "Early childhood experience does seem the probable foundation for subsequent psychopathology, be it intrapsychic or interpersonal, which may serve to aggravate and perpetuate the asthmatic illness granted its specific basis of physiological vulnerability." But they go on to say, "Studies (of parental attitudes in asthma) are inconclusive. To the extent that they generate tension, parental attitudes will be relevant to the course of the disorder, but this is far from claiming that certain maternal prototypes may actually 'cause' or 'exacerbate' the child's asthma" (p. 90). These authors seem to contradict themselves, however, when they refer to an earlier study by the senior author: "Pinkerton (1967) was able to show, in fact, that emotional factors operate throughout the whole range of physiological severity in childhood asthma with a definite tendency for the more negative or rejective attitudes to be correlated with the severe end of the physiological spectrum, where the steroid-dependent cases are located" (p. 90). They also refer to their own, more recent, study of asthmatic children; again, one of their observations appears to contradict their earlier assertion quoted above: "In 182 cases (88 percent) there was a significant deviation in attitude; 107 were of the overaccepting, cosseting type; 75 demonstrated nonaccepting intolerant attitudes" (p. 94).

Franzini states most emphatically, "Mothers of asthmatic children did not differ from mothers of other seriously ill children, contradicting the literature on the subject" [50]. Since only an abstract was available for review, it is impossible to assess the validity of this author's conclusion.

Gauthier and coworkers are the only "dissenters" I was able to discover whose conclusions appear to be supported adequately by their data. In two related and highly sophisticated studies of a group of asthmatic children and their parents [54, 55], these authors were unable to confirm Sperling's hypothesis [136] of a particular "psychosomatic type" of mother-child relationship. They investigated, among other things, the assumption (derived from Sperling [136]) that the mother of the asthmatic child "does not easily accept . . . tendencies toward autonomy and assertion; she tends to foster dependency in him . . . and to reject him when he is well, independent, and expressing oppositional tendencies" (p. 113) [55]. Their results would seem to refute this assumption: They note [54], "As a group, the mothers . . . appeared very adequate in their reactions to their children's strivings for autonomy and their oppositional tendencies" (p. 687). As a result of their findings, these authors conclude [54], "A disturbed mother-child relationship does not appear to be as frequent and manifest in childhood asthma as originally thought, nor does it appear to be primary" (p. 691).

The sources reviewed above constitute only a small fraction of my sample of the literature. All the other investigators conclude, either explicitly or implicitly, that there is a definite correlation between parental character structure and psychosomatic illness in the child.[3]

There is also general agreement that the mother's role is the crucial one in the genesis of psychosomatic diseases. Mohr and colleagues [95] observe, "It is probable, however, that important as the father's role may be, the more immediate and direct dependency of the child on the nursing care provided by the mother more heavily weights the importance of her personality and reactions in influencing the healthy or abnormal responses of the child" (p. 260). And Sperling [138] comments: "It does not seem, in these cases in which the preoedipal symbiotic relationship with the mother is the determining factor, that the neurosis of the father constitutes a major hazard in the child's development" (p. 548). The fathers, when they are mentioned at all, are generally described as passive, ineffectual, dominated by the mother, and relatively uninvolved with the child [8, 20, 31, 42, 68, 69, 76, 92, 94, 114, 128, 133, 141, 151, 152]. In contrast to the mothers, who appear with clarity and vividness, the fathers remain shadowy and ambiguous [14, 57, 128, 142].

---

[3] An interesting variant of this thesis should be mentioned. Several investigators [30, 41, 64, 65, 98, 143, 146, 150] have proposed a correlation between familial *psychopathology* and anorexia nervosa. Kay and Leigh [64, 65] and Dally [41] have demonstrated a significantly higher than expectable incidence of discrete psychopathological symptoms and syndromes in the families of anorectic patients. More specifically, Warren [146], Theander [143], Morgan and Russell [98], Cantwell and coworkers [30], and Winokur, March, and Mendels [150] report an increased incidence of depression in anorectic families. Cantwell and coworkers [30] conclude, "A family history of affective disorder was extremely common in these families (of children with anorexia nervosa), *particularly in the mothers*" (italics mine) (p. 1093). Similarly, Winokur, March, and Mendels [150] observe, "The data we have reported indicate that primary affective disorder is more frequent in relatives and families of patients with anorexia nervosa than in relatives and families of matched normal control subjects" (p. 697).

Certain specific features, traits, and attitudes are described or alluded to with sufficient frequency in the literature, then, to be considered characteristic for the mother of a psychosomatically ill child, no matter what the child's disorder may be. It should be borne in mind that, since I am concerned with complex behavioral configurations, precise definition and distinction are often difficult, and some blurring of boundaries is inevitable.

A typical mother may be described as follows:

1. *Domineering.* She attempts to dominate and control every aspect of the affected child's life [1, 4, 6–8, 11, 15, 26, 27, 32, 35, 36, 40, 42, 45, 46, 48, 53, 57, 58, 68, 74, 78, 81, 83, 84, 94, 98, 100, 103, 110, 111, 114, 128, 131–134, 136, 138, 139, 141, 142, 145, 148, 151, 152]. Sperling [134] observes, "The mother, in every one of these cases, had an unconscious need to keep the child in a helpless and dependent state" (p. 377). Finch and Hess [48] state, "In all cases, the mother appeared dominating and controlling toward the patient" (p. 820). Prugh [110] states, "The mother dominates the child, in some instances by forceful methods, and others by overindulgence, and still others by a combination of both techniques" (p. 695). And Gifford, Murawski, and Pilot [57] describe the mothers of anorectic children as having "an intense need to maintain control over their child's every bodily function, item of dress, and everyday behaviour. The strong need of these mothers to impose their own external regulations upon the developing self-regulatory tendencies of the patients in infancy is characteristically found in all psychosomatic disorders" (p. 152).

2. *Overly involved and intrusive.* (This descriptive phrase is a reasonably close synonym for the many adjectives found in the literature. These include: "overprotective," "oversolicitous," "entangled," "overindulgent," "overly concerned," "engulfing," and "overly close" [1–4, 8, 9, 13, 15–18, 20, 23, 26, 31, 35, 36, 38, 53, 59–61, 63, 68, 71–75, 78, 82, 84–86, 89, 91, 93, 98, 99, 101, 103, 106, 113, 119, 120, 122, 125, 128, 130, 131, 133, 144–146, 148, 151]. Meijer [83], in describing the mothers of the asthmatic children included in his study, refers to their "dominating overinvolvement, irrespective of these children's needs" (p. 217). Minuchin and coworkers [89] describe the "pathologically enmeshed family system," one of the five transactional patterns that they believe are characteristic for the "psychosomatic family," as follows: "Intrusions on personal boundaries, poorly differentiated perception of

self and other family members . . . a lack of privacy, and excessive 'togetherness' and sharing" (p. 1033).[4]

3. *Exceedingly demanding.* She insists on unquestioning compliance and submission [18, 22, 48, 111, 132], and she presses the child to perform and to achieve, but only in those areas that she, herself, values [15, 22, 25–28, 34, 48, 52, 53, 57, 73, 78, 96, 110, 111, 126, 131–133, 149]. On the basis of evidence derived from their studies of asthmatic children, Selesnick and Sperber [126] draw the following inferences: "Sometimes in his childhood the asthmatic's mother begins to provide love 'conditionally.' The child perceives that, if he is to receive affection, he has to meet certain maternal demands for performance. These demands are set up to meet his mother's need rather than his own. . . . As demonstrated by the level-of-aspiration experiment of Little and Cohen [73], the standards the asthmatic mother sets for her child are often not easy to meet. In comparison with mothers of normal children, the asthmatic child's mother was significantly more prone to raise her aspiration level well above the child's performance level" (p. 329). Sours [131] in his discussion of the developmental history of four anorectic patients writes, "(During) the toddler stage . . . the patients were prematurely encouraged to conform to parental models of compliant and socially acceptable behaviour" (p. 252). Bruch [28] draws attention to the unconscious demand by parents of anorectic children for "special achievement" thereby to fulfill their "dreams of having a perfect child" (p. 170). Williams [149] also refers to this issue, but from the child's perspective. He concludes, "In fantasy behaviour asthmatic children display a higher need for achievement than normal children and *perceive their mothers as having a higher need for them to achieve*" (italics mine) (p. 214).

4. *Clinging and smothering.* She tries to keep the affected child bound firmly to herself and vigorously opposes the child's efforts to separate from her and to individuate [1, 16, 17, 20, 33, 39, 40, 42, 44, 62, 70–72, 83, 87, 89–92, 97, 100, 103, 104, 114, 120, 127, 128, 139, 145]. Thus, Minuchin and Fishman [90] state, "Transactions (in psychosomatic families) are marked by intrusiveness, with the net effect being an interference with the development and functioning of the members' autonomy"

---

[4] Minuchin and coworkers use a transactional model in their approach to psychosomatic diseases in children, a model that they contend is "markedly different from the individually oriented approach" (p. 78) [90]. I would agree that there are major differences between these two theoretical models. Despite these differences, however, much of Minuchin's data seems to be compatible with data derived from the "individually oriented" approaches employed by other investigators.

(p. 83). Crisp and associates [39] refer to the "intensely enmeshed family (of anorectic patients) with concrete domestic boundaries smothering individuality and wider social freedom" (p. 229).

Since independent assertion may threaten the symbiotic bond, the mother emphatically. . .

5. *Discourages any behavior or affective expression by the child that may even remotely suggest autonomous strivings* [1, 5, 8, 21, 24, 26, 29, 35, 36, 79, 83, 86, 89, 91, 99, 125, 131–133, 139]. Thus, for example, aggressive behavior in the form of overt antagonism, belligerence, or defiance is not tolerated by the mother [17, 48, 89, 126, 139]. Sperling [139] comments, "This unresolved symbiotic relationship turns into a psychosomatic relationship in those cases in which the mothers do not permit overt expression of aggression or self-assertion" (p. 558). Abramson [1] maintains, "It is the mechanism of engulfment by the parent which stifles independence, maturity, and the physical and mental health of the child" (p. 36). Meijer [86], in his study of maternal attitudes toward the eating habits of asthmatic children concludes: "The child's innate striving towards autonomy becomes a source of friction and resentment if the mother insists on imposing her will on the child in the choice and handling of food. In this case the likes and dislikes of the child represent a threat to the mother's need for closeness and intimacy, which she imposes on the child by asserting pressure toward dependency and compliance with resulting feelings of depression" (p. 106). He continues, "The need of the mothers for closeness makes it easier to tolerate dependency than self-assertive and autonomous behaviour of the child" (p. 108). Bruch [21] observes, "(In anorectic children) there had been a conspicuous deficit in encouragement of self expression or in reinforcement of what the children wanted to do" (p. 193).

In her zeal to suppress independent initiative, the mother sometimes resorts to harsh measures [15, 56, 102, 110]. The mother's opposition to the child's individuation may also take the form of . . .

6. *Rejection of the child, either covert or overt* [5, 10, 15, 19, 20, 31, 51, 53, 54, 56, 57, 60, 62, 68, 76–79, 88, 95, 104–106, 123–125, 130, 148]. But I have earlier described the mother as clinging and oversolicitous, characteristics that seem to be exactly opposite to what is conveyed by the word "rejection." This apparent contradiction may be resolved in the following way: The mother regards her child as very precious, but only

so long as he or she remains a compliant extension of herself. She becomes enraged and pushes the child away whenever an initiative distinct from her own is demonstrated [136, 139]. At these times she hates her child and wishes to destroy him or her [12, 51, 80, 92, 94, 96, 114]. But she cannot permit herself to become conscious of her rage or her destructive impulses. Her engulfing solicitude for the child, then, serves to protect her against any awareness that she hates him or her.

Gifford, Murawski, and Pilot [57] describe the alternations in attitude displayed by the mothers of anorectic patients as follows: "The underlying ambivalence of these mothers then emerged in violent, sometimes unpredictable extremes of attitude or behavior, alternating between periods of constant attendance on the patient followed by total absence, or between excessive indulgence and abrupt coercion" (p. 152). These authors later expand on the above statement: "The early maternal behavior of *the mothers of children with various psychosomatic disorders* suggests an oscillation between extremes, from guilt-ridden closeness and overcontrol to abrupt withdrawal and abandonment" (italics mine) (p. 184).

Based on the traits and attitudes previously described, it would follow that the mother must be . . .

7. *Unempathic and insensitive.* (As in 2, above, a number of other terms found in the literature seem to have approximately the same meaning as my descriptive phrase. These include "cold," "aloof," "remote," "unaffectionate," and "emotionally distant" [18, 19, 21, 22 – 24, 26 – 29, 31, 35, 36, 44 – 46, 53, 56, 80, 94, 95, 103, 121, 126, 129, 130, 145, 148]). Bruch, in her description of the personality structure of patients with anorexia nervosa, asserts [23]: "This personality structure is conceived of as the outcome of childhood experiences lacking in appropriate responses to child-initiated cues" (p. 51). She continues, "Detailed analysis reveals . . . an all-pervading attitude of doing for the child and superimposing the parents' concepts of his needs, with disregard of child-initiated signals" (p. 53). In a separate report [24] she elaborates as follows: "These parents (of anorectic children) appeared to be impervious to the emotional needs and reactions of their children" (p. 795). Similarly, Sours [131] observes, "The (anorectic) patients' individual needs had been subordinated to the needs, strict moral codes and rigid, ambitious and narcissistic ego ideals of their mothers" (p. 252). The mother is capable of perceiving, understanding, and responding appropriately to her child's communications only when her own preoccupations are in tune with the child's needs. Failures in empathy also result

from the mother's tendency to project her own tensions, affective states, and anticipations onto the child [47, 62, 66, 134, 153].

Taking all the preceding points into account, I assume that the mother's characteristic attitudes and approaches to the child are manifestations of a specific personality organization, which might be described as . . .

8. *Narcissistic.* Most authors use the term "narcissistic" in a descriptive sense — as a synonym for "self-centered" and "self-absorbed." But a broader, dynamic meaning, basically in accord with Kohut's [66, 67] use of the word, can be inferred from the statements of a number of authors [17, 20, 27, 29, 32, 37, 53, 57, 62, 81, 83, 86, 118, 125, 128, 131, 134, 137, 148]. Thus, Meijer [86] points out that a "self-oriented approach of the mother has . . . often been described in childhood asthma studies, whereby the mothers often get satisfaction from the child's dependency and from the resulting proximity and closeness, which fulfills a need of the mother at the expense of the child's autonomous development. In order to maintain this closeness, the mother behaves in a controlling and over-protective or indulgent manner" (p. 105). Jessner and associates [62] observe, "This special closeness of mother to her child leads to an inability to see the child as a separate individual" (p. 369). These authors further state, "She (the asthmatic mother of an asthmatic child) unconsciously regards the child as a part of herself without which she feels incomplete" (p. 374). Shafii, Salguero, and Finch [128] refer to a "pseudosymbiotic fusion" (p. 631) between a mother and her two anorectic daughters. Bruch [20] describes the attitude of a mother toward her obese son as follows: "Her concept of a child was that of a concrete possession for herself with no inkling or regard for his basic needs, that he is to grow up into an independent and self-reliant new individual" (p. 63). In a separate paper, Bruch explains the mother's need for this "concrete possession," this fantasized "perfect child" [26]: "Often a mother (of an anorectic child) needs this child to feel complete and as proof of her own perfection" (p. 3). Gifford, Murawski, and Pilot [57] describe "an early incomplete differentiation between the mother and her (anorectic) daughter, a reciprocal ego defect in both. As a result, the mother unconsciously experienced her child's physical attributes and intellectual accomplishments as a part of herself, to be used as narcissistic extensions of her own ego, as pleasurable acquisitions or painful losses depending on the child's success or failure" (p. 152). Cohler [36] writes, "The anorectic patient feels swallowed up by her controlling mother who incorporates

her daughter into her psyche and uses her for her own ends. Seldom does the future patient exist as a person in her own right; she exists only as a means for satisfying her mother's needs" (p. 378). "Narcissistic," in the sense used by these authors, refers to a solipsistic world view in which objects are experienced either as part of the extended self or as segments of a universe over which the subject expects to exert absolute control.

Even in oversimplified form, the construct "narcissistic personality" provides an integrating focus for the characterological configuration I have been attempting to delineate: The mother experiences her child as a "selfobject" [66, 67]. As such, the child is expected to remain an integral part of the mother's self-system, to submit to her absolutarian control, and to function in accord with her wishes and requirements. If the child's needs conflict with the mother's, the mother's needs always take precedence. And if the child attempts to break away from the suffocating union with the mother, or rebels against the mother's authoritarian regime in any way, she excludes the child from her safe, warm, protecting presence until he or she capitulates.

It must be emphasized that this "typical" characterological configuration and the specific approach to the child that it engenders were constructed entirely from diverse and sometimes fragmentary data derived from the literature; they are, therefore, artificial constructs — abstractions that might have no basis in demonstrable fact. However, data from two sources, both detailed studies of psychosomatic children and their parents, suggest that these constructs are more than empty abstractions. The clinical investigation of children with peptic ulcer referred to at the beginning of this paper yielded extensive data indicating that the personality organization of these mothers is much like that of the "typical composite psychosomatic mother" as described above. Two monographs, "The Mother-Child Interaction in Psychosomatic Disorders" by Garner and Wenar [53] and "Origins of Psychosomatic and Emotional Disturbances" by Wenar, Handlon, and Garner [148], provide even more convincing support to the concept of a "psychosomatic mother." These monographs are reports of two related research projects that, in design and execution, are models of ingenuity and thoroughness.

Four groups of child-mother pairs were studied by Wenar, Handlon, and Garner; these groups were designated the Psychosomatic Group, the Neurotic Group, the Non-Psychosomatic Illness Group, and the Severely Disturbed Group. A variety of techniques were used to investigate these several populations and, thereby, to test the authors' basic hypothesis, which they summarize as follows [148]: "There is a common denominator in all psychosomatic disorders — namely, faulty caretaking by the mother in earliest infancy" (p. 1). They further state [53]: "The early susceptibility to psychosomatic illness flourishes within a field of a particular sort of mother-infant interaction, where the mother is lacking in what we here call 'motherliness'" (p. 11).

The results of the studies confirm the authors' basic hypothesis. In addition, their interpretation of the data pertaining to the group of "psychosomatic mothers" is entirely in accord with the major thesis proposed in this paper. Garner and Wenar [53] state:

The psychosomatic mothers might be epitomized as follows: they are ambitious, controlling women who have high expectations for their child during pregnancy but find the actual caretaking of the infant unrewarding or disagreeable; because of their emotional investment, however, they are irresistibly drawn to this ungratifying activity to the point of becoming entangled in a close, mutually frustrating relationship. . . . (They) seem to be intense women in that they tend to be driving, rigid, and to expect conformity; moreover these qualities are relatively unrelieved by tenderness or spontaneous enjoyment or casualness. Their heightened anticipation during pregnancy cannot be regarded solely as an intensification of a healthy desire for fulfillment through motherhood; rather, it represents an overinvestment in specific goals ulterior to those of giving and receiving gratification from the infant. (P. 160)

In spite of the fact that the mother finds infant care unrewarding and unpleasant, she cannot relinquish her closeness to the infant. In all probability the strength of the ulterior needs plus the rigidity in her personality make her persist tenaciously in her efforts to make the infant serve her purposes. (P. 162–163)

The general atmosphere of the relationship is one of discomfort, with a minimum of empathy and a maximum of irritability and anger. More important, domination and competition keep both mother and child tightly enmeshed in the antagonistic relation. (P. 164)

In summary, I have reviewed the literature on psychosomatic disorders in children, and have made the following inferences:

1. Most authors agree that there is a correlation between the character structure of the parents and the development of a psychosomatic disorder by the child.
2. The mother's role is the crucial one in the genesis of psychosomatic disease.
3. The mother's personality is organized primarily around narcissistic attitudes, motives, and behaviors, a configuration that determines and shapes her characteristic approach to the child and thus the specific form of the mother-child interaction.
4. The father's contribution is less clear. It is probable that his relative

lack of involvement with the child and with the mother is, in and of itself, an important predisposing factor. His absence might directly affect the child's development in some adverse fashion, or it might produce its effects indirectly, in that the mother's influence on the child will be exaggerated if the father is not available as a counterbalance.

5. I am not proposing a linear, one-to-one causal relationship between the character structure of the parents and the development of a psychosomatic disease by the child. Rather, I am proposing, in accord with Pollock's "combinatorial specificity hypothesis" [108, 109], that these factors are predispositional and, in combination with other predispositional factors (biological, psychological, environmental), will render the child vulnerable to the effects of those specific precipitating factors that will produce the onset of the disease. As Pollock [108] states succinctly: "The outcome (a psychosomatic disease) is the interaction and resultant of these many variables, no single one being causal" (p. 157).

References

1. Abramson, H. A. Some Aspects of the Psychodynamics of Intractable Asthma in Children. In H. J. Schneer (Ed.), *The Asthmatic Child: Psychosomatic Approach to Problems and Treatment.* New York: Harper & Row, 1963.
2. Abramson, H. A., and Peshkin, M. M. Psychosomatic group therapy with parents of children with intractable asthma. XI: The Goldey family. Part I. *J. Asthma Res.* 17:31, 1980.
3. Abramson, H. A., and Peshkin, M. M. Psychosomatic group therapy with parents of children with intractable asthma. XII: The Goldey family. Part II. *J. Asthma Res.* 17:81, 1980.
4. Abramson, H. A., and Peshkin, M. M. Psychosomatic group therapy with parents of children with intractable asthma. XII: The Goldey family. Part III. *J. Asthma Res.* 17:123, 1980.
5. Ammon, G. Psychosomatic illness as a result of a deficit in egostructure under consideration of the genetic, dynamic, structural, and group dynamic point of view. *Psychother. Psychosom.* 31:179, 1979.
6. Baraff, A. S., and Cunningham, A. P. Asthmatic and normal children. *J.A.M.A.* 192:99, 1965.
7. Bell, A. I. Some thoughts on postpartum respiratory experiences and their relationship to pregenital mastery, particularly in asthmatics. *Int. J. Psychoanal.* 39:159, 1958.

8. Bemis, K. M. Current Approaches to the Etiology and Treatment of Anorexia Nervosa. In S. Chess and A. Thomas (Eds.), *Annual Progress in Child Psychiatry and Child Development.* New York: Brunner/Mazel 1979.

9. Bergmann, T., and Freud, A. *Children in the Hospital.* New York: International Universities Press, 1965.

10. Berlin, I. N., Boatman, M. J., Sheimo, S. L., and Szurek, S. A. Adolescent alternation of anorexia and obesity. *Am. J. Orthopsychiatry* 21:387, 1951.

11. Biermann, G. Psychosomatics of bronchial asthma in childhood and youth. *Prax. Kinderpsychol. Kinderpsychiatr.* 18:33, 1969.

12. Blitzer, J. R., Rollins, N., and Blackwell, A. Children who starve themselves: Anorexia nervosa. *Psychosom. Med.* 23:369, 1961.

13. Block, J. Parents of schizophrenic, neurotic, asthmatic, and congenitally ill children. *Arch. Gen. Psychiatry* 20:659, 1969.

14. Block, J., Harvey, E., Jennings, P. H., and Simpson, E. Clinicians' conceptions of the asthmatogenic mother. *Arch. Gen. Psychiatry* 15:610, 1966.

15. Block, J., Jennings, P. H., Harvey, E., and Simpson, E. Interaction between allergic potential and psychopathology in childhood asthma. *Psychosom. Med.* 26:307, 1964.

16. Blom, G. E., and Nicholls, G. Emotional factors in children with rheumatoid arthritis. *Am. J. Orthopsychiatry* 24:588, 1954.

17. Blom, G. E., and Whipple, B. A Method of Studying Emotional Factors in Children with Rheumatoid Arthritis. In L. Jessner and E. Pavenstedt (Eds.), *Dynamic Psychopathology in Childhood.* New York and London: Grune & Stratton, 1959.

18. Boswell, J. I., Jr., Lewis, C. P., Freeman, D. F., and Clark, K. M. Hyperthyroid children: Individual and family dynamics. *J. Am. Acad. Child Psychiatry* 6:64, 1967.

19. Botella, C., and Botella, S. Two cases of anorexia nervosa. *J. Child Psychother.* 4:119, 1978.

20. Bruch, H. Psychosomatic Approach to Childhood Disorders. In N. D. C. Lewis and B. L. Pacella (Eds.), *Modern Trends in Child Psychiatry.* New York: International Universities Press, 1945.

21. Bruch, H. Perceptual and conceptual disturbances in anorexia nervosa. *Psychosom. Med.* 24:187, 1962.

22. Bruch, H. Anorexia nervosa and its differential diagnosis. *J. Nerv. Ment. Dis.* 141:555, 1966.

23. Bruch, H. Psychotherapy in primary anorexia nervosa. *J. Nerv. Ment. Dis.* 150:51, 1970.

24. Bruch, H. Anorexia Nervosa. In S. Arieti (Ed.), *American Handbook of Psychiatry,* Vol. 4. New York: Basic Books, 1975.

25. Bruch, H. Anorexia Nervosa. In S. C. Feinstein and P. L. Giovacchini (Eds.), *Adolescent Psychiatry: Developmental and Clinical Studies,* Vol. 5. New York: Jason Aronson, 1977.

26. Bruch, H. Psychological Antecedents of Anorexia Nervosa. In R. A. Vigersky (Ed.), *Anorexia Nervosa.* New York: Raven Press, 1977.

27. Bruch, H. Developmental deviations in anorexia nervosa. *Israel Annals of Psychiatry and Related Disciplines.* 17:255, 1979.

28. Bruch, H. Preconditions for the development of anorexia nervosa. *Am. J. Psychoanal.* 40:169, 1980.

29. Bruch, H. The Sleeping Beauty: Escape from Change. In S. I. Greenspan and G. H. Pollock (Eds.), *The Course of Life: Psychoanalytic Contributions to Understanding Personality Development, Vol. II: Latency, Adolescence, and Youth.* Washington, D.C.: Government Printing Office, 1980.

30. Cantwell, D. P., Sturzenberger, S., Burroughs, J., et al. Anorexia nervosa: An affective disorder? *Arch. Gen. Psychiatry* 34:1087, 1977.

31. Chapman, A. H., Loeb, D. G., and Young, J. B. Psychologic aspects of pediatrics: A psychosomatic study of five children with duodenal ulcer. *J. Pediatr.* 48:248, 1956.

32. Chediak, C. The so-called anorexia nervosa: Diagnostic and treatment considerations. *Bull. Menninger Clin.* 41:453, 1977.

33. Cohen, D. J. Competence and biology: Methodology in studies of infants, twins, psychosomatic disease, and psychosis. *The Child in His Family.* 3:361, 1972–73.

34. Cohen, P. An eating disorder in adolescence: A preliminary report. *Bull. Hampstead Clin.* 3:49, 1980.

35. Cohler, B. J. The Residential Treatment of Anorexia Nervosa. In P. L. Giovacchini (Ed.), *Tactics and Techniques in Psychoanalytic Therapy,* Vol. 2. New York: Jason Aronson, 1975.

36. Cohler, B. J. The Significance of the Therapist's Feelings in the Treatment of Anorexia Nervosa. In S. C. Feinstein and P. L. Giovacchini (Eds.), *Adolescent Psychiatry: Developmental and Clinical Studies,* Vol. 5. New York: Jason Aronson, 1977.

37. Coolidge, J. C. Asthma in mother and child as a special type of intercommunication. *Am. J. Orthopsychiatry* 26:165, 1956.

38. Crisp, A. H. Clinical and therapeutic aspects of anorexia nervosa: A study of 30 cases. *J. Psychosom. Res.* 9:67, 1965.

39. Crisp, A. H., Hsu, L. K. G., and Harding, B. The starving hoarder and voracious spender: Stealing in anorexia nervosa. *J. Psychosom. Res.* 24:225, 1980.

40. Crisp, A. H., Hsu, L. K. G., Harding, B., and Hartshorn, J. Clinical features of anorexia nervosa: A study of a consecutive series of 102 female patients. *J. Psychosom. Res.* 24:179, 1980.

41. Dally, P. *Anorexia Nervosa.* London: William Heinemann Medical Books, 1969.

42. Dikowitz, S. Anorexia nervosa. *J. Psychiatr. Nursing.* 14:28, 35, 1976.

43. Dubo, S., McLean, J. A., Ching, A. Y. T., et al. A study of relationships

between family situations, bronchial asthma, and personal adjustment in children. *J. Pediatr.* 59:402, 1961.

44. Ehrensing, R. H., and Weitzman, E. L. The mother-daughter relationship in anorexia nervosa. *Psychosom. Med.* 32:201, 1970.

45. Eissler, K. R. Some psychiatric aspects of anorexia nervosa, demonstrated by a case report. *Psychoanal. Rev.* 30:121, 1943.

46. Engel, G. L. Psychological Aspects of Gastrointestinal Disorders. In S. Arieti (Ed.), *American Handbook of Psychiatry,* Vol. 4. New York: Basic Books, 1975.

47. Falstein, E. I., Feinstein, S. C., and Judas, I. Anorexia nervosa in the male child. *Am. J. Orthopsychiatry* 26:751, 1956.

48. Finch, S. M., and Hess, J. H. Ulcerative colitis in children. *Am. J. Psychiatry* 118:819, 1962.

49. Fitzelle, G. T. Personality factors and certain attitudes toward child rearing among parents of asthmatic children. *Psychosom. Med.* 21:208, 1959.

50. Franzini, B. S. A Multilevel Assessment of Personality and Interpersonal Behavior of Mothers of Asthmatic Children as Compared with Mothers of Non-Asthmatic Children (Abstract). New York University, 1965.

51. Frazier, S. H., Faubion, M. H., Giffin, M. E., and Johnson, A. M. A specific factor in symptom choice. *Proceedings of the Staff Meetings of the Mayo Clinic* 30:227, 1955.

52. Galdston, R. Mind over matter: Observations on fifty patients hospitalized with anorexia nervosa. *J. Am. Acad. Child Psychiatry* 13:246, 1974.

53. Garner, A. M., and Wenar, C. *The Mother-Child Interaction in Psychosomatic Disorders.* Urbana, Illinois: University of Illinois Press, 1959.

54. Gauthier, Y., Fortin, C., Drapeau, P., et al. Follow-up study of 35 asthmatic preschool children. *J. Am. Acad. Child Psychiatry* 17:679, 1978.

55. Gauthier, Y., Fortin, C., Drapeau, P., et al. The mother-child relationship and the development of autonomy and self-assertion in young (14–30 months) asthmatic children: Correlating allergic and psychological factors. *J. Am. Acad. Child Psychiatry* 16:109, 1977.

56. Gerard, M. W. Genesis of Psychosomatic Symptoms in Infancy: The Influence of Infantile Traumata Upon Symptom Choice. F. Deutsch (Ed.), In *The Psychosomatic Concept in Psychoanalysis.* New York: International Universities Press, 1953.

57. Gifford, S., Murawski, B. J., and Pilot, M. L. Anorexia nervosa in one of identical twins. In C. V. Rowland (Ed.), *Anorexia and Obesity.* Boston: Little, Brown, 1970.

58. Hall, R. A., and Dobrow, B. Psychogenesis in ulcerative colitis. *J. Nerv. Ment. Dis.* 125:388, 1957.

59. Harley, M. Panel report: Resistances in child analysis. *J. Am. Psychoanal. Assoc.* 9:548, 1961.

60. Harris, I. D., Rapoport, L., Rynerson, M. A., and Smater, M. Observations on asthmatic children. *Am. J. Orthopsychiatry* 20:490, 1950.

61. Hodas, G. R., and Liebman, R. Psychosomatic disorders in children: Structural family therapy. *Psychosomatics* 19:709, 1978.
62. Jessner, L., Lamont, J., Long, R., et al. Emotional impact of nearness and separation for the asthmatic child and his mother. *Psychoanal. Study Child* 10:353, 1955.
63. Kalucy, R. S., Crisp, A. H., and Harding, B. A study of 56 families with anorexia nervosa. *Br. J. Med. Psychol.* 50:381, 1977.
64. Kay, D. Anorexia nervosa: A study in prognosis. *Proc. R. Soc. Med.* 46:669, 1953.
65. Kay, D., and Leigh, D. The natural history, treatment and prognosis of anorexia nervosa, based on a study of 38 patients. *J. Ment. Sci.* 100:411, 1954.
66. Kohut, H. *The Analysis of the Self.* New York: International Universities Press, 1971.
67. Kohut, H. *The Restoration of the Self.* New York: International Universities Press, 1977.
68. Krakowski, A. J. Psychophysiologic gastrointestinal disorders in children. *Psychosomatics* 8:326, 1967.
69. Launay, C., Trélat, J., Daymas, S., et al. The role of the father in the development of juvenile anorexia. *Neuropsychiatr. Infant* 13:740, 1965.
70. Lesser, L. I., Ashenden, B. J., Debuskey, M., and Eisenberg, L. Anorexia nervosa in children. *Am. J. Orthopsychiatry* 30:572, 1960.
71. Liebman, R., Minuchin, S., and Baker, L. The role of the family in the treatment of anorexia nervosa. *J. Am. Acad. Child Psychiatry* 13:264, 1974.
72. Liebman, R., Minuchin, S., and Baker, L. The use of structural family therapy in the treatment of intractable asthma. *Am. J. Psychiatry* 131:535, 1974.
73. Little, S. W., and Cohen, L. D. Goal setting behavior of asthmatic children and of their mothers for them. *J. Pers.* 19:376, 1951.
74. Loeb, L. Anorexia nervosa. *J. Nerv. Ment. Dis.* 131:447, 1960.
75. Long, R. T., Lamont, J. H., Whipple, B., et al. A psychosomatic study of allergic and emotional factors in children with asthma. *Am. J. Psychiatry* 114:890, 1958.
76. Lorand, S. Anorexia nervosa: Report of a case. *Psychoanal. Q.* 5:282, 1943.
77. Marmor, J., Ashley, M., Tabachnick, N., et al. The mother-child relationship in the genesis of neurodermatitis. *Arch. Dermatol.* 74:599, 1956.
78. Masserman, J. H. Psychodynamisms in anorexia nervosa and neurotic vomiting. *Psychoanal. Q.* 10:211, 1941.
79. Masterson, J. F. Primary Anorexia Nervosa in the Borderline Adolescent: An Object-Relations View. In P. Hartocollis (Ed.), *Borderline Personality Disorders: The Concept, the Syndrome, the Patient.* New York: International Universities Press, 1972.
80. McDermott, J. F., Jr. Resolving a therapeutic impasse: The mother of a child with ulcerative colitis. *Am. J. Psychiatry* 120:815, 1964.

81. McDermott, J. F., Jr., and Finch, S. M. Ulcerative colitis in children: Reassessment of a dilemma. *J. Am. Acad. Child Psychiatry* 6:512, 1967.

82. McNichol, K., Williams, H., Allan, J., and McAndrew, I. Spectrum of asthma in children: III. Psychological and social components. *Br. Med. J.* [Clin. Res.] 4:16, 1973.

83. Meijer, A. Generation chain relationships in families of asthmatic children. *Psychosomatics* 17:213, 1976.

84. Meijer, A. Sources of dependency in asthmatic children. *Psychosomatics* 19:351, 1978.

85. Meijer, A. Emotional disorders of asthmatic children. *Child Psychiatry Hum. Dev.* 9:161, 1979.

86. Meijer, A. Conflictual maternal attitudes towards asthmatic children. *Psychother. Psychosom.* 33:105, 1980.

87. Millar, T. P. Peptic ulcers in children. *Can. Psychiatr. Assoc. J.* 10:43, 1965.

88. Miller, H., and Baruch, D. W. Psychosomatic studies of children with allergic manifestations. I. Maternal rejection: A study of sixty-three cases. *Psychosom. Med.* 10:275, 1948.

89. Minuchin, S., Baker, L., Rosman, B. L., et al. A conceptual model of psychosomatic illness in children: Family organization and family therapy. *Arch. Gen. Psychiatry* 32:1031, 1975.

90. Minuchin, S., and Fishman, H. The psychosomatic family in child psychiatry. *J. Am. Acad. Child Psychiatry* 18:76, 1979.

91. Minuchin, S., Rosman, B. L., and Baker, L. *Psychosomatic Families: Anorexia Nervosa in Context.* Cambridge: Harvard University Press, 1978.

92. Mitchell, R. G., and Dawson, B. Educational and social characteristics of children with asthma. *Arch. Dis. Child.* 48:467, 1973.

93. Mogul, S. L. Asceticism in adolescence and anorexia nervosa. *Psychoanal. Study Child* 35:155, 1980.

94. Mohr, G. J., Josselyn, I. M., Spurlock, J., and Barron, S. H. Studies in ulcerative colitis. *Am. J. Psychiatry* 114:1067, 1958.

95. Mohr, G. J., Richmond, J. B., Garner, A. M., and Eddy, E. J. A Program for the Study of Children with Psychosomatic Disorders. In G. Caplan (Ed.), *Emotional Problems of Early Childhood.* New York: Basic Books, 1955.

96. Mohr, G. J., Tausend, H., Selesnick, S., and Augenbraun, B. Studies of eczema and asthma in the preschool child. *J. Am. Acad. Child Psychiatry* 2:271, 1963.

97. Monsour, K. J. Asthma and the fear of death. *Psychoanal. Q.* 29:56, 1960.

98. Morgan, H. G., and Russell, G. F. M. Value of family background and clinical features as predictors of long-term outcome in anorexia nervosa: Four-year follow-up study of 41 patients. *Psychol. Med.* 5:355, 1975.

99. Nemiah, J. C. Anorexia nervosa: A clinical psychiatric study. *Medicine* (Baltimore) 29:225, 1950.

100. Olds, S. Say it with a stomachache. *Today's Health* 48:41, 88, 1970.

101. Parker, G., and Lipscombe, P. Parental overprotection and asthma. *J. Psychosom. Res.* 23:295, 1979.
102. Perkins, G. L. Discussion: Anorexia nervosa in the male child. *Am. J. Orthopsychiatry* 26:770, 1956.
103. Piazza, E., Piazza, N., and Rollins, N. Anorexia nervosa: Controversial aspects of therapy. *Compr. Psychiatry* 21:177, 1980.
104. Pinkerton, P. Correlating physiologic with psychodynamic data in the study and management of childhood asthma. *J. Psychodynamic Res.* 11:11, 1967.
105. Pinkerton, P. Depression v. Denial in Childhood Asthma: Equipotent Fatal Hazards. In A. Annel (Ed.), *Depressive States in Childhood and Adolescence.* New York: Halsted Press, 1971.
106. Pinkerton, P. The enigma of asthma. *Psychosom. Med.* 35:461, 1973.
107. Pinkerton, P., and Weaver, C. M. Childhood Asthma. In O. W. Hill (Ed.), *Modern Trends in Psychosomatic Medicine,* Vol. 2. New York: Appleton-Century Crofts, 1970.
108. Pollock, G. H. The psychosomatic specificity concept: Its evolution and re-evaluation. *Annu. Psychoanal.* 5:141, 1977.
109. Pollock, G. H. Combinatorial specificity and the complemental series. Unpublished, 1981.
110. Prugh, D. G. Variations in attitudes, behaviour and feeling-states as exhibited in the play of children during modifications in the course of ulcerative colitis. *Res. Publ. Assoc. Res. Nerv. Ment. Dis.* 29:692, 1949.
111. Prugh, D. G. The influences of emotional factors on the clinical course of ulcerative colitis in children. *Gastroenterology* 18:339, 1951.
112. Prugh, D. G. Toward an Understanding of Psychosomatic Concepts in Relation to Illness in Children. In A. J. Solnit and S. A. Provence (Eds.), *Modern Perspectives in Child Development.* New York: International Universities Press, 1963.
113. Rahman, L., Richardson, H. B., and Ripley, H. S. Anorexia nervosa with psychiatric observations. *Psychosom. Med.* 1:335, 1939.
114. Rampling, D. Single case study: Abnormal mothering in the genesis of anorexia nervosa. *J. Nerv. Ment. Dis.* 168:501, 1980.
115. Rees, L. The significance of parental attitudes in childhood asthma. *J. Psychosom. Res.* 7:181, 1963.
116. Rees, L. The importance of psychological, allergic and infective factors in childhood asthma. *J. Psychosom. Res.* 7:253, 1963.
117. Rees, L. A reappraisal of some psychosomatic concepts. *Psychother. Psychosom.* 31:9, 1979.
118. Rhode, M. One life between two people: Some themes from the analysis of a nine-to-fifteen-year-old anorexic girl. *J. Child Psychiatry* 5:57, 1979.
119. Rogerson, C. H., Hardcastle, D. H., and Duguid, K. A psychological ap-

proach to the problems of asthma and the asthma-eczema-prurigo syndrome. *Guy's Hosp. Reports* 85:289, 1935.

120. Rose, J. A. Eating inhibitions in children in relation to anorexia nervosa. *Psychoanal. Q.* 5:117, 1943.

121. Rosenthal, M. J. Psychosomatic study of infantile eczema: I. Mother-child relationship. *Pediatrics* 10:581, 1952.

122. Rosman, B., Minuchin, S., Liebman, R., and Baker, L. Input and Outcome of Family Therapy in Anorexia Nervosa. In S. C. Feinstein and P. L. Giovacchini (Eds.), *Adolescent Psychiatry: Developmental and Clinical Studies,* Vol. 5. New York: Jason Aronson, 1977.

123. Sandler, L. Child rearing practices of mothers of asthmatic children (1). *J. Asthma Res.* 2:109, 1964.

124. Sandler, L. Child rearing practices of mothers of asthmatic children (2). *J. Asthma Res.* 2:215, 1965.

125. Sandler, N. Working with families of chronic asthmatics. *J. Asthma Res.* 15:15, 1977.

126. Selesnick, S. T., and Sperber, Z. The Problem of the Eczema-Asthma Complex: A Developmental Approach. In N. S. Greenfield and W. C. Lewis (Eds.), *Psychoanalysis and Current Biological Thought.* Madison and Milwaukee: The University of Wisconsin Press, 1965.

127. Senn, M. J. E., and Solnit, A. J. *Problems in Child Behavior and Development.* Philadelphia: Lea & Febiger, 1968.

128. Shafii, M., Salguero, C., and Finch, S. Psychopathology and treatment of anorexia nervosa in latency-age siblings. *J. Am. Acad. Child Psychiatry* 14:617, 1975.

129. Shainess, N. The swing of the pendulum: From anorexia to obesity. *Am. J. Psychoanal.* 39:225, 1979.

130. Sontag, L. W. The genetics of differences in psychosomatic patterns in childhood. *Am. J. Orthopsychiatry* 20:479, 1950.

131. Sours, J. A. The anorexia nervosa syndrome: Phenomenologic and psychodynamic components; clinical heterogeneity in four cases. *Psychiatr. Q.* 43:240, 1969.

132. Sours, J. A. The anorexia nervosa syndrome. *Int. J. Psychoanal.* 55:567, 1974.

133. Sours, J. A. *Starving to Death in a Sea of Objects: The Anorexia Syndrome.* New York: Jason Aronson, 1980.

134. Sperling, M. The role of the mother in psychosomatic disorders in children. *Psychosom. Med.* 11:377, 1949.

135. Sperling, M. Children's interpretation and reaction to the unconscious of their mothers. *Int. J. Psychoanal.* 31:36, 1950.

136. Sperling, M. Asthma in children: An evaluation of concepts and therapies. *J. Am. Acad. Child Psychiatry* 7:44, 1968.

137. Sperling, M. Psychologic desensitization of allergy. *Bull. NY Acad. Med.* 44:587, 1968.

138. Sperling, M. Ulcerative colitis in children: Current views and therapies. *J. Am. Acad. Child Psychiatry* 8:336, 1969.
139. Sperling, M. The Clinical Effects of Parental Neurosis on the Child. In E. J. Anthony and T. Benedek (Eds.), *Parenthood: Its Psychology and Psychopathology.* Boston: Little, Brown, 1970.
140. Spitz, R. A. The psychogenic diseases in infancy: An attempt at their etiologic classification. *Psychoanal. Study Child* 6.255, 1951.
141. Szyrynski, V. Anorexia nervosa and psychotherapy. *Am. J. Psychother.* 27:492, 1973.
142. Taipale, V., Larkio-Miettinen, K., Valanne, E. H., et al. Anorexia nervosa in boys. *Psychosomatics* 13:236, 1972.
143. Theander, S. Anorexia nervosa. *Acta Psychiatr. Scand.* [Suppl.] 214, 1970.
144. Wall, J. H. Diagnosis, treatment and results in anorexia nervosa. *Am. J. Psychiatry* 115:997, 1959.
145. Waller, J. V., Kaufman, M. R., and Deutsch, F. Anorexia nervosa: A psychosomatic entity. *Psychosom. Med.* 2:3, 1940.
146. Warren, W. Clinical Psychiatry: A Study of Anorexia Nervosa in Young Girls. In S. Chess and A. Thomas (Eds.), *Annual Progress in Child Psychiatry and Child Development.* New York: Brunner/Mazel, 1969.
147. Weiner, H. The Psychobiology of Human Disease: An Overview. In G. Usdin (Ed.), *Psychiatric Medicine.* New York: Brunner/Mazel, 1977.
148. Wenar, C., Handlon, M. W., and Garner, A. M. *Origins of Psychosomatic and Emotional Disturbances: A Study of Mother-Child Relationships.* New York: Paul B. Hoeber, 1962.
149. Williams, J. Aspects of dependence-independence conflict in children with asthma. *J. Child Psychol. Psychiatry* 16:199, 1975.
150. Winokur, A., March, V., and Mendels, J. Primary affective disorder in relatives of patients with anorexia nervosa. *Am. J. Psychiatry* 137:695, 1980.
151. Wolff, E., and Bayer, L. M. Psychosomatic disorders of childhood and adolescence. *Am. J. Orthopsychiatry* 22:510, 1952.
152. Ziegler, R., and Sours, J. A. A naturalistic study of patients with anorexia nervosa admitted to a university medical center. *Compr. Psychiatry* 9:644, 1968.
153. Zylberszac, F. Research for a better understanding of the psychological problems posed by the asthmatic child: Clinical study of fifty-three cases. *Psychiatr. Enfant* 15:149, 1972.

Bibliography

Anthony, E. J. The state of the art and science in child psychiatry. *Arch. Gen. Psychiatry* 29:299, 1973.
Baraff, A. S., and Cunningham, A. P. Interpersonal concepts of rapidly remitting and steroid dependent asthmatics. *J. Psychosom. Res.* 10:291, 1966.

Beumont, P. J. V., George, G. C. W., and Smart, D. E. "Dieters" and "vomiters and purgers" in anorexia nervosa. *Psychol. Med.* 6:617, 1976.

Bliss, E. L., and Branch, C. H. H. *Anorexia Nervosa: Its History, Psychology, and Biology.* New York: Paul B. Hoeber, 1960.

Bruch, H. The Tyranny of Fear. In K. A. Frank (Ed.), *The Human Dimension in Psychoanalytic Practice.* New York: Grune & Stratton, 1977.

Bruch, H. *The Golden Cage: The Enigma of Anorexia Nervosa.* Cambridge: Harvard University Press, 1978.

Christodoulou, G. N., Gargoulas, A., Papaloukas, A., et al. Primary peptic ulcer in childhood: Psychosocial, psychological and psychiatric aspects. *Acta Psychiatr. Scand.* 56:215, 1977.

DeBenedetti Gaddini, R. Psychosomatic Disorders in Children. In E. D. Wittkower and H. Warnes (Eds.), *Psychosomatic Medicine: Its Clinical Applications.* Hagerstown, Maryland: Harper & Row, 1977.

Friedman, M. H., and Anderson, J. Body-image variability in peptic ulcer. *Arch. Gen. Psychiatry* 16:334, 1967.

Garma, E. The predisposing situation to peptic ulcer in children. *Int. J. Psychoanal.* 40:130, 1959.

Garner, D. M., and Garfinkel, P. E. Social-cultural factors in the development of anorexia nervosa. *Psychol. Med.* 10:647, 1980.

Gerard, M. W. Bronchial asthma in children. *Nervous Child* 5:327, 1946.

Goetz, P. L., Succop, R. A., Reinhart, J. B., and Miller, A. Anorexia nervosa in children: A follow-up study. *Am. J. Orthopsychiatry* 47:597, 1977.

Goodsitt, A. Narcissistic Disturbances in Anorexia Nervosa. In S. C. Feinstein and P. L. Giovacchini (Eds.), *Adolescent Psychiatry: Developmental and Clinical Studies,* Vol. 5. New York: Jason Aronson, 1977.

Hill, O. W. Anorexia nervosa. In O. W. Hill (Ed.), *Modern Trends in Psychosomatic Medicine,* Vol. 3. London: Butterworth, 1976.

Jessner, L., and Abse, D. W. Regressive forces in anorexia nervosa. *Br. J. Med. Psychol.* 33:301, 1960.

Krakowski, A. J. Treatment of psychosomatic gastrointestinal reactions in children. *Dis. Nervous System* 27:403, 1966.

Maurer, E. The child with asthma: An assessment of the relative importance of emotional factors in asthma. *J. Asthma Res.* 3:25, 1965.

McLean, J. A., and Ching, A. Y. T. Follow-up study of relationships between family situations and bronchial asthma in children. *J. Am. Acad. Child Psychiatry* 12:142, 1973.

Meyer, B. C., and Weinroth, L. A. Observations on psychological aspects of anorexia nervosa: Report of a case. *Psychosom. Med.* 19:389, 1957.

Mohr, G. J., Selesnick, S., and Augenbraun, B. Family Dynamics in Early Childhood Asthma: Some Mental Health Considerations. In H. J. Schneer (Ed.), *The Asthmatic Child: Psychosomatic Approach to Problems and Treatment.* New York: Harper & Row, 1963.

Mutter, A. Z., and Schleifer, M. J. The role of psychological and social factors in the onset of somatic illness in children. *Psychosom. Med.* 28:333, 1966.

Neuhaus, E. C. A personality study of asthmatic and cardiac children. *Psychosom. Med.* 20:181, 1958.

Pinkerton, P. The influence of sociopathology in childhood asthma. *Psychother. Psychosom.* 18:231, 1970.

Pinkerton, P. Symptom formation reconsideration in psychosomatic terms. *Psychother. Psychosom.* 23:44, 1974.

Purcell, K., Bernstein, L., and Bukantz, S. C. A preliminary comparison of rapidly remitting and persistently "steroid-dependent" asthmatic children. *Psychosom. Med.* 23:305, 1961.

Purcell, K., Brady, K., Chai, H., et al. The effect on asthma in children of experimental separation from the family. *Psychosom. Med.* 31:144, 1969.

Purcell, K., and Metz, J. R. Distinctions between subgroups of asthmatic children: Some parent attitude variables related to age of onset of asthma. *J. Psychosom. Res.* 6:251, 1962.

Purcell, K., Muser, J., Miklich, D., and Dietiker, K. E. A comparison of psychologic findings in variously defined asthmatic subgroups. *J. Psychosom. Res.* 13:67, 1969.

Reinhart, J. B., Kenna, M. D., and Succop, R. A. Anorexia nervosa in children: Out-patient management. *J. Am. Acad. Child Psychiatry* 11:114, 1972.

Ross, J. L. Anorexia nervosa; An overview. *Bull. Menninger Clin.* 41:418, 1977.

Seidenberg, R. An unusual oral symptom-complex. *Psychosom. Med.* 21:247, 1979.

Smart, D. E., Beumont, P. J. V., and George, G. C. W. Some personality characteristics of patients with anorexia nervosa. *Br. J. Psychiatry* 128:57, 1976.

Sturzenberger, S., Cantwell, D. P., Burroughs, J., et al. A follow-up study of adolescent psychiatric inpatients with anorexia nervosa: I. The assessment of outcome. *Am. J. Child Psychiatry* 16:703, 1977.

12

Maternal influences in creating fetishism in a two-year-old boy

Robert J. Stoller

Though it may be doubted that a genuine perversion is possible in a small child, the following case lets us imagine it could. In doing so we must be careful. First, we may be facing a problem with no more substance than a matter of definition. Second, there is the question of whether a rarity is simply an inconsequential event or if it hides generalities. (We know the latter is usually the case in biology, including psychology.) Third, we should not use "perversion" loosely, as is often done in analytic theory: perversion, with its strong connotations of willful badness, becomes something else when made synonymous with any erotic or gender aberration. This is too undynamic a position: If there is any caution that analysis has given to those who study behavior, it is that behavior not be judged only by its surface, but by its meaning, at all levels of awareness, to the behaving person.

Mac was 2½ years old when his fetishism first appeared: he was frantic to put on his mother's stockings. I shall say he is perverse because he was so preoccupied with the act, became visibly erotically excited, and developed his fetishism as the result of specific traumas imposed, from earliest infancy, on character structure emerging in his relationship with his mother. There are those [2, 6] who, following Sigmund Freud, say that perversion is not possible until one has passed through oedipal conflict; in the perversions of later childhood, adolescence, and adults, one finds clear evidence of (perversion-related) damage from oedipal conflicts. The recent consensus in the literature, however, adds that preoedipal issues also count.

A second problem in definition must also be faced before I report Mac's dilemma. Take the word "fetishism." (Let us ignore its common meaning in anthropology, with its nonerotic connotations.) Undue focus on an inanimate object (e.g., a piece of cloth) is very different depending on whether or not it is accompanied by genital excitement, though the two may share some dynamic and etiologic features. To use the same word to label experiences that are subjectively and dynamically so different invites confusion.

427

I wish to show that this little boy, Mac, was truly erotically perverse from age 2½. He did not just have preoedipal precursors of perversion, but, because of a precociously induced, erotically soaked, mutually needful, ambivalence-loaded relatedness between Mac and his mother that led to his developing an erotic fetishism, he deserves to be assigned as perverse. Nonetheless, we cannot say his disorder is the same fetishism as in the adult perversion.[1]

Case Material

Mac and his parents were first seen for evaluation when he was 3½ years old. Here is the statement his mother (L) gave in the first moments after we met.

L: About a year ago, my little boy was under some pressure. He was 2½ then. He had a 6-month-old brother, and we had just moved him into his bed, out of his crib; and I had started him in nursery school. He was not happy because he is very shy with strangers; he doesn't want to be too far from me even now. He started pulling my legs and my feet and my stockings. I didn't pay too much attention to this at that time. I was nursing the baby, and I thought he just wanted to touch me. He really liked my hose and my stockings. He did not put them on, but he would always feel my legs. One day, my mother was visiting me; he started rubbing up against her legs. He was aroused, and it bothered me.

I thought at the time it could be just because of the baby: maybe if I paid more attention to him, he would find more creative things to do and it would stop.

So I tried that, and it did. Then a year later—two months ago—one day I saw him with my panty hose with his clothes off. I was shocked. I told him to take them off, that they were mine, that girls wear them and he wasn't a girl; he was a boy and wore socks like Daddy did.

It didn't happen again until two weeks later. I was tired and took off my slippers with no stockings on. My baby came in; he is now 1½, and he grabbed my slippers and ran off with them. My oldest son, Mac, saw me without my stockings on, and he started rubbing up against my leg and feeling my feet. I turned around and said, 'Stop it, Mac'; and he did not.

---

[1] The diagnosis need not have heavy prognostic significance: Children's psychic structures are more malleable than adults, and should the dynamic process we call "family" redistribute its forces, the perversion may no longer serve any of the parties.

He wouldn't stop. I turned around and whacked him and said, 'Stop it.' So he did. He went off, and later on he said he wanted to go play in his room. That's kind of funny because he normally does not ever say that. He likes to be very close to where my husband and I are, with the family. I was putting the baby to bed, and I thought, 'He is very quiet.' I did not understand. I went into his room, and he had a pair of my stockings. He had hidden them under his bed. I asked him what he was doing, and he just said, 'What?' So I took them away from him and said, 'These are my stockings. They don't belong to you, and you are not supposed to play with them.' The next day I was tired and said to the boys, 'Come on; let's go lie down and relax.' My baby was jumping up and down on top of me, and my older son all of a sudden became very aroused. I could tell. I got up and tried to change the subject of whatever he was thinking, and it stopped. The next morning I woke up later than usual. He came in bed with me; he doesn't usually do that; I don't allow that. He was touching me where my nightgown was, and I said to him, 'Go play in your room, Mac. I'm trying to sleep.' So he went in his room, and I fell asleep—I normally don't do that.

When I woke up, I found my nightgown, my underwear, and my stockings in his room. He had gotten them from a pile of clothing. He had hidden them—not really, but he thought they were hidden. Behind his chair.

Since then, he has been in my drawer and into my hose. Finally, I became so upset that I just took them and hid them. He would not listen to me. One day, I was sitting in the kitchen, and I thought he was taking a nap. I was concentrating. I got up to check if he was asleep. He was in my bedroom. He tore the whole place apart looking for my stockings, and he found them and he had them on with my boots, this time not just my stockings but my boots. Now I finally realized that he is aroused when he puts them on. This time his sexual organ was aroused. This time I saw it. He had my stockings, and he had no underwear on. He takes all his clothes off, and he puts on my stockings. He had an erection. . . . The very first time I ever saw him aroused was when he rubbed up against my mother's legs; that was the first, the very first time [at 2½].

L noted that his erotic behavior then subsided for a year when she got him interested in other things. But during that year she observed he had erections when, in clothing stores, he sat under the mannequins and rubbed their legs. His mother found this embarrassing; on one occasion a saleswoman asked him to stop it. She wondered if she did not wear stockings often enough, and I told her it was not that simple.

METHODOLOGY

Since the mother allowed our sessions to be audiotaped, a verbatim account is available. Different treatment sessions are numbered in sequence, and the excerpts are subsumed under categories that help to organize a clearer understanding of the onset and nature of the little boy's fetishism.

OVERALL PERSPECTIVE ON THE CASE

Let me quickly summarize these findings. The infant (Mac) was adopted three days after birth. His adoptive parents had been unable to conceive, and my patient, L (the boy's mother), had been hungry for a child. The very fact of adoption stirred in her an intense process of identification with the infant, the result of her sense of having also been abandoned in childhood by her parents. A fiercely felt symbiosis was thereby set in motion; both mother and son responded to each other with intense love, frustration, and rage. By 9 months, L reports her son was already sensually focused on her skin, perhaps her legs, since he could reach them easily and since she at first allowed him his pleasure.

When Mac was 1 year old, a circumcision — traumatic to them both — was performed. Following this, he never was seen to touch his genitals, until, at 2½, he was observed sexually excited, rubbing on his grandmother's (L's mother) foot.

L conceived and delivered another son when Mac was about 2. This, of course, threw pressure on the L-Mac symbiosis.

When Mac was 2½, he and his mother were traumatically separated in a restaurant. Immediately after this event, the fetishism began. It went underground after some weeks and emerged a year later, again immediately following another traumatic separation when he was lost in an elevator.

Therapy Sessions

CIRCUMCISION

THERAPY HOUR 1. L: Mac was circumcised when he was a year old. He should have been circumcised when he was first born; I did not realize that he wasn't circumcised. The adoption agency didn't tell me, and I was in such a state of shock: with a brand new baby, it didn't occur to me that he wasn't circumcised. When I went to the doctor and he was 6 weeks old, the doctor said, "You realize he isn't circumcised, don't you?" And it just hit me. By the time I could get an appointment at the hospital with the urologist, he was 3 months old. It was too late for him to have it done in the office. They said they couldn't do it. Well anyway, he was circumcised when he was a year old: we went to the hospital for the day. After, it was very painful.

It wasn't healing correctly somehow, and I went back to the urologist. He recircumcised him in the office. Without an anesthetic. With me holding him down. With the baby screaming. And me, I was hysterical. I was. I didn't expect it. And I was mad as hell; I really was. I thought he should have had a nurse to hold the baby. He just said, "Hold the baby." When I turned around to look, he had a knife in his hand. Then he was cutting him, and it was very painful to him. I had to keep pulling the foreskin back. And he was screaming.

THERAPY HOUR 2. L: The circumcision. The first one [when 1 year old]. He came out of surgery, very groggy. He finally woke up and started to cry. I started to pick him up, and the nurse ran in and said, "Don't touch him! Don't touch him! He's still under the anesthetic." I couldn't lift him up so I didn't. He had to urinate, and it must have been excruciating, because he went into a screaming, bloody fit, which is only natural. I know it must really, really hurt.

And we took him home. It was pretty hard for a couple of days. Every time he would urinate, he would really, really cry. I would change his diapers right away and put vaseline on it to protect it. They never told me what to do. The doctor never said a word to me. And three weeks later, we went in for the checkup, and I said to the doctor, "It looks funny to me; it just doesn't look like a circumcision." I was standing, holding Mac. The doctor looked at it. And he went over to the side. And I was looking at Mac. And he came back and he was holding a scissors. I looked at him, and it didn't dawn on me what was going to happen; I just blanked out. I stood there, and he said to me, "Hold him." I should have opened my mouth and said something to him; why I didn't, I don't know.

I don't know whether it went too fast or whether I was scared or whether . . . I should have opened my mouth and said, "Let the nurse do it: I don't want to be in here." But I didn't. I held him. And he cut him. I didn't look. I was sobbing. And Mac was screaming. In fact, I looked out of the corner of my eye, and I couldn't believe that he was doing that in front of me. So . . . I was hysterical. I couldn't believe that he would do that. Mac took it better than I did; he stopped crying after a couple of minutes. I was still crying. The doctor said I should have pulled the foreskin back [during the weeks after the first procedure] and I said,

"Why didn't you tell me that I was supposed to do that after the circumcision was over?" The skin had just grown back.

So I left. I was really upset. I called my husband and said, "Come and get me; I can't drive home." I was hysterical. I couldn't get myself together. I said, "What the hell is going on around here? I don't understand what he's doing. I don't know why he did it. He never told me a thing." When I got home, I called the doctor. He was very terse, saying it had grown back and he had to do it. I called him a butcher. He didn't do a normal circumcision; he did some new type. I said, "Why?" and he said, "After a man becomes 50 years old, they lose their sensitivity there; by leaving more skin there, he won't lose the sensitivity." I don't give a damn about his sex life when he's 50. I said he just doesn't look like he's been circumcised. He went through all that, and he doesn't look like he's been circumcised.

I didn't understand why he hadn't told me what to do. I had to continually pull back that foreskin, and he would go into a screaming, bloody fit every time I did. I had to continue that for two or three months. It hurt him every time. Well, I don't know if it hurt him every time, but I think he just expected it to. So he cried. I was supposed to pull the foreskin back every day, but I didn't. I was so upset by having to do it that I would avoid it. And I would try to do it when he was in the bathtub playing in the water. I would sneak it in. Pretty soon, he never thought about it. But one thing I can really say: he has never played with himself, never touched himself too much. Much less than Billy [youngest son]. Maybe that's why he is so attracted to my stockings. Because the only time I have seen him with an erection is with my stockings. It felt good. He never otherwise has shown sexual interest in his penis. I think maybe he would have come out of it if the nurse had been there, if I hadn't seen it, if I hadn't been so hysterical. He must have known my reactions. He was only a year, but gee whiz.

I was leaning over him, holding him down, and I was sobbing, just absolutely sobbing, sobbing when I left the office.

THERAPY HOUR 3. L: When he gets hurt, that's another thing altogether. He would get into a state of absolutely going hysterical when he got hurt, when he bumped his knee or saw blood or fell down or the baby hit him. I think about the circumcision and how much that hurt him, when the doctor redid it. When he is hurt now, he becomes uncontrollable, absolutely uncontrollable, just absolutely screaming at the top of his voice. I try to calm him down and end up getting angry with him. I know it's a terrible reaction, but I can't help it. And then he will cry and cry and cry and cry and cry. I try to comfort him again, and it goes round and round and round in circles. I feel bad that I got angry, and then I try to comfort him. Then he keeps going, and then I get angry at him. And it will stop. I tell him he has to be a big boy because he likes firemen and firemen don't do that. Even just a little scratch, he isn't able to accept at all. But before the circumcision, he would fall down, and I would say, "Boom, boom," and he would pick himself up and go toddling on his way.

With the baby, I don't do that at all. With Mac, before the circumcision, I could see myself clear about what I thought of how he should react. Later on, after the circumcision, I changed too.

PRECIPITATING EVENTS

The Birth of a New Baby

THERAPY HOUR 1. L: When he was a year and 3 months, we moved to our new house. All of a sudden, I had lots of things to do and I pushed Mac into the background: "Mommy wants to do this, and now you have to play by yourself." I don't think he was prepared for that. All of a sudden no Mommy — not all day long. And I was pregnant. When I went to the hospital, he went to stay with my mother. He had never been to my mother's, he had never been away from home. Then all of a sudden there was a baby, and all of a sudden there was not very much time with Mommy. [He was 2 years and 1 month old.]

The day after the baby was born, I developed a migraine headache. [She did not have a spinal.] It lasted a week; I had never had a migraine before in my life. No matter what they gave me, I could not get rid of that headache. I know what it was from: I was so worried about Mac being at my mother's. I would call her on the phone, and I could hear Mac crying in the background. Here I am having a baby, and I adopted another one. I felt I betrayed him. A month after we were cleared by them and were just waiting, my gynecologist said he can do an exploratory on me. And when I came out of surgery, there was a 100 percent chance of my getting pregnant; I never used anything to not get pregnant. I didn't get pregnant until Mac was 15 months old. And I feel guilty. I feel he should be a pampered child. I had another baby; I don't spend that much time with him [Mac] because of the other baby. But he [Mac] got whiney, and I dislike whininess intensely. I am not whiney, and I dislike it in others.

Traumatic Separations

THERAPY HOUR 1. L: The time when he was 2½ really started it. We were separated. It wasn't for hours, only for maybe 15 minutes. But it seemed hours. And I'm sure it did for him, too. It was horrifying to me and to him. Before that, he had never been interested in panty hose, except maybe to touch them while I was getting dressed, but he wasn't interested in touching me anywhere else or touching me intensely.

It was a big community party, hundreds of people. We went into a restaurant and waited an hour. Mac was having a good time with the other kids. Then we went outside, and I turned around to find Mac. And I couldn't find him. A little boy said that he went around the building. So we went around the building, and we couldn't find him at all. There was nobody back there. We went to the front, and there must have been a hundred cars in the parking lot. People were coming and going on a huge highway on the other side of the parking lot. And my first thought was, "My God, he's going to get killed. He's going to go out in that parking lot, and he's going to get hit." We all fanned out to try and find him. I went back toward the restaurant and heard this horrendous screaming from the inside. And he ran through all these tables and all these people. And he ran toward me, and he cried hysterically. He was crying at the top of his lungs, "Mommy, Mommy!" I grabbed him and hugged him and kissed him. And he calmed down. He didn't cry continuously after that, but he was petrified. I felt guilty as hell. I was terrified he would be hit by a car or someone would take him. This was a beautiful child. There are lots of nuts in this world that would just pick up a child like that and take him. I felt — because my mother has told me that for years — "Stay near me; stay close to me because someone might take you." I can remember that distinctly. It was a terrible feeling to ever have gotten lost from her.

I ran toward him with my arms open: "Here I am, Mac." Because he was so hysterical that he did not see me at first. I ran toward him, and I picked him up, and I hugged him and kissed him, and I said, "Where did you go? Why did you leave me? Why didn't you stay by my side?" Because I am always telling him, "Stay here beside me." I didn't say it that day because I was distracted.

It was right after that that he masturbated on my mother's foot and started with the clothes. Within a few days. A week prior to that he had been moved out of his crib and put into a bed. In a room separate from us. He was very excited about that, but it was a great strain for him too. That's why I delayed so long. I waited until Bill was 6 months old to make the transition as easy as possible. And that same month Bill was baptised. So there was a lot of attention for the baby.

And for two and a half months he was excited about the panty hose. Then it went away. It died away for a year.

It began again the next time we got separated; that was a year later. We were in the hospital for Bill's 11-month routine appointment. We came out of the office, walked down the hall, and went to an elevator off to the side. We waited and waited for the damn elevator. I sat Bill in his carrier. Mac was standing by my side, the elevator door opened, and Mac walked into it. I had turned to pick up Bill. And the door slammed shut. There was no one else in the elevator, and I could hear him screaming all the way up the elevator shaft. It was — my blood was curdling — it was horrible. Honest to God there was nothing I could do to stop that goddamn elevator. Then it went down; I don't know where it went. And I pushed a button, and I waited and I waited, and I began to cry. Like I am now. I could hear him all the way down that elevator shaft, crying for me. And when the door finally opened, it was empty. It was empty! It was like that goddamn dream I had with doors opening, and I walking down the hallway and that dreadful thing is trying to suck me into it. I got on the elevator with Bill, and I didn't know where to go. I didn't know where he could have gone. My first reaction was that it went down to the main floor and that he had gotten off and gone out to the parking lot. I'm always afraid he's going to get hit by a car.

I went down to the first floor and walked over to some people and said, "Did you see a little boy who got off the elevator?" I said, "He got lost from me." And everyone said, "No." I felt like the earth swallowed me up; I couldn't figure where a little boy could be. I just stood there. I was beginning to get hysterical, not screaming and yelling, but I must have looked panic-stricken. Then the elevators opened, and a nurse came off. I said to her, "Have you seen a little boy?" And I said, "I can't find him; he got lost on the elevator." She said, "He may have gotten off on the second floor." So I got back into the elevator and went up to the second floor. And there he was sitting behind a desk on a nurse's lap. He wasn't crying, but the minute he saw me, he came to me, and he was crying, and I was crying, both of us there crying.

I know what it's like to be lost. I know the feeling.

THERAPY HOUR 2. L: One morning when he [Bill, not Mac] was about 2 months old, I wanted to cut his fingernails. I took my husband's clippers and cut a little flesh on each finger. I looked at it and — you know — part of his finger was gone. I was so absolutely hysterical my husband had to stay home from work. I was just so hysterical; I couldn't believe it — that I would act that way. Bill wasn't crying; I was crying. It was bleeding. It was like I took a little portion of each end off his fingers with the clippers. It grew back right away. I never react that way about anything except with the children.

FETISHISM

THERAPY HOUR 1. Dr.: What's his preference: to touch you or to hold stockings?

L: Putting them on. And when he was a baby and I was getting dressed — 9 months or following — he would come into the bathroom and crawl around my legs. (My 18-month-old does that; they hug your legs. And they put their little head there. So I never thought much about it.)

And he started doing this to me when he was 2½ years old, and he wouldn't leave me alone — for an instant. We went out to dinner one day. He was under the table the whole time — it was a nightmare — rubbing my legs. I couldn't believe it. And then it stopped a few weeks later. Only one time has he been interested in my bare legs. If it is cold and I am wearing slacks, he will say, "Do you have any stockings on, Mommy?" And I will say, "Yes, I am wearing them because I am cold." I tried to explain that stockings are to keep me warm, like men's pants to keep them warm.

Dr.: He knows something about stockings that we don't know.

L: Obviously. He is so bright. He said to my mother, when he was rubbing up against her that first time . . . She said, "Macky, you don't know what you are doing." He said to her, "Oh, but Grandma, I do."

THERAPY HOUR 2. L: These little occasions [panty hose episodes] occur when there has been — not upheaval but tension. He and I had been sick for weeks on end and we never left the house. I was talking on the phone; he was in bed for his nap. I was on the phone for 10 or 15 minutes, and I saw him go back to his room, sneakylike — not crawling but low so he might have thought he was out of my vision. When I went into my bedroom, my whole closet — all my shoes, were just a shambles. Everything was completely ripped up. I went into his room. He was awake but he had his shorts off. I wondered: why does he have his shorts off? Then I saw underneath the bed were my ballet slippers from high school. Then I realized he had had an erection. Not then, but he had had — it looked very red.

There was another incident two days ago. I was sitting bare-legged in my shorts. All of a sudden, Mac turned around, and he looked at me very peculiarly. Nobody else sees this but me. I don't know if it was in my head or whether it's really there, but all of a sudden I just felt a little stiff . . . [pause]. He walked between my legs, and he looked at my legs funnylike. He didn't touch me. I think it's sexual. To me it is. I've had that look before, from men. And from my 4-year-old son! . . . After that he touched himself. He had on shorts, but he had taken his underwear off. I don't know when. Later, when I took his shorts off, he was all red.

THERAPY HOUR 3. L: He exhibits no femininity at all. That's not the problem. It's the panty hose. He touches me or looks at me peculiarly: lustful. He does that to my mother at times. Today she had on Bermuda shorts. She was sitting there, and he stroking across her legs. Mother gave me a look like: "What's going on here?" But he loves my mother very much, and I know he loves me. I know that. He's very verbal about it too. He'll come over to me and say, "Oh, Mommy, I love you." The other day, we were at the grocery store, and he saw, way down the aisle, the panty hose advertised on TV. And he's yelling at his brother Bill, "Oh, Bill. Panty hose! Panty hose!" And Bill doesn't know or care what panty hose is.

So Mac grabbed one, and I said, "Put that back, now!" He was giddy and laughing, and I was trying to get at the core of what he was saying. He said, "Let's buy panty hose; let's buy panty hose." And I said, "Oh, I have lots of them; I don't need any." And he said, "Well, we need some." And I said, "Who?" and he said, "Baby and me." And I said, "Oh." And I said, "You're a boy. You don't need panty hose." And he said, "Oh, no. I'm a girl." And he kind of looked at me, and I just completely ignored that statement. I wasn't going to give him an inch to go on that. So I just turned around and said, "Let's go."

But it's there; something's there about that. I had some clothes piled on a couch. One was a pink silk dress. Mac was playing with the tie of it. I wondered what he was doing with it, if he was just horsing around. But in actuality he was playing it was a fireman's rope, tying it around his waist and saying, "Put me on something so you can hoist me up." Like firemen do.

Dr.: Is other cloth stimulating for him — whether for his penis or not — other textures or garments?

L: No. The only thing is the panty hose and my shoes and boots, I caught him once long ago in the panty hose with my boots on. He's not interested in my underwear, just the panty hose.

Dr.: Does anything else turn him on?

L: No. I would say not. No.

THERAPY HOUR 4. L: I'm thinking of when I used to be getting dressed, and he was just standing there, like babies do. But I had stockings on. He was just caressing me, saying, "Mommy, Mommy." He was about 9 months, just starting to stand. He could already talk. And he had a vocabulary of maybe 20 words. It scared me because he was so smart. He's so intelligent that I think to myself, "How am I going to cope with it?"

I can remember one incident specifically. I was getting dressed to go out. It was the first time I had a baby-sitter. Naturally he didn't know that, 9 months old. Anyway, he crawled into the bathroom. I was standing there in my nylon slip, and I had my panty hose on. He sat there and played with my feet for a little while. And then he had my leg. He just kind of felt it for a while. I was putting on my makeup, and I didn't pay any attention to him. I thought it was just sort of normal. Most babies touch their mothers. Then he stood up — managed to pull himself up — and he managed to stand there for a while, just touching me. I thought maybe he just wanted my attention, because he was all the time babbling, saying, "Oh, Mommy; oh, Mommy." I picked him up, gave him a hug and a kiss, and I talked to him. I always brought toys with me, wherever I was with him. But no. He'd never play with the toys; he always wanted to be closer to me. He'd sit there and touch my legs.

Dr.: Now this is at other times as well?

L: Yeah. At other times. But this one I am remembering was the first. It would happen anytime I would get dressed. The other times around the house. I wore pants or shorts. If he touched me then, I don't remember it as well as when I was getting dressed to go out in a dress and panty hose.

Dr.: Excuse me: I want to get it right. The first time it happened, he was 9 months old. He comes in and is feeling your legs, and you gradually realize that it goes on longer and is more intense than you expected. From then on, whenever you were in your stockings, he would try to touch them. And while doing this, from the start, he would say, "Oh, Mommy," as if he were having a glorious experience?

L: Yeah. And especially when I was going out. I wear panty hose only when I go out.

Dr.: Suppose you had panty hose on and were not going out when he was 9 or 10 months old, would he still be interested?

L: No. I don't think so. But he has developed an eye for it. Say, for instance, I've gone to the grocery store and have panty hose underneath my slacks. He will come by and make sure. He will just touch. He is checking up on me. And then at 2½ years it became different. He had on a very wet diaper that I should have changed and didn't. It was exciting to him, I suppose. He was laying across my mother's foot and moving up her leg, masturbating on her foot. And I thought to myself, "What is he doing?" I knew what he was doing, but I didn't want to realize what he was doing. I should have picked him up and changed his diaper, but I thought it was good that he was having a good feeling, because, prior to that time, he had always been afraid of himself from the pain after the circumcision. That was the first time I had seen him get pleasure from his penis. The "Oh, Mommy" pleasure was not with an erection, only after this time with my mother. Before that he was avoiding touching his penis.

THERAPY HOUR 5. L: He hasn't been interested in panty hose for a long time. Then yesterday, he pulled a chair up to my dresser and got into my panty hose. Because he was away from school for two days and did not want to go back. He wanted to stay home with Mommy. "I don't want to go to school. I'll stay home, Mommy." It's my problem, too. He wouldn't go back to school with the car pool. So I took him. He toddled off and waved good-bye. When I picked him up, everything seemed fine. But when we got home, he was in my bedroom a long, long time. It did not occur to me he was in the panty hose. I called him, and finally he came; he looked a little sheepish. He had pushed a chair against the dresser. So I said, "When I kept calling you, were you in here with my panty hose?" He said, "Well, I did open your hamper up there. I touched them." I tend to think it was the crisis of going back to school.

THERAPY HOUR 6. L: We went to this restaurant. Mac got under the table and he was rubbing his hands up and down my stockings till I was ready to—not kill him—I was ready to lose my mind. I really was. . . . Yesterday I was wearing stockings. I was wearing a dress. Mac found any possible way to get near me. He'd joke and go around the table and touch my legs. Or he'd go under the table and say, "I see a toy" and make all kinds of excuses because he knows that it gets to me. And I cannot hide it.

THERAPY HOUR 7. L: I picked up his pillow, and my panty hose dropped from inside the pillowcase. He no longer hides them under the bed; now he hides them under the pillow. Today I said to him, "Mac, I found my panty hose in your pillow the other day." And he said, "Yeah, Bill is doing that now." I said to him, "I don't think Bill is doing that. I think you're doing it. Why do you hide them in there?" He said, "I put them there so I can put them on." And I said, "Why do you have to put them on?" He never really answered me. He went back to saying it was Bill who got them and put them in there and that he — Bill — was wearing them. I said, "I know Bill wasn't wearing them: you're putting them on." And he said, "Oh, I never put them on." I said, "Well, one day Daddy caught you with them on." And he said, "That was only one day." I said, "I would appreciate it if you'd leave my panty hose alone." Which I am not sure was good. But at least he and I were talking about it; he opened up that much about it, where before if I would even mention the subject, he would scream at me. We had a nice conversation.

MASCULINITY: MASCULINE INTERESTS, SEXUAL ADVANCES TOWARD MOTHER, EARLY IDENTIFICATION WITH FATHER

THERAPY HOUR 1. L: He never had had a lot of pain before in his life. Then he did [circumcision]. And now, all of a sudden, he realizes he has a nice sensation. I am confused. I feel threatened. Here is my son, my adopted son at that. He is making — not really — sexual advances toward me. Maybe it is — I don't know — but it's not right. And it frightens me that I don't know how to stop it without . . . because I am angry. I am angry at him. I don't understand what he's doing. And I don't think I'm controlling the situation correctly. I have tried to think what I am doing wrong in my reactions toward him: maybe I am angry at him too often. I know he is much too dependent on me. My youngest isn't that way at all. Because Mac is so smart, he gets bored easily and that makes him more dependent on me. He has a lot of toys and creative things. I will put his things on the kitchen table, and he will paint for five or ten minutes. Then he is bored. He loves books. I read books to him a lot. But lately he is smothering me. He wants me to kiss him all the time, and he wants me to carry him, and then he gets mad at me. Then he talks to me in a mad tone of voice all day long, very angry with me and I get angry with him because he is bored and under foot. He follows me around the house and gets into whatever I am doing. Then he won't play; he won't go out and play unless I really tell him, "Go outside and play." I could understand that if he didn't have a good father who didn't spend a lot of time with him.

When my husband is home, he will go with him to the garage together. He loves tools. He will work on the truck with my husband. He will work in the yard with my husband. He loves being with my husband. When Jim [husband] is home, I could be long lost; but when Jim isn't, then I'm the one who he sticks around with. Other 3½-year-olds are more independent than he is. I have never tried to push him. I know he will go at his own speed, like playing in the yard or in the park. He never gets into anything dangerous at all; he's very careful about himself. He wouldn't climb up the ladder to go on the slide until he was with another boy his age who did it. Now he does it and goes down stomach first. I am happy to see that. I want him to be a real boy. He doesn't have any feminine characteristics, though: he doesn't want to play with dolls; he doesn't want to play with girls.

THERAPY HOUR 2. L: He was beautiful physically. Gorgeous. I never saw a baby with such a head of hair in my life. He never lost it. Beautiful features. Very fine skin. He looks very much like my husband. I think he is going to be a very handsome man. I don't think it is a homosexual thing, but I have heard of men who cannot get aroused with women because they have fetishes. I want him to be a normal man. I don't want him to . . . I cannot figure it out. I have finally just taken and hidden the stockings in the closet. He shouldn't go to my clothes like that, although he hasn't touched my nightgowns or anything else. It's just my stockings and my shoes, my boots.

He doesn't like girl's clothes. In fact, he is very interested in firemen and fire trucks. He likes his one red shirt because he thinks it's a fireman's or a ranger's. He plays with fire trucks a lot, and he's a forest ranger; and he has never played with feminine things. I have a doll, and I gave it to him one day, and I said, "Would you like to play with this?" And he said, "That's dumb."

THERAPY HOUR 3. L: Mac, age 5, said something odd to me yesterday. It took me off guard; I didn't know how to take it. He said, "I have a great dream, Mommy. That I will marry you." The night before, he had had a nightmare. Sometimes, when he has a nightmare, he climbs into bed with us for five minutes and calms down. Then I put him back in his own bed. But this time, because Jim was having a hard time sleeping, I told Mac, "Let's be quiet." And instead, I got into his bed with him. It was just going to be a couple of minutes, but I fell asleep and woke in the morning. Mac had had a nightmare. I don't know about what. After Jim left for work, Mac came back to bed with me. I was so tired I just fell asleep and he fell asleep. And when he said, later on, that he wanted to marry me, I thought of that. I shouldn't let him do that; I shouldn't have gotten into bed with him. Not that it's sexual; maybe it is a little bit with him that he's taking Daddy's place. He kept saying to me all day, "Oh, boy! Tonight I'm going to have a nightmare, and you're going to sleep in bed with me." I said to him, "No nightmares tonight; if you have a nightmare, I'm not coming to bed with you. That's it!" When I went to check him the next night, he said, "Hey, Mommy; no nightmares." I said, "You're a good boy," and he went to sleep.

He never slept a whole night with us, never even stayed a long time in the bed. I never wanted to start that business. But Jim has a new schedule, and he gets up so early. It wakes Mac, and he comes into bed with me. I'm half asleep, really. Really, that time of the morning I'm very, very deep asleep and sometimes don't even know he's in bed with me until I awake later. I don't think that's such a wise idea. It's been off and on for three weeks now.

Dr.: When he was a baby, how much, if at all, did you have him in bed or hold him?

L: I always made it a point when I gave him his bottle to never prop it up. Even when he was a year old. I still held him. I don't ever remember putting him in his crib and giving him his bottle. I always held him, walked him, and sang to him and held him. He would climb into bed with us if he had a nightmare, but it would never be for long. I always held him and cuddled him an awful lot. That's not so with my baby now. I always held him and rocked him when I was reading to him when he was little. Now we sit on the floor in his bedroom propped up against his bed next to one another: and I read to him. He's getting to be a big kid, and I don't think he finds Mommy's lap helpful unless he really hurts himself.

THERAPY HOUR 4. Jim (Mac's father): He is a very inquisitive boy; he is always inquisitive, always wants to know why things work. And I encourage that. I think it is good. He is always trying to help me. Like, today I was in the garage. I needed some textbooks for the office and was going through the books. He wanted to go through the books. He was looking at the photographs of the buildings and architectural details. He is just interested, and I let him look at it. I have a bunch of boxes; he will go through them and pull stuff out and scatter it around. He is with me when I am working around the house with tools; he will be with me until his interest runs out. Sometimes I'll go after him, because he'll leave the tools around and drag off stuff. They lose interest and go out and play. I can see where it would be easy to tell him, "Don't bother me; go play," when you really had to get something done right away. But sometimes he will come back and bother you, hang around. Just hang around until you are forced to say it a half dozen times. His mother doesn't have the patience I do. She is home all day and has to do the work. I can come home; it's easier. Sometimes I lose patience with him, too. When I come home, I just want to sit there. But it's easier for me, because I look forward to seeing the kids. I play with them for a half hour or so; it's kind of new with me and takes my mind off things. I enjoy playing with the kids and get a kick out of it. But with her, you are there all day long. There is a difference.

THERAPY HOUR 5. L: When Jim's home, Mac leaves me alone. He only wants Dad. He only wants to be in the garage, in the car, or working in the yard, down the hill, across the street, just Dad, Dad.

But not when Dad's gone.

THE ADOPTION PROCESS

THERAPY HOUR 1. Dr.: How did you happen to adopt him?

L: My husband and I had been married for some years and no baby. I had taken birth control pills for the first years. Then I stopped and had no period for years and finally had surgery, became regular, and my obstetrician said I could get pregnant. That was two months before we applied to the adoption agency. They said we would have to wait nine months. I never told them that I had the surgery. Six weeks after surgery they called and said they had a baby boy and gave us 24 hours to make that hard decision: Should we wait and see if I could get pregnant or should we take this baby? I say maybe I'll never get pregnant. So we adopted him when he was 3 days old. We were very lucky. He was a beautiful baby, very healthy.

THERAPY HOUR 2. L: Thursday was one of the most horrendous days I ever had. Not only as a mother but just as a person. My day started at 6:00 A.M., and the boys were into everything all day long. My husband wasn't coming home until midnight. Billy was sick, I couldn't get out of the house — I was stuck with two kids. I was an absolute, total, unbelievable bitch to Mac the whole day. I never felt that way before. I really recognized that I hated him. That day, anyway, I did.

I didn't handle them well. I was lousy. I yelled at them all day. I called Mac a little bastard all day, not to his face but to myself or when he walked out of the room. And I don't think I have ever said that about my kid before. Because he *is* adopted.

Dr.: All right, let's hear about that.

L: He was conceived by a bastard. And that's the best I can think about him. His father was married twice. Not to Mac's mother. I guess they had an affair — he found out that she was pregnant and he took off. Then she fell in love with someone else and decided she wanted to start a new life without this baby that she was still carrying, which I think is shitty.

When I think of their having an affair, I don't even picture it was in a motel. It was in the back seat of a car, something like that. I figure that because what they told me about her — that she — I don't know how they got that information — but somehow I have the idea that he was the first man she had ever gone to bed with. From what they told me, he was very, very extremely handsome, and she was beautiful . . . a very sensual relationship. And she got pregnant. She was Catholic and so she wouldn't — very dumb — she wouldn't have an abortion. So she gave the baby up. She had the affair because she was in love with him. Because he wooed her. All I can say is I feel extremely sorry for her. He was a bastard.

Dr.: 'He was a bastard; she was a virgin; he was a handsome guy who really didn't care.' Isn't that right?

L: Yeah. He didn't give a shit about her. He just used her. She was used. She had more guts than I did.

Dr.: So she's abandoned. She has to go to the hospital. She has to go through the delivery alone. And she has a baby. And he takes off which — incidentally — not at all incidentally — recapitulates your childhood.

L: Yes. My father. [See later section about L's father.]

Dr.: What about the baby?

L: He's my baby. It's just as if he is, and what I imagine happened with his father and mother is what I always imagined would happen to me if I had had an affair before Jim.

Dr.: But the baby. Why do you get enraged at the *baby*?

L: I was just thinking that he was left like I was left.

Dr.: Why would you get angry at him? What's he done wrong?

L: He was my baby till Billy came. Then he was no longer my baby. Then I abandoned him.

Dr.: Then you're like your father?

L: Uh-huh. [dead pause] I've lost my train of thought.

Dr.: Don't look for it. What are you feeling?

L: Horror. . . . I feel sick. I feel like a bad seed. That's what I feel like. I feel like I'm getting back at him [Mac] for what they did to me. I want to get back at him. I really want to get back at him. I really want to make him sick and scared. And I feel unloved. Because he's a boy. I don't know why I said that. Because he's a boy. I'm scared that he's going to turn out like his father. He's going to abandon me; so I'm going to have to abandon him first. He's going to find out that he's adopted, and then he'll take off. That's what I'm afraid of. He's going to take off and leave. Because I love him too much. He was the most beautiful thing that I ever saw. Jim and I had a big fight the night before. I had had surgery [ovarian wedge resection] six weeks before, and I went back to work. I was back to work three days and I got a call from the adoption woman. She said that she had a baby boy. She didn't know I had the operation; I never told her about it [and within the year, L had become pregnant as a result]. She said we had to come down the next day and make up our minds if we wanted him. I talked to Jim, and he said no. He said that the doctor told us we could have our own child, so let's wait and have our own child. I thought maybe he was right, maybe.

I just cried and cried and cried. I said I wanted the baby. I didn't give a damn if I ever had any of my own. At that point, I didn't think I ever would anyway. Finally, he changed his mind. Because he knew how much I wanted that baby. So why did he not want it? Well, we got to the adoption agency, and she came in with him. He was absolutely gorgeous. He was the most beautiful baby I ever saw.

But his face was all red [indicating to her that he had sheet burn and therefore had been abandoned by the hospital personnel]. They said he had been laying on his stomach, turning back and forth. And they said he had a caul. [That is, completely enclosed at birth by intact fetal membranes, and therefore, she once said, isolated from the world.] I always thought about that, this being taken immediately from his mother, who never saw him (because when I read a lot about those first hours of newborns). I knew he was so alone. Nobody to nurse him or come in [to visit]. He was there three days.

He was so beautiful. A very serious little boy. Didn't smile or laugh. My period came that day — the first period I had had in five years. I was in agony, like I was in labor. [It was] the first period I had after the operation. And . . . we went home, didn't have anything for him but a blanket. And . . . I laid down on the bed with him beside me, and Jim went to the store. And it was like I had [borne] him. I was in such pain. That's why I feel that he's mine. He *is* mine. And I don't want to tell him. Because when I do, he's just going to look his mother up and go back to her. He will. I know he will. I know he will. Just as I went back to see my father's family years later and my mother didn't want me to. But I did. I wanted to see them. I wanted to know them. I wanted to hold them. I know that he wants to do that, too. He's going to want to look at them. And after I saw my father's family, I liked them better than my own; I like them better than my own family. And he's going to do that to me. I know he will because I've been so awful to him.

THERAPY HOUR 3. L: I always thought I was adopted. I felt alienated, different. . . . My mother said that it was because of the incubator [she was premature; Mac's caul equals her incubator], which was a bunch of hogwash. I would sit and think about it for hour upon hour when I was a child. I really wasn't my mother's child. I was my father's. . . . I think I felt that my [dead twin] sister was my mother's child but that I wasn't. By some fluke, she was the real child and I wasn't.

THE NATURE OF THE MOTHER-CHILD RELATIONSHIP

THERAPY HOUR 1. L: I felt so sorry for him [Mac] Tuesday. [He was very ill.] Wednesday, when I took him into the doctor, when I saw he was in such pain, and he was so good, he was so good. And I knew what pain he was in, I knew what pain he was in. And he was so happy, he was happy, really happy. I have never seen him like that in a long time because he had me in that reception room by himself. He and I were together. And I knew what kind of agony he was in, and I held him and loved him and . . . [pause].

Dr.: Then we are left with the paradox: you love him so much that it is almost supernatural and at the same time you're turning on him and thinking, "My God, what a fiend I am!" What happens to the impulse not to turn on him?

L: Where is it? Oh, it's lost. It's like I'm an enraged animal. The rage is absolutely, totally uncontrollable. I could kill him. I could literally kill him. Not beat him or stab him or shoot him. But shake him, shake him, shake him. Just shake him. I've only done it a couple of times to where it's been enough to rattle his teeth. I never slap him across the face. He's never gotten slapped; it's been on the fanny or maybe on the hand. That doesn't mean I haven't had the urge to slap him across the face. Tuesday I had that urge. I know mothers who have done that, but I think that's totally degrading. I have spanked him pretty darn hard on the ass. I shook him Tuesday. I wanted him to leave me alone. I wanted him to go away. I wanted to call up the adoption agency and tell them to take him back.

I'm frightened that I love him. So why not do it first? How can I love somebody so much and hate them so much at the same time? Is it possible for two people to be like that? I've never done that before. My mother said as a kid I would go around the house leaving her little notes: "I hate you, I hate you, I hate you." But I never told her to her face. I remember that. I hated her because she left me everyday to go to work. When I was little, I was alone, alone; lonely. I had nobody to play with. Just my grandmother in the house, who would yell at me and scream. But my hating my mother was not very sharp. More dull, more . . . not that she would ever leave me, but that she would die, up and die on me. Her and her goddamn Kotex. [See section on Mother's Fear of Traumatic Abandonment.]

Dr.: What are you waiting for Mac to do to make it all all right?

L: I don't know. To tell me that he really wants me, that he loves me. I hate him because he's hers [natural mother] and he's not mine: He's not really mine. He's a fantasy; it's a horrible, horrible, horrible, horrible, unbelievable fantasy. It's because I took those goddamn pills [contraceptive, before discovering she was sterile]. He'll go back there, and he'll find her.

THERAPY HOUR 2. L: I just love Mac; I love him passionately. I love him like I would have loved my father, I suppose. I know I did love my father. I saw him until I was 5. I was the same age as Mac is. It makes me so goddamn angry, because I feel Mac knows me better than anyone else does. I feel that I am never faithful to him, that he has seen me in all kinds of horrible, miserable, terrible moods. I know this because I hate him so much for this. He has seen me at my worst. My husband never does. When Mac and I get into these things, we're alone.

When I get angry at Bill, he jolts back when he sees me that way. But I never get angry that way at him; it's that he sees me that way with Mac. When Mac gets that anger thrown at him, his eyes get big. Most of the time, he comes at me with his own anger, or he'll joke around or he'll tease me. But he does not pull back the way Bill does.

Dr.: He is more your equal than anyone else on earth?

L: Yes. But I feel he is that way because he has lived with me. He knows me better than anyone else.

Dr.: But there's no dishonesty in the relationship?

L: No. None at all. He lies like all kids lie at 5. But that is completely different.

THERAPY HOUR 3. L: Last night I was with Mac and Bill, in a bookstore with them, and they were sitting and reading. I was across the room, hidden by a bookshelf, and Mac came out and called to me. And I moved from behind the bookshelf and said, "I'm right here, Mac." And he said, "Oh, don't move from there. I want to make sure that you're there." Ten million times — when I *was* there, I did not move — he'd come back and check on me. Bill couldn't have cared less; he was so busy looking at those books. We were there half an hour with Mac continually asking, "Where are you, where are you, where are you?" And I tell you — continually: "Are you there?" It drives me batty. I swear to God it does. I don't know what I've done to do it but . . . I remember when we first got him, he was very unsmiling, a very serious baby. I always tried to make him happier. I always talked to him and cooed to him and sang to him. I don't mean that I held him every minute, because I didn't do that. I was thinking, the other day, that whenever I picked him up, I kissed him, and whenever I put him down I kissed him. Up and down into the crib a million times to change his diapers to put him into the crib. I probably did it just to pick him up, to kiss him. I love him — a truly dear, dear baby. Just give him a hug and a little kiss on his cheek. You know, kiss him. I always kissed him that way. I always kissed Billy that way, too. I think I kissed Bill more, because I nursed him. I held him more than I did Mac. With Mac, it was less touching him, because I was holding the bottle. And holding him and holding the bottle wasn't easy. With Bill, it was just I was nursing and I had a free hand. I could touch his hand, his little arm, or his face. But with Mac, I couldn't manage both. And I always felt I wish I had a third hand to touch him more. But I never propped a bottle with him. I always held him until he was 14 months.

When I wasn't feeding him, I put him in his playpen or in the infant's seat. I didn't carry him around all day. I didn't want him to get into the habit of that. But he was always near me, because he always fussed if he wasn't. I don't mean right next to me but in the same room. Sometimes when he got older, he would come and crawl into bed with me. But he always had his own room, and we had ours.

THERAPY HOUR 4. L: The intensity came not with me but with him. I can remember when he was maybe 9 months, a year, sitting in the car with him. I would be driving, and he would grab me and he would put his arms around my neck and he would hold my *[sic]* head very close to my chest. He always did that to me.

THERAPY HOUR 5. L: I'm afraid I won't do it — treat Mac the way I can Bill. Because I'm unable to: to push him away. But I don't mean totally. I feel that I have hurt him so much that the only way I can make up to him is by not pushing him away. Not in the slightest. The way I can with Bill. Do all children grow up feeling abandoned? I don't think Bill does.

Yesterday I took Mac for his 5-year-old physical exam. The nurse came in and gave him a shot. . . . he's a big kid now, and here he was crying, every inch of the way, and I had to help her hold him down. It was just like I wanted that. I wanted that sensation. He didn't see my reaction; he was laying on his stomach, but I could. . . . and immediately afterwards, I felt this horrendous migraine headache. It was so bad I could barely focus. Then they were going to take blood tests. He was sitting on my lap. That kid was so good, but he was so scared. And I was angry, because any time anything happened to me like that when I was a kid, I was always alone. But with Mac, I was always there. And it seems that I'm angry with him for my having to take the brunt of what's happening to him. I don't mean that I don't want to be with him. I want to be with him, and I want to share things with him. But it's almost that I've taken too much. Do you understand? [Crying.] I'm putting out for him what I never got myself.

SEPARATION ANXIETY

THERAPY HOUR 1. L: He went to nursery school for the first time this week [age 4]. A big boy. I said, "I'm going now, Mac." And he said, "Bye." You know like, "O.K. I'm O.K. And I'm safe." But every once in a while — we went to the county fair yesterday, my husband, the boys, and me. And I sat down on a bench, and Mac walked a little far away from me and didn't see me for a couple of minutes. He screamed bloody murder. "Mommy! Mommy!" It was just half a yard away from me. And I thought to myself, "Holy cow, he really is afraid of being lost."

Dr.: He does not feel lost in nursery school, and so he can just wave you good-bye, but he is lost when an unexpected break in the contact between you occurs?

L: Very much so. Yes. He spoke to me this morning. "What would happen if you forgot to pick me up at nursery school?" And I said, "Well, I don't think I would ever forget to pick you up at nursery school." And he said, "Well, what if you did? Would I live there forever?" And I said, "No, if something happened and I was late, I would call them and they would take care of you until I got there." But he worried; he worried about that in the back of his head.

Dr.: How do you know?

L: When we go to strange places, he will always hold my hand. I don't have to ask him to hold my hand. Bill won't; he's a little rascal, that one.

He is extremely independent and he'll just take off and . . . "Bye, Mom." But not Mac. He'll always be there to hold my hand. I can just see him thinking, when we go to some place far away, he just never really goes too far from us. It's just something I know. I can't really explain it to you. It's just something I feel, I don't know. He's always been that way since a baby, very close to me more than Bill. I nursed Bill for almost a year, yet Mac has always been more physically close to me. Holding on to me or clutching me or — he never let me out of his sight. I couldn't leave him in the front room in his playroom. He would always want to be where I was, in the kitchen. This was at 6 weeks, 3 months. Yeah, sure; he just didn't want to be alone. I always had to bring his playroom into where I was so he could see me working. Not physically wanting to hang onto me all the time but just to know where I was.

He was always a very serious child. I never got that kid to laugh. I was looking through his baby book and every picture I have of him is serious. Whenever I took him to a photographer, he would never give them a smile. It was a terrible thing, he would scream and cry and never want me away from where the photographer was in order to get a picture; just was always very glum.

Dr.: What if you were separated from him around the house?

L: He'd cry. Well, he could stay by himself for maybe a total of 15 minutes or something like that if I was out of sight. I had to keep all kinds of baby toys in the crib so he would be busy and occupied. He'd be quiet for 10 or 15 minutes, and then I'd have to bring him in to where I was. But Bill played for a long time by himself; not Mac. But I don't think I ever treated them differently.

Dr.: How long would he keep crying?

L: It was not a question of how long he would keep it up but it was how long I would let him keep it up. The longest was probably 10 minutes. Not sitting there screaming his lungs out but just fussing.

And when he grew older, maybe 18 months, he would whine because he couldn't follow me around the kitchen or from room to room. It drove me up the wall. Maybe some mothers can take that but . . . I could never do any work until he went to bed. Like if I was cleaning the bathroom, he would get into the tub-scouring powder; that stuff's poison.

THERAPY HOUR 2. L: Jim and I are going away for a few days, and Mac was a little worried. Perhaps he thinks I won't come back. The last time I was gone for a few days was when he was a baby and Bill was born. And what I did to Mac was something awful, so god-awful. I left him. And I had a baby. I wasn't supposed to have a baby. When we signed up to adopt a baby, we had been married for so many years and couldn't have a baby. That was why they let us sign up. That was why they let us have Mac. So I promised them — and it was like I had promised *him* — that I would not have my own baby from inside me. I promised the adoption agency, or Mac, or whoever that I would never have a baby of my own. He would be the only baby I could ever have. And the day after Bill was born, I developed a migraine headache, and it was horrendous. I couldn't move my head off the bed. Mother called me at the hospital. She had Mac. He was crying on the phone. She told me she was having a terrible time with him. He would not do anything she said; he wasn't eating and he wasn't sleeping. She managed to lay it on me right there: Why wasn't he doing what he was supposed to be doing? Here I am, just six hours after having Bill. And she pulled that. I just wanted her to stay home and take care of him. I wanted someone to just stay home and take care of him. But no one would listen to me. After I came home from the hospital with Bill, Mac seemed so forlorn and lost. Two days later, he came down with a herpes virus; his entire mouth was filled with sores. He was so sick, God, he was sick! He couldn't eat anything. He cried and cried and cried. And when I came home from the hospital, two days later Mother left and Jim went back to work. And there I was. Mac was sick, and I was trying to learn how to nurse the baby. It was awful; it was horrible. And it continued like that for months, months, and months. I never left the house. I was angry at Mac. I was tired. Sick. It was horrible, horrible. And I handled it absolutely awful. Mac took the brunt of it. I didn't want him to. It was like I abandoned him; it really was. I was caught in between — one son who was adopted and one who wasn't. I couldn't decide if I should love my natural-born son or Mac. I was thinking that I loved Bill and that I didn't love Mac. After all those years, I had Bill, my own.

I would be nursing Bill, and Mac would hang around. He would hang around every single minute. And I'd think, "Why doesn't he leave me alone; why can't I be alone with my own baby?" I just wanted to be alone with him. "Why can't he just stop it, why can't he just go and play a little bit?" And then I would feel horrendously guilty for feeling or thinking that. Mac would be around continually. He wouldn't leave me alone, not for an instant. I was trying to sort out how I felt about him, and I couldn't. There was no time. All the time I had no time, no time to be away from him, no time to be alone with my baby, no time to understand, no fun. No time to love him or care for him. Every time it went wrong, I'd just pile up the guilt on top of me. When I yelled at Mac, I'd go in the bathroom and cry because I didn't want to do that. But I wasn't able to control myself.

But when I put him to bed at night, I'd touch him and read to him, and I would love him greatly. Or he'd be asleep, and I'd go in and look at him. And I'd feel that I really loved him in spite of everything he had done during the day. But the thing during the day—that he was on me so much, yelling and screaming and crying. It wasn't that I didn't love him at those times. I was only angry at him. Horrible anger. I just wanted to—I just had to leave him alone. So I'd just be silent. I can only remember once losing my cool. Bill was lying on the couch and Mac was standing on the couch, jumping up and down. I told him to stop or he might fall on Bill. But he kept doing it and he fell on Bill. I thought he had crushed the baby's head in. I went really nuts. I spanked him, and I put him into his bed, yelling at him the whole time.

THERAPY HOUR 3. L: I dropped a can of cream on my foot and thought I had broken my toe. I was in absolute agony. So I lay down and was crying. I couldn't stop. Mac became so upset. Bill just stood there and looked at me, but Mac became so upset that he went into his room and he cried. After he finished crying, he came back in and got ice and put it on my foot. And he sat there for half an hour and kept putting ice on my foot and kept saying, "Is that better?"

THERAPY HOUR 4. L: A bee bit me on the face—it didn't sting me. And Mac became very upset. So Jim said, "If I die, I'll never have to worry about someone to take care of you, because Mac will always take care of you." That's very nice for a mother to know about her child. I want him to love his mother, to be responsible for me. But I don't want him to live his life worrying about me. My cousin remembers what Mac was like when he was little. She remembers that he never left my side, never let me go anywhere without him.

MOTHER'S RELATIONSHIP WITH HER PARENTS

THERAPY HOUR 1. L: And he's [Mac] going to leave me. And there's going to be so much heartache for me. It's going to be just like my Dad did. He's going to grow up and leave me. Because I've been a crappy mother to him. Because I've wanted to leave my mother's and find my father's family, Mac must too. He must. He must want to know about them. Because I wanted to know so much about my father's family. I know that feeling. I know it desperately. I know that he's going to know it. I wanted to know them. I wanted to leave my family and go to them. But there was no way when I was young. They hated one another. My mother hated my father's family. To this day, she hates them, and they hate her.

When my mother married my dad, she married him. She stayed home, and she was his wife. If anybody did the running around, it was Dad. He took off six months after they were married and went on a job far away. He took off for a year and left her. My mother's version was that he went because of the good pay. I don't know my father's version. But he was an adventurer. He was truly an adventurer. He took off and did what he damn-well pleased. When he was 13, he joined the merchant marine and did not come back until he was 18, and his family did not know where he was for five years. He moved all around the world. He could do anything he put his mind to. And he made money at it. He was good. And he was sneaky as hell. Either he was not sneaky and my mother was dumb, or I can't understand how she managed to go from place to place with him and not really understand. She must have. Either that or she just didn't want to understand. But *my* husband wouldn't cart me around unless *I* knew what the hell was going on.

THERAPY HOUR 2. L: I was always by myself for everything. My mother was there, physically, but I don't remember her holding me. It's like I've taken all the pain of my children upon myself. I don't want to do that but I have to, out of my own misery. I don't want to go through that anymore. I'm mad as hell at my mother, because she didn't go through it for me.

I'm thinking about when I was 5. My mother took me to the county clinic, because I had bad tonsils, and they were going to do a tonsillectomy. There must have been 25 or 30 other kids in the room, and they were just sitting there [i.e., abandoned also]. It was early in the morning. I remember my mother taking me, but I don't remember her being there. The nurse and doctor came, looked at all the kids, pointed at me, and said, "Let's take this one; she's little and so skinny." So they took me first. And she wasn't there. Mom wasn't there. She took me there, but she didn't hold me. She wasn't there when I woke up from the ether.

And I can still remember the dream: of being in a tunnel or hole—black—and calling for her. And I can remember around that age playing on the ground. The wind was blowing very hard through the trees. And it blew a beehive right down beside me. I can remember screaming for my mother. And she didn't come. Daddy finally came. I don't remember him coming any other time but that time. He got me out of the bees. It seems that I have always called for her. And she has never been there.

Never been there. I've always been there for her, always taken care of her, always. [Crying.] As a little girl, I sat by her bed when she was sick. I sat by her bed hour after hour and never went out to play. I always stayed with her and brought her water, took care of her. It was like I was the mother, and she was the child. All my life like that. I feel I was taken away from him by my mother, always taken away from him. He never abandoned me. Not till the end. But it was always her. She had to run back to her damn family. And her family would always say to me, "You're lucky you have a good mother." Saying, I suppose, that a mother is better than a father.

When I leave Mac and Bill with my mother to come here, I look at them: he's so afraid. And it's me all over again, waiting for my mother, looking out the window, feeling a horrible knot in the bottom of my stomach until she came home, so afraid that she'd never come back. I think of that every time I leave Mac. I do. It is like I was left again all over again. That's why it's so hard for me. With Bill it isn't hard, but with Mac it is. [Crying.]

Dr.: Your feeling transmits itself, doesn't it?

L: Yeah. He's so damn perceptive.

Sometimes, in my brain, I think of coming and going on airplanes and ships and never staying in one place or being in one bed for long enough. I've always worried about where the kids are going to sleep. Are they going to sleep well. Now I know why; because I've slept in so many beds myself.

THERAPY HOUR 3. L: I can remember standing every night at the window when I was little waiting for my mom to come home thinking what if anything happened to her. . . . It was bad. . . . I was scared something would happen to her and I'd be left with my grandmother.

I already had feelings of being abandoned by my father; so feelings of losing my mother were horrible. I don't know why I was so afraid to live without her; your mother's your mother. I love my mother very much, although she's acted very stupidly in many ways. She puts her heart before her mind.

She was always bleeding heavily. Extremely. All the time. One night I woke up, and my aunt was there. And she had gone into the hospital and was losing blood by the gallon. They did a hysterectomy.

I don't want to think that she abandoned me. Well, I think I felt that when I was little. I would go to bed and cry, feeling that Daddy didn't love me and that's why he left me. Mother had to work and support us but didn't abandon me. I was always with her even on vacations. There was never a physical abandonment, just in my stupid little mind, and I think just her going to work every day was an abandonment. I was left alone with my grandmother. I was always terrified of Mother being in an automobile accident, or someone hurting her, or her dying.

She was terribly sick. She told me that she was so sick when I was 4 or 5 that she would lie in bed for days on end. I would never leave her side — hemorrhaging. I knew she was sick. I dream about that in myself: If I die, what would happen to the children?

MOTHER'S FEAR OF TRAUMATIC ABANDONMENT

THERAPY HOUR 1. L: I can remember when I was a kid my family's joke about my mother's Kotex. My uncle would say that if he grabbed a box of Kotex and threw it out the door I would be enraged because they belonged to my mother. And she needed those [pause]. . . . or she would die. I was always afraid she would die. When I was 6, we had twin beds and my mother always slept in one. But this time my aunt was there. I don't know where my mother was. I said to her, "Where's Mommy?" And she said, "You'd better be a good girl because Mommy went to the hospital and she was hemorrhaging." My mother had had surgery six weeks before, a hysterectomy. The night before, she picked my big baby cousin up, and she ripped her stitches. And I guess during the night she started hemorrhaging in the bathroom. And they didn't wake me up until she was at the hospital. They stuffed a sheet between her legs. I can remember seeing the sheet. . . . it was in the kitchen. And it was — they couldn't stop her bleeding and rushed her to the hospital. They got her out of the car, and she fainted from the loss of blood. And the sheet was loaded with it. I never saw so much blood in all my life, and it was my mother.

I can't imagine my aunt saying that. I wouldn't say that to my child. It scared the shit out of me. And for all of my life I was afraid that she would die — not so much when I was growing up. . . . I was with my grandmother. . . . I was an only child, the only one in the neighborhood, and all I had was my grandmother.

I'm just sorry about my twin sister [who died at birth]. My mother named me after her dead sister . . . pretty tough to take. She died at 18 of leukemia. And I never thought I would live past the age of 18. I thought since she named me after her that the same thing was going to happen to me. All of the children in my family are named after dead sisters and brothers.

A Note on the Treatment of Mother and Son

Data are, of course, the product of the treatment, and so theories and explanations are at the mercy of what happened in treatment and what we decide is worth reporting. Let me say a few words about the treatment. L was in treatment with me for about three years. It could not be analysis for logistical reasons, such as the long distance between her home and UCLA and the difficulty in getting regular baby-sitters (not only because they were hard to find during the daytime hours but because the family could not afford them regularly, not to mention the expenses of transportation). Instead, L saw me twice a week, sitting up. She would have been a good analytic patient and in fact allowed me to work with interpretations that were effective; she had no difficulty in associating freely enough; I felt almost always immersed in a comfortable and creative analytic atmosphere. A transference neurosis developed, and it was dealt with via interpretations and reconstructions (though I was more restrained in this work than I would have been had she been seen more often). There was, therefore, interpretation in depth of her oedipal situation, but less exploration of her earliest life. There was far more to the treatment than Mac; however, that material is not pertinent here.

Though L first came for evaluation because of Mac's fetishism, her relationship with me converted almost immediately, because of her needs, from an evaluation to treatment. The greatest part of our time was not spent on Mac but flared out into all the other areas of her life. Unfortunately, her therapy was effective; she changed so much that her marriage was thrown out of balance. Her comfort in accepting the role of wife and mother, as drawn and commanded by her husband—to whom she had been grateful for rescuing her from an unanchored life—gave way as she discovered how much more she needed and was able to seize from the world. His demands that she break off treatment became so dangerous that she had no choice. Unfortunately, from the start, he stated that he not only had no interest in joining the family's therapeutic process but that he found the whole effort absurd. Mac should simply be told to stop it, and if that failed, he should be properly disciplined. It was only L's failure of nerve and toughness, he felt, that allowed Mac to persist in this dirty habit.

Mac was in analytically oriented treatment for a year and a half, which, in brief, confirmed L's descriptions of Mac in every way. Mac's treatment failed to change the fetishism, though his therapist felt that, in other ways, Mac was coming along very well.

Following the therapist's leaving our training program, Mac was referred to a behavior modification program. That treatment seemed to have failed. L reported, at the end of her work with me, that Mac had not changed. But now, years later, when she read this report, she told me that she believes the fetishism is gone and that she saw no evidence of it after the behavior modification procedures. L, on reading the manuscript, added:

Going through the report, I still feel the loneliness of waiting for mother. I suppose I still haven't worked it out or I wouldn't act so scared inside when I am an hour late getting home and the boys are alone. I wish I could be rid of that horrible anxiety. I cried a lot when I read the report for the second time, as I am crying now while I write you this. I think the one line, "She loves him the way she feels her mother could not love her and hates him the way she hates herself" is very true, yet devastating. It says it all.

Can a 2½ Year Old Be Perverse?

Erotic fetishism has been an important subject for psychoanalysts, containing in its structure mechanisms of defense central for understanding all human relationships. The capacity to substitute part for whole, nonhuman for human, and inanimate for animate helps make life bearable —even enjoyable— when intimacy, insight, and lovingness would be too intense. So it does not surprise us that adolescents and adults turn to this complex construction; that a child of 2½ can also create the fullblown symptom is impressive.

A child may get genitally aroused, but can the arousal be sophisticated enough to fill his or her excitement in the ways arousal does from later childhood on? Such behavior in a small child should not be; in fact, we must question—as does the next quote by A. Freud [6]—if it can be.

. . . diagnostic categories which cannot be used outright for children are perversions such as transvestitism, fetishism, addictions. In these as in the cases of all *perversions,* the reason is an obvious one. . . . Since infantile sexuality as such is by definition polymorphously perverse, to label specific aspects of it as perverse is at best an imprecise usage of the term, if it does not imply a total misunderstanding of the development of the sex instinct. Instead of assessing certain childhood phenomena as perverse, as even analysts are apt to do, the diagnostic questions must be reformulated for these cases and we must inquire which component trends, or under which conditions part of the component trends, are likely to outlast childhood, i.e., when they have to be considered as true forerunners of adult perversion proper. (Pp. 197–198)

Three problems come to mind. First, "Infantile sexuality as such is by definition polymorphously perverse" [14]. Although a classical position in analysis from 1905 on (Freud), this statement confuses me. First, knowing the history of the word "sexuality" in the development of analytic drive theory, I do not know to what experiences it refers. It can mean such things as "erotic," "masculinity and femininity," or precursors to these; it can mean "sensual," "life force" (as in Eros), or defenses against all these. It can also mean pleasure or pain, activity or passivity, love or hate, and excitement or boredom. With such a load of meanings, the word scarcely has meaning. What, therefore, is "infant sexuality," or perhaps we should ask what is not?

Second, enjoying sucking or playing with feces are, in the classical analytic view, examples of polymorphous perverse behavior because such infantile pleasures may or may not be part of adult erotism and may or may not play a part in later neuroses: there is too much slippage in a theory built on such logic.

Third, "polymorphously perverse" is part of the language of a clinically incorrect theory that equates *awareness* ("cathexis," "hypercathexis") with *erotism* ("perversion") of body parts or body functions in the infant/child as if it were all the same, whether that awareness is consciously erotic, becomes erotic only in later life, is sensual but not erotic, or is simply an aspect of relations with others. One thereby manages to call infants perverse when they do what comes naturally and, as above, one also denies that perversion can exist in infants.

We are well warned that, as is found daily in work with children and adults, precursors are not full-blown pictures, and a full-blown picture in a child may be gone by adolescence [6, 7]. Yet I have trouble with the idea that a boy of 2, 3, 4, or 5 who gets erections from his mother's stockings and who is masturbating while fondling or putting on these stockings is not perverse. When a behavior starts in childhood and persists into adult life—a not so rare occurrence—is it perversion only from adolescence on? For instance, over half of the children with significant gender disorder in childhood—some starting as early as a year or two of age—are found to still have a gender disorder in adolescence [15, 16]. And if a psychotic child grows up to become an adult psychotic, we do not question that the child was truly psychotic.

Should "perversion" identify only those excitements that result from a failed passage through oedipal conflict? As A. Freud [6] stated:

With regard to manifest behavior some clinical pictures in children are almost identical with those in adult perverts. Nevertheless, this overt similarity need not imply a corresponding metapsychological identity. With adults, the diagnosis of perversion signifies that primacy of the genitals has never been established or has not been maintained, i.e., that in the sexual act itself the pregenital components have not been reduced to the role of merely introductory or contributory factors. Such a definition is necessarily invalid if applied before maturity, i.e., at an age when intercourse does not come into question and while equality of the pregenital zones with the genitals themselves is taken for granted. Accordingly, individuals under the age of adolescence are not perverts in the adult sense of the term, and different viewpoints have to be introduced to account for their relevant symptomatology. (P. 198)

Again we have the problem of those whose aberrant behavior carries through from childhood to adulthood. Is the behavior "metapsychologically" different at 6 and 26, though behaviorally the same?

Bak [2] is another who denies that a child can be a fetishist. "According to a strict definition of the clinical concept of fetishism, it is a male sexual perversion and belongs to adulthood. *Formes frustes* may appear in childhood from the age of 4 or 5, with experiences of diffuse sexual excitement, but they do not necessarily lead to adult fetishism" (p. 193). I cannot call Mac's fetishism a *forme fruste,* nor is it an experience "of diffuse sexual excitement." "There can be a childhood—but not an infancy—fetishism that is transitory. . . . Genetically, the *sine qua non* of fetishism is its phase-specific castration anxiety during the phallic phase in an oedipal setting. . . . It is absolutely necessary to emphasize the phase-specific position of fetishism in order to clarify its relation to aggression. The destructive and castrative wishes of the male child reach their peak at the phallic-oedipal phase with their consecutive retaliatory fantasies of heightened castration anxiety. In contrast, the so-called pregenital fetishes defend against separation, object loss, deprivations, and total loss of body integrity, at a phase when the destructive wishes toward the parental objects play a different and less important role" (pp. 194–195) [2]. An essential feature of perversion for Bak is regression: "This regressive feature is common to all perversions and involves the denial of heightened castration anxiety and marked bisexual identification" (p. 195). It is regression for Mac, if we feel he crawls into his mother's skin when he puts on her panty hose, but it is not regression if we grant him the genius to create such a dynamically rich neurosis when so young.

Though we must heed the warnings of A. Freud and Bak that we look beneath surface phenomena to underlying structure[2], theory should suggest, not command. Can we not say Mac is perverse and a fetishist and still not consider him identical to an adult fetishist?

---

[2] I think, however, it is closer to the facts to say "meanings" or "fantasies" than "structure."

The Psychoanalytic Understanding of Fetishism and its Origins

Another problem arises when we turn for help to the rest of the analytic literature. Some use "fetish" to refer to an object that is erotically exciting, some to an object that is not. For example, some feel a transitional object is a fetish (or prefetish) and some do not. Though erotic and nonerotic fetishes may share similar origins and dynamics, there are also great and wonderful differences between a state of erotic excitement and one that, though intense, does not feel erotic. Once the definition is open to include the nonerotic fetish, one's explanations can go anywhere. Many authors contribute many theories, however, few are testable. I shall list them here without pause so that the reader can get a sense of how many there are, how they often contradict each other, and how far we have to go to make order out of such disarray: pregenital identification with the phallic mother, separation anxiety, anal erotic fixation, scopophilia, symbolic representation of the female phallus, identification with the mother with the penis, identification with the penisless mother, castration anxiety, compromise between separation anxiety and castration anxiety, intense submission to castration, father's penis fantasized in the female genital, the last object (e.g., a piece of clothing) seen before the recognition that females do not have penises, congealed anger, splitting of the ego, displacement of the female penis onto another body part, interference with the distinction between self and nonself, physical trauma in infancy, the fetish as representative of the feeding function, suffusion of the entire body with aggressive stimulation, diffusion of aggression resulting in frozen immobility, susceptibility to active irritability, a kind of automatic reversal of reaction at a psychophysiological level, topical unreality, flowering of protective screen memories, prolongation of the introjective-projective stage, nasal congestion, turning away from the primary object, annihilating sadistic love, the unresolved wish in the male to have a child plus the consequent fear of pregnancy, persistence of attachment to a transitional object, fetish as a substitute and/or symbol for mother's breast (good or bad), mouth, uterus, vagina, anus, or swollen pregnant abdomen plus their products, early motility disturbances, illness in infancy, illness in the mother, inconsistent mothering, envy, seeing female genitals too frequently in early childhood, very close visual contact (type undescribed) with a female, a state of primary identification with mother or sister, blurred sense of one's own body dimensions, hypertrophy of visual activity, subjective sensations of sudden changes in body size, defense against homosexuality, substitute for criminality in cowards, depreciation of females, the female genital as a wound through which a woman could empty herself out, dentate vagina, denial of parental intercourse, defense against suicide, defense against homicide, defense against psychosis, defense against incest, focal disturbance in sexual identity, infarct in the reality sense, the fetish as a substitute for excrement, passive homosexual submission to one's own sadistic and castrating superego, fetish as a symbol of one's own castrated self, defense against rejection, splitting of the object, weakness of the ego structure that may be inherent or may come about secondarily through physiological dysfunctions or disturbances in the mother-child relationship that threaten survival, the mother's body, oneself as pregnant and at the same time as mother's fetus in the womb, defense in homosexuals against heterosexual impulses, inverted oedipal relationship with the father, passive anal relationship with the phallic mother, oral sadism, anal sadism, unsuccessful olfactory repression, erotization of the hands and predilection for touching, an exquisitely sensitive body-phallus equation, observing the primal scene, inborn weakness of ego integration, an executive weakness of the sexual apparatus, defense against fear of annihilation, respiratory incorporation, respiratory introjection, alien smells that stand for archaic superego elements, massive overstimulations (e.g., frequent body massages) that throw the infant into states of extreme excitement with abrupt termination, the conflict between anal giving and withholding, pleasant tactile sensations, to find the object identical with one's own fantasized penisless state, transferring of sensual sensations to an indifferent object by association, bisexual splitting of the body image, witnessing a particularly mutilating event in childhood, the mother's unconscious need to resist separation from her child, a deprived or violent family atmosphere, mothering that is not good enough or at least not quite good enough, inability to accept weaning, mother's conscious or unconscious encouraging the child to take a fetish, all the significant instinctual part-objects of the prephallic years, mother's abdominal skin which the fetishist penetrates, identification with the maternal feces, identification with the bad mother and at the same time to feel the elation of the introjected good object, the fetish as symbol condensing breast-skin plus buttocks-feces plus female phallus, identification with the partial object (the breasts) of the total object (the mother), the fetish as a symbol of mother's milk devaluated and subsequently commuted into excrement, a replacement of a combination of breast and penis, an effort not to avoid castration anxiety but rather the outcome of pregenital disturbances, fixation not regression, and disturbance in the formation of the body image in infancy. The fetish undoes the separation from the mother and the fetish creates an independence from the love object. (I spare the reader and printer the citations for this long list, most of which are exact quotes.) No data (often not even a well-honed anecdote) for any of the numerous explanations are given.

Though these explanations do not each contradict all the others, it would take some artistry in theory making to shape them, even after debridement, into a synthesis. Besides, we know that most of these have been used to explain many conditions examined by analysts and that many are so nonspecific that they fit the description of the genesis of almost any behavior of almost anyone.[3]

Nonetheless, and less disheartening, *there is general agreement that the fetish — erotic or nonerotic, in child or adult — stands for some aspect of the separated mother, and that the precipitant to creating it is castration anxiety.* At any rate, a fetish is a thing that has become a story.

Having recently immersed myself in the data and thinking of ethnography, I join with those who wish we analysts would temper our *furor theoreticus* and at least muse on other societies. If a glimpse of pudendum — the cause of fetishism in classical theory — is enough to derail a boy for life in New York or London, does the same occur in primitive societies? Ethnographers may not be good clinicians and perhaps therefore do not report on individuals with erotic fetishism. But it may be the case that there is more to castration anxiety — secrecy, prudery, and the promise of the forbidden unknown, for instance — than our theories provide, and that there really is less erotic fetishism in societies in which genitals are less covered. In the one tribe with which I am personally familiar, despite intimate observation [24], no perverse fetishism is known. The skeptic also wonders why, when the trauma of seeing a female without a penis occurs in childhood, does the overt perversion first occur shortly thereafter in a few boys, not until latency, puberty, and adolescence in some children, decades later in some adults, or — as is almost always the case — never.

We can legitimately use "fetish" for either erotic or nonerotic objects so long as we appreciate the clinical differences (as do, for instance, Roiphe and Galenson [34, 35]). Though "fetish" can indicate either an

---

[3] Other than the psychodynamic, there are two general types of explanatory systems for fetishism. The first is the learning theory model, in which the aberrant erotism is said to result from an otherwise neutral object (e.g., a shoe) being perceived by chance at a time of high erotic excitement, with the object and the drive then fused (e.g., [44]). The second is an organic explanation, as exemplified in the following: "The state of increased organismic excitability is considered the primary disturbance in fetishism. This state is regarded as a product of cerebral pathophysiology. Some of the major manifestations of this state appear to be related to seizure and other episodic phenomena found in temporal lobe dysfunction" (p. 107) [5].

erotically exciting or nonerotically exciting object, I shall use it to refer only to the former.[4] Bak [2] is especially helpful here. (Varieties of positions are stated by Freud [8, 9], Gillespie [11, 12], Friedjung in Wulff [49], Bak [1], Greenacre [17–22], Winnicott [47], Weissman [45], M. Sperling [39], Dickes [4], A. Freud [6], Roiphe and Galenson [34, 35], and Silverman [37]). This not only sharpens the clinical description leading toward theory, it also highlights how unusual Mac's behavior was. There are mighty few fetishists, in age and form of the fetishism, like Mac.

Mac had a security blanket, used only in early infancy and held only while he nursed. He gave it up easily. Disagreeing with Sperling [39], I feel it is clinically inept to call it a fetish (especially, as we sense, the fetish — different from the usual transitional object — is a densely compacted tangle of sadomasochistic fantasies).

Early Childhood Fetishism: A Very Rare Condition

In some reports of fetishism, the interest in the fetish goes back to childhood, but rarely before age 4 or 5 (Friedjung in Wulff [49], Sterba [40], Lorand [29], Idelsohn in Wulff [49], Wulff, [49]; of course we cannot be sure the need did not start further back. Unfortunately, the failure of a patient's memory keeps us from knowing of a very early fetishism. Practically no cases report that the object that is erotic for the adult was erotic in early childhood. However, Dickes [4] does report a case of a woman with a nonerotic fetish that had been erotic in childhood. It is not clear in this case to what extent the object — a teddy bear — was in itself erotized; we only know that it was used for rubbing the genitals, which may not be the same as being a fetish.

If we restrict ourselves to preoedipal children with a clear-cut erotic fetish, there are few reports (I have not attempted a survey of the nonanalytic literature.) To what extent, when we are dealing with adults talking about their childhood, we are dealing with a childhood amnesia or with a truly absent behavior cannot be determined. At any rate, I am not surprised to hear transvestites report that their earliest memory of erotic cross-dressing is in childhood, though none remembered this activity before approximately age 6.

---

[4] And, believing that the clearest possible clinical definition is the best approach in looking for explanations, I distinguish between objects that themselves erotically excite and those that only clear the way to an exciting object. The latter include such things as amulets held in the hand or looked at, without which one is impotent in erotic use. The shared psychodynamic features of the two types should not blind us to the differences.

I am not familiar with the detailed report of erotic fetishism in another child as young as Mac. In fact, the analytic literature has few reports even of adults who remember early childhood erotic fetishism (Garma [10], Socarides [38], Wolf [46]). In addition, I have reported [41] on a man with a fetish for women's stockings, who remembers excitement when he was 3 or 4 (his father reports seeing the boy in nylons at age 2½). I also evaluated a very feminine boy whose mother said she saw him, at age 3, with erections while fondling his *father's* clothes, never his mother's (cf Zavitzianos [50] who says this homeovestism is not fetishism); this behavior disappeared spontaneously in a few months (see also Socarides [38]). These reports are clinically thin, and, when the child is reported to be sexually excited, we are not told enough to be sure what was experienced. Even the next quotation, more explicit than most reports, could tell us more. "Around 4 or 5, the experience of being left alone at home when his mother went out shopping had been unbearably frightening, and the patient recalled seeking relief through creating a state of sexual excitement by running into his mother's bedroom and excitedly feeling her smooth, silky underclothes" (p. 109) [46].

The following case, by Lombroso in 1883 in Krafft-Ebing, suggests that other cases like these have been around a long time. "A boy of very bad heredity, at the age of four, had erections and great sexual excitement at the sight of white garments, particularly underclothing. He was lustfully excited by handling and crumpling them. At the age of ten he began to masturbate at the sight of white, starched linen. He seemed to have been affected with moral insanity, and was executed for murder" (p. 254).

The Synergy of Trauma, Excessive and Focal Identification, and Separation Anxiety

In line with Greenacre's observation that marked physical trauma may contribute to fetishism, we can note that Payne [31], Peabody, Rowe, and Wall [32], Hunter [25], Hamilton [23], and Socarides [38] also report on the significance of circumcision in a fetishistic patient; Lorand [29] links his patient, who had a nonerotic interest in shoes, to a circumcision at age 2. Though we cannot build a case for childhood (not postnatal) circumcision as an expected feature in erotic fetishism, a more careful study might show that the conjunction sometimes is not coincidental.

Putting aside the question (because I cannot answer it) to what extent the transitional object, the nonerotized infantile fetish, the erotized infantile fetish, and the adult erotized fetish are related, we have uniform agreement, based on observations, that these objects stand as a bridge between the infant's wanting to stay merged with mother and wanting to become an independent person. No one writing in recent years disagrees that "the background of the development of the infantile fetish is a chronically disturbed relationship to the mother, with individuation delayed and incompletely achieved" (p. 452) [22]. The second common feature with which most concur, one that can help explain why erotic fetishism is unreported in female infants and children, is castration anxiety.[5] "The fetish . . . is the product of need for reparation because of the persistence of an illusion of defect in the body, which has become fixed through its association with certain concomitant disturbances invading self-perception. The adoption of the fetish makes it possible for development to proceed though under a burden" (p. 455) [22].

No one has suggested as strongly as Greenacre [17–22] that severe physical trauma in infancy, as was the case with Mac, can precipitate fetishism (though the absence in most reports of a history of such trauma cautions us not to generalize). "It is my impression that early fetish formation does not develop unless the accompanying disturbances have been so undermining as to produce a severe preoedipal castration problem, whether through illness, operative procedure, or severe parental mishandling. It is significant that at the early age of 1 to 2 years there is a general body responsiveness to discomfort or physical insult, and discharge of tension may occur through whatever channels are available at this special time. If the disturbance is so severe, however, that ordinary discharge mechanisms are inadequate, premature genital stimulation may be induced. This is most likely to occur during the second year" [22].

In Mac's case, we have, as in no other reports, his mother as an articulate witness. She not only dates and describes the circumcision and separation traumas, but she also lets us know how she maximized Mac's trauma by her shocked, terrified, and enraged behavior (perhaps heightened by her own experiences in childhood with her hemorrhaging mother). Recall the ambience of their relationship and contrast it with the way, from birth on, she related to Bill, her younger son.

Mac's mother is permanently stamped with grief and fear because of her abandoning mother plus the remembered terror during her mother's

---

[5] I hesitate to use "castration anxiety" here because that term has historically implied an oedipal (as Freud felt to the end [9]) rather than preoedipal-stage danger. But in these infant erotic or nonerotic fetishists, castration threat *in the classical sense of threat from father* is not part of the picture. In addition, if we did not use the classical term, we might more easily sense connotations of more profound danger — separation anxiety, dissolution of self, loss of existence [34, 35].

bloody, life-threatening episodes. Her father was literally a deserter of the family. Mac, as an adopted child, is, in his mother's eyes, another creature abandoned by mother and father, and so he and she resonate to each other, fears and rages locking them into an excessively close though jittering mother-infant symbiosis. So now she sees herself treating her child as her mother did her, leading her to more hatred of herself. Greenacre [17] talks of "those infants who are held in a state of appersonation—especially guilty, hostile, or anxious appersonation by the mother, who may touch the child little, and when she does so, handle it as though it were a contaminating object" (p. 90). This describes only half of the ambivalence L laid on Mac. She experiences herself as a fusion of an unlovable child and a failed mother. She hates herself in the body of herself and herself in the body of the son with whom she identifies. Therefore, she must undo that hatred and its visible effects on Mac. Powered by her identification with him, she tries to prevent his being mother-abandoned as she was, but the effort to save him from suffering as she did when she was a child exhausts her, as do Mac's efforts to separate himself, alternating with his nestling in to her intermittent engulfments. I hope you can see in the transcript material, as was powerfully present when she talked with me, the anguish L suffered as she kept failing to come close to her maternal ego ideal, although she strove to do so because she felt that was her most important aspect [3].

Mac was to be L's eternal cure. Now she would no longer be alone, abandoned, anatomically incomplete, and endangered (as her mother was by her father). It was to be just the two of them, but, after promising him symbiosis forever, she became pregnant and had a different sort of infant—one she could only define as "normal," a complex of lovely qualities that intensified her sense of the frenzy in her self-Mac relationship. Making the ambivalence more wonderful and more awful, Mac really was a beautiful, intelligent, precocious child who in those ways lent himself to her being drawn to him as her equal, a part of herself that, though outside, she was constantly drawing back into herself. As if all this were not enough, she is the person who left behind at birth — or was left behind by — her dead twin sister. (Incidentally, with the present interest in bonding as an innate mechanism, Mac and his mother show us how, even in the absence of chance for bonding in the first three days, a fiercely intense symbiosis can occur with an adopted infant.)

I do not think that L actively and consciously helped Mac choose his fetish or encouraged its use [39]: Mac did not need her to assist him in creating his fetishism [4].

The Fantasy of Parthenogenesis

I want to note (but not discuss herein) the fantasy of parthenogenesis. It is probably at work in the pregnancies and postpartum periods of all mothers (an aspect of Winnicott's "primary maternal preoccupation" [48], I suppose). Its more intense and prolonged forms put children at great risk, whatever its roots (e.g., a mother's thought: I don't need you anyway, Father, where "Father" means both her father and her "child-as-father"). This fantasy can be so intense it swamps children's development. Though it harms gender and erotic development, it may, depending on a mother's needs, lead to precocity intellectually and artistically [41, 43].

Let me suggest, as a further twist to parthenogenesis, that women also get themselves pregnant with themselves — themselves as an infant. The issue, as we see in Mac's case, is not that the dynamic is there but how powerful it is.

We cannot get into Mac's mind; he could not put in words the signals arcing between him and his mother, and his therapy was not psychoanalytically illuminated. Still, we can imagine how her silky smooth, skin-like panty hose — a garment closer to being her than any other can be — fit his needs to have her with him — part of him, covering him, protecting him, and comforting him more reliably than she, a full person, did. The garment, as is true with fetishes [2, 12, 17, 30, 38], was better than his real mother in so many regards that it was really delectable. Panty hose were infinity (as long as he could keep the adults from meddling). Once in his possession, they were always available; he could control their presence. They did not scold, become enraged, threaten with abandonment, go crazy, excite and frustrate, or have a mind of their own. They did not have to be shared with father or brother. They could cover him as if he were still inside his mother. They did not complain when he put them aside. With them, he mastered the trauma of the symbiosis.

Perhaps we should emphasize more the function of mother's skin as a recognized, perceived, wanted part of an infant's relation with his or her mother and not just equate skin, breath, belly, face, hair — for the sake of theory — as all being "the good breast." The same oversimplifying makes the fetish equal mother's phallus, thereby keeping us from seeing that other parts of mother (e.g., skin, breast, voice) are also incorporated in the fetish.

Yet we are left with the same question we have with all psychic constructions, neurotic or other: Who and/or what put together all the pieces so that the perversion resulted? The boy who experiences himself as Mac did not do it, nor did Mac's "self" or "ego."[6]

Nor do we know—it is no slight question—why and how Mac connected his mother's panty hose/skin to his *erotic* machinery so that he not only got comfort, safety, and peace from his fetish, but also had that much more highly experienced, focused, uncontrolled, tight, hard tension that a *motivated* erection has for a child, who does not have the physical means for gratifying it or the psyche for dealing with not having the means. (Nor can the physiologists tell us how his still unformed body could mobilize its response so efficiently. Colleagues recalling that hearty erections are available to infants from birth on will wonder why there is a question here. Perhaps there is not, but, although no more than a hunch, I think these mindless erections of infants are little more erotic than the reflex erection of "spinal preparations" such as quadriplegics. I do not belong to the school that believes that a nursing infant with an erection wishes — let me use the most evocative word possible — to fuck his mother. [Or even the good breast.] (But Mac did, sort of.)

Why, at that age, does Mac's need involve his genitals? To reach for a brain/spinal cord explanation as we do with vague biologic explanations such as "constitution" and "diathesis," is premature. Such explanations may have value, but we do not yet know how; we do not even have procedures for testing them. (Still the old question: How is the mind connected to the brain?) Let me guess: Mac's physical trauma, the circumcision—which was certainly terrible psychic trauma as well— was to his penis, that most primary erotic apparatus. And the psychic trauma—the jolting symbiosis—threatened his developing sense of separateness as a male. The cure he invented—fetishism—should therefore be directed to the anatomy of maleness and its consequence, masculinity.

Discussion

This paper, as different from the others on fetishism, is written more from the point of view of the mother than the fetishist. Partly this is due to the fact that the data from Mac's treatment were thin and not filtered through an analyst-therapist. However, I want to emphasize a point of research methodology not available when the analyst has only the patient—adult or child—as the partner in the search for childhood

---

[6] I find the usual analytic answer that "the unconscious" does the work begs the question completely.

experiences. Though the analyst fills up with and interprets the transference, we still do not get a full picture of childhood, though it may be good enough for the therapeutic success. For research into the external and psychic events of childhood, transference data must be augmented by information from parents — the deeper the better.

In joining those who believe this, I also repeat the position (at times forgotten in the heat of theorizing) that some of what is intrapsychic starts from the outside world. In other words, what mothers, fathers, siblings, and others actually do to an infant/child counts in the psychic structure that develops. Fetishism is not due simply to castration anxiety, splitting, fantasies of the female phallus, separation anxiety, symbolization, fixation, identification, or fantasized good and bad breasts — the view from inside the infant. We should see those mechanisms as defenses raised to deal with traumas inflicted by the outside world. What parents and others really do really counts.

In Mac's case, Freud's explanation of fetishism [9] — the conjunction of the boy seeing female genitals and later being threatened with castration by his father for masturbating — does not fit. That being, as Freud believed, every boy's experience does not tell us why every boy is not as fetishistic as Mac.

How interesting that Mac's masculinity developed in the face of traumas strong enough to produce fetishism and was not grossly eroded as time passed [27, 36]. He is not an excessively feminine boy [41] and will not, I think, become transsexual. Will he become a transvestite, a nontransvestic fetishist, or a homosexual? Will he exchange his erotic defense for a nonerotic neurosis? I dare not predict. From Freud on, our theory of fetishism says that perversion serves males to protect their sense of maleness against the threat of castration, but no report gives data making clear why in one case the outcome of that threat is fetishism and in others it is homosexuality, narcissistic personality, fear of flying, Don Juanism, voyeurism, a successful career as a painter, masochistic heterosexuality, or a need to kill prostitutes. One cannot even decide, from the reports, why one boy will grow up to be a fetishist of the transvestite type while another's fetish is rubberized garments or dead bodies.

There are two clues as to why Mac is masculine. First, his father, though tough, taciturn, and unempathic, was masculine, present, admired, and supportive of Mac being masculine. Second, his mother encouraged masculine behavior. (The mothers of some very feminine boys have an excessively close identification/symbiosis with the son who will be too feminine, but those mothers — as opposite to Mac's — try to promote an unending blissful closeness and encourage all behavior that society reads as being feminine.) Yet, most present-day theorists do not argue, as does Freud, that the fetish is used to protect masculinity, but rather, that its primary purpose is to prevent traumatic disruption of the mother-son symbiosis. At least in Mac's case, inventing the fetish seems a matter between mother and son, without father playing a major part in the interpersonal dynamics. (I think, however, there are fetishistic cross dressers — transvestites — for whom the damaged relationship with father is powerfully important. For example, "If I was a girl, you'd love me; so I'll be one even if I am also, and shall always be, a male." We should probably not look for identical explanations in the fetishism of a child as young as Mac and the fetishisms that surface later.) Mac is not repairing castration anxiety as a result of observing a castrated object — mother — but is repairing his own direct experiences with terrifying separations and literal castration (i.e., circumcision).

Renik, Spielman, and Afterman [33] report the case of an 18-month-old boy with a bamboo phobia. This child has much in common with Mac, though phobia and fetish — even infantile phobia and infantile fetish — do not intuitively seem connected. In both cases there is: intense genital erotism [33]; a markedly premature erotic relationship between mother and son; disruption of "the orderly and sequential unfolding of psychosexual phases" (p. 262); mothers who are intensely interested in their son's masculinity; mothers with a great need to identify with this son, who is to repair traumas of their infancy; intense and precocious motor development; direct or indirect fear of the genitals being literally cut off (e.g., the boy with the bamboo phobia observing his father trimming bamboo [33]), not just castration anxiety from observing an absent penis (i.e., femaleness); mothers who "re-enacted situations in which she considered herself stranded and left behind by an adventurous and self-centered male. The pleasure she received from her identification with [his] aggression and confidence was denied by her ostensible feelings of being neglected and victimized" (p. 257); a boy in whom "the particular emphasis on his penis led to a dominantly phallic organization of . . . sexuality at a time when conflicts pertaining to the oral and anal impulse had not yet been resolved or mastered" (p. 262); a boy with a mother who, "out of her own needs, met the wish for increased closeness with a certain impatience and rejection" (p. 276); a boy with precocious sexual and cognitive development, "while the development of his *object relations* was not [precocious]" (p. 277).

We have a clue that can fit the clinical facts of Mac's perversion with the insistence by Bak and A. Freud that perversion cannot occur before oedipal development:[7] he is cognitively and genitally erotically precocious so that he moved into a full-blown phallic phase — "premature genitalization" (p. 152) [34] — epigenetically out of kilter with the rest of his development. Then, because his mother was excessively identified with him and treated him in many ways as an equal, a precociously "adultified" relationship was established between mother and son. This poor, crazy little wise man was driven, by his inner — innate and learned — precocities and by his mother, beyond what his body, his experience, and his phase-disrupted development could handle. Renik, Spielman, and Afterman [33] hint at this in saying, "Considering the sophistication of Ted's phobia, his case demonstrates that capacity for symptom formation is not easily correlated with level of psychosexual development" (p. 267). In treating their sons as equals, these mothers encouraged the boys to identify with the aggressor (mother); that process became part of the symptom.

Renik, Spielman, and Afterman [33] feel that the mother of the boy they studied "actually treated him in many ways as a phobic object" (p. 265). Perhaps we could also say that these mothers, who try to cure their own lifelong unhappiness by overidentifying with a son, use the boy as a (nonerotic) fetish. (I have found, in extremely feminine boys and men, that their mothers handled them as *things,* the mothers' lifelong sense of worthlessness as a female repaired by having brought forth this penis from their own bodies. As adults, these transsexuals are more like things than people capable of interpersonal relationships [43].)

Though I do not believe that neurosis is the negative of perversion — I believe, rather, that perversion is an erotic neurosis — there is sense in a similar idea: Phobia is the negative of fetishism [13].

I see Mac's fetishism, then, as a frantic precocity (see [22]). His mother treats him as an equal and wants him too much, but she also cannot bear him. She hits him and then hugs him. He is to undo her infantile trauma, but she sees him as being just like her and thus not to be trusted, respected, or found lovable. She loves him the way she feels her mother could not love her and hates him the way she hates herself. Every day he is thrown from one extreme to the other — merged with and extruded by his mother — hardly the best ambience in which to develop a stable body image and sense of self. Driven by these unmanageable demands, Mac does what everyone does: Without training or experience, as if for the

---

[7] They would be more accurate, I think, if they stated that perversion cannot occur before a fully experienced phallic stage, with or without triangular oedipal conflict.

first time in the world's history (he certainly has no genes for panty hose fetishism and no center for it in the limbic system), he invents neurosis. He condenses his problems and their solutions in one efficient, ever-ready, exciting, gratifying act. Themes that are loving, hostile, defensive, and reparative to himself and to his mother now exist in a fiercely intense instant, a wondrous collecting of unconscious and yet purposive — logical, effective, creative — elements that give mastery of formerly uncontrollable traumas, frustrations, and threats.[8]

What we do not know is how Mac ever managed it. The rest of us need years more of development, experience, and conscious and unconscious intrapsychic experiments in childhood and beyond before we can impact such scattered debris into the densely massed experience we call erotic excitement.

Conclusions

Is Mac so rare a case that he does not tell us much of anything? (I must be careful not to overstate his value for theory or to extrapolate freely from him to fetishists in general and, beyond that, to what seems a whole race of erotic minifetishists — most males of most cultures [42].) Yes, in a way. Mac's case is too rare to be a model for fetishism in general. On the other hand, the reasons he is rare contain clues for wider application.

We do not know enough yet to make firm statements on the causes and dynamics of fetishism. However, below are some ideas emphasized by Mac's case.

1. When the word "fetish" is used loosely enough, it fits any interesting object (or theory).
2. Though identification with each parent is inevitable and essential for identity development, a mother's excessive need (e.g., in a parthenogenetic fantasy) to encourage that identification in her son is dangerous for both.
3. Mothers with a badly damaged sense of worth about their femaleness are likely to misuse a favored son as a cure to their lifelong sense of defectiveness.
4. Castration threat is not just a father's prerogative.

---

[8] "This way of dealing with reality, which almost deserves to be described as artful. . ." (p. 277) [9]. Or, "One is impressed and almost awed by the degree of condensation" (p. 449) [22].

5. The combination of intellectual and libidinal precocity can upset the natural pace of gender and erotic development.
6. A true perversion — a true fetishism — can develop in very little boys, though perhaps only if the boy is erotically and intellectually precocious.
7. The perversion of fetishism at any age is not just an oedipal matter in the classical sense but is especially a consequence of a mother-infant symbiosis in disarray.
8. Erotic fetishism in a little boy is as much the result of a primeval separation anxiety as of the more sophisticated, more cognitively recognized experience of castration threat.
9. Intense physical trauma, especially when augmented by a terrified mother, can be a precipitant to fetishism.
10. Early boyhood fetishism is the consequence of a constellation of events, not a single event. It is therefore very rare since few boys are exposed to the whole constellation. To explain any case, much less all cases, as a splitting of the ego in the effort to substitute the fetish for mother's absent penis leaves out too much.

Though he is statistically rare because so young, Mac paradoxically confirms the belief of A. Freud and Bak that perversion does not occur in so young a child, for, in his intellectual and erotic precocity, Mac appeared much older. But in their saying that perversion — by which they mean erotic and gender aberrance — required triangular oedipal tensions they are wrong, for lifelong disorder in either or both these spheres is found as early as the first year or two of life. Also, we do not want (nor do they) their emphasis on oedipal matters to obscure the fact, as has been described by most recent workers, that the preoedipal relationship between mother and son — with father not playing much of a part — is crucial.

References

1. Bak, R. C. Fetishism. *J. Am. Psychoanal. Assoc.* 1:285, 1953.
2. Bak, R. C. Distortions of the concept of fetishism. *Psychoanal. Study Child* 29:191, 1974.
3. Blum, H. P. The Maternal Ego Ideal and the Regulation of Maternal Qualities. In S. I. Greenspan and G. H. Pollock (Eds.), *The Course of Life, Vol. III: Adulthood and the Aging Process.* Maryland: U.S. Department of Health and Human Services, 1981. Pp. 91–113.
4. Dickes, R. Fetishistic behavior. *J. Am. Psychoanal. Assoc.* 11:303, 1963.

5. Epstein, A. W. Fetishism: A study of its psychopathology with particular reference to a proposed disorder in brain mechanisms as an etiological factor. *J. Nerv. Ment. Dis.* 130:107, 1960.
6. Freud, A. *Normality and Pathology in Childhood.* New York: International Universities Press, 1965.
7. Freud, S. Three Essays on the Theory of Sexuality. In J. Strachey (Ed.), *The Standard Edition of the Complete Psychological Works of Sigmund Freud.* London: Hogarth 1905. Vol. 7.
8. Freud, S. Fetishism. *Standard Edition.* 1927. Vol. 21.
9. Freud, S. Splitting of the ego in the process of defence. *Standard Edition.* 1938. Vol. 23.
10. Garma, A. The meaning and genesis of fetishism. *Int. J. Psychoanal.* 37:414, 1956.
11. Gillespie, W. H. A contribution to the study of fetishism. *Int. J. Psychoanal.* 21:401, 1940.
12. Gillespie, W. H. Notes on the analysis of sexual perversions. *Int. J. Psychoanal.* 33:347, 1952.
13. Glover, E. On the aetiology of drug-addiction. *Int. J. Psychoanal.* 13:298, 1932.
14. Glover, E. The relation of perversion-formation to the development of reality-sense. *Int. J. Psychoanal.* 14:486, 1933.
15. Green, R. Childhood cross-gender behavior and subsequent sexual preference. *Am. J. Psychiatry* 136:106, 1979.
16. Green, R. Personal communication. 1982.
17. Greenacre, P. Certain relationships between fetishism and the faulty development of the body image. *Psychoanal. Study Child* 8:79, 1953.
18. Greenacre, P. Further considerations regarding fetishism. *Psychoanal. Study Child* 10:187, 1955.
19. Greenacre, P. Further notes on fetishism. *Psychoanal. Study Child* 15:191, 1960.
20. Greenacre, P. Perversions: general considerations regarding their genetic and dynamic background. *Psychoanal. Study Child* 23:47, 1968.
21. Greenacre, P. The fetish and the transitional object. *Psychoanal. Study Child* 23:144, 1969.
22. Greenacre, P. The transitional object and the fetish with special reference to the role of illusion. *Int. J. Psychoanal.* 51:447, 1970.
23. Hamilton, J. W. Preoedipal factors in a case of fetishism. *Bull. Menninger Clin.* 42:439, 1978.
24. Herdt, C. H. *Guardians of the Flutes.* New York: McGraw-Hill, 1981.
25. Hunter, D. Object-relation changes in the analysis of a fetishist. *Int. J. Psychoanal.* 35:302, 1962.
26. Idelsohn. In M. Wulff, Fetishism and object choice in early childhood. *Psychoanal. Q.* 15:450, 1946.
27. Katan, M. Fetishism, splitting of the ego, and denial. *Int. J. Psychoanal.* 45:237, 1964.

28. Krafft-Ebing, R. v. *Psychopathia Sexualis*. Brooklyn: Physicians and Surgeons Book Co., 1932.
29. Lorand, A. S. Fetishism in statu nascendi. *Int. J. Psychoanal.* 11:419, 1930.
30. Mittlemann, B. Motor patterns and genital behavior: fetishism. *Psychoanal. Study Child* 10:241, 1955.
31. Payne, S. M. Some observations on the ego development of the fetishist. *Int. J. Psychoanal.* 20:161, 1939.
32. Peabody, G. A., Rowe, A. T., and Wall, J. H. Fetishism and transvestitism. *J. Nerv. Ment. Dis.* 118:339, 1953.
33. Renik, O., Spielman, P., and Afterman, J. Bamboo phobia in an eighteen-month-old boy. *J. Am. Psychoanal. Assoc.* 26:255, 1978.
34. Roiphe, H., and Galenson, E. The infantile fetish. *Psychoanal. Study Child* 28:147, 1973.
35. Roiphe, H. and Galenson, E. Some observations on transitional object and infantile fetish. *Psychoanal. Q.* 44:206, 1975.
36. Scharfman, M. A. Perverse development in a young boy. *J. Am. Psychoanal. Assoc.* 24:499, 1976.
37. Silverman, M. A. Cognitive development and female psychology. *J. Am. Psychoanal. Assoc.* 29:581, 1981.
38. Socarides, C. W. The development of a fetishistic perversion: The contribution of preoedipal phase conflict. *J. Am. Psychoanal. Assoc.* 8:281, 1960.
39. Sperling, M. Fetishism in children. *Psychoanal. Q.* 32:374, 1963.
40. Sterba, B. An important factor in eating disturbances of childhood. *Psychoanal. Q.* 10:365, 1941.
41. Stoller, R. J. *Sex and Gender*. New York: Science House, 1968.
42. Stoller, R. J. *Sexual Excitement*. New York: Pantheon, 1979.
43. Stoller, R. J. *Perversion*. New York: Pantheon, 1975.
44. Storms, M. D. A theory of erotic orientation. *Psychol. Rev.* 88:340, 1981.
45. Weissman, P. Some aspects of sexual activity in a fetishist. *Psychoanal. Q.* 26:449, 1957.
46. Wolf, E. Ambience and abstinence. *Annual Psychoanal.* 4:101, 1976.
47. Winnicott, D. W. Transitional objects and transitional phenomena. *Int. J. Psychoanal.* 34:89, 1953.
48. Winnicott, D. W. Primary Maternal Preoccupation. In *Collected Papers*. London: Tavistock, 1958.
49. Wulff, M. Fetishism and object choice in early childhood. *Psychoanal. Q.* 15:450, 1946.
50. Zavitzianos, G. The perversion of fetishism in women. *Psychoanal. Q.* 51:405, 1982.

13

The sins of the father: notes on fathers, aggression, and pathogenesis

John Munder Ross and James M. Herzog

In this chapter, we will present our converging and current thinking regarding a father's gender-specific function in exciting and modulating aggression in his children. We will briefly review the existing psychoanalytic literature on fathers and turn to our own previous contributions on the subject. We will then consider some specific paternal failures either in the stimulation or in the containment of aggressive displays in children (primarily sons but daughters as well) within the total family matrix, presenting case material in some depth to illustrate two opposing pathogenic constellations. We will evaluate the consequences of optimal paternal aggressivity for such various adaptational achievements as the establishment of impulse control and the consolidation of sexual identity. Finally, we will raise questions regarding an unfolding of aggression along a developmental line and a father's unique relation to this progression.

Backdrop

Sigmund Freud wrote to Wilhelm Fliess — alter ego and father figure — that the death of a man's father looms as the most "significant event" in a man's life. He had lost his own father, and while he witnessed his father's dying and death, he also sired a whole new science — psychoanalysis. Indeed, Mahl [56] points out, psychoanalysis began as a father-son psychology. Fathers, certainly, played a central role in Freud's personal drama and in the intellectual revolution to which this gave rise. Who were they, these fathers of the mind? Were they real? And how did they impinge on the inner lives of all the analysands to follow?

Struggling to come to terms with the death of Jakob Freud in 1896, and the "little hysteria" this engendered in him during the year that followed, Freud uncovered the universality of the Oedipus theme [14, 16, 21]. In the process he did away — if tentatively — with his newfound "seduction theory," in which he had inculpated the fathers of neurotic sufferers as molesters and Svengalis, the disavowal of whose

477

transgressions bred denials of reality, strangulation of emotion, and all sorts of symptomatic contortions. He replaced this emphasis on actual trauma with a theory of psychic reality, wherein the adult's unconscious inhibitions were seen to spring from the child's own impulses and fear of castration at the father's hands. This fear was to be understood, in its turn, basically as a projection of the child's own hostility, as a creation, that is, of the individual's own conflictual imaginings. The genital seductions reported by patients were not real events, then, but rather by-products of wishful thinking, of unconscious fantasy. Evidently their unreality mattered not at all as far as a patient's unconscious convictions were concerned. We were, Freud told Fliess, all "budding Oedipuses" in our irrational hearts, where desire and deed were confounded.

Surprisingly, as Mahl has demonstrated, Freud's dream book reveals not one direct reference to fear of the father or of his motives in the manifest content of and associations to Freud's dreams. Nor, for that matter, does Freud remark on the role of Oedipus' pederastic and filicidal father, Laius, in setting the whole Greek tragedy in motion (see [10, 32, 66, 69]). Thus it might be most accurate to say that psychoanalysis unfolded as a psychology simply of sons and, secondarily, of daughters, one in which, theoretically at least, the actions and inner lives of the parents were not considered as causative agents.

Freud's immediate disciples followed suit. The analysis of instinct theory and the Oedipus complex focused on the father, albeit a father of fantasy. The specter of punishment at his hands, the by-now proverbial "paternal castration threat," was held to be the prime organizer of early development and of evolving psychic structure. An externalized prototype of the superego [23, 24, 26], it prompted the relatively belated formation, between 4 and 6 years of age, of sexual identity, self-direction, and guiding ego ideals and values.

Freud's case histories [15, 17, 18, 19, 22] chronicled at length the indiscretions and manipulations of duplicitous fathers. At the same time, however, their children's difficulties were ascribed not to these misbehaviors but rather to the work of overactive and peremptory imaginations. The contradictions persisted, and Freud never quite articulated the dovetailings he described between his patient's inner and outer reality.

Mothers, in the way of whom fathers stood, tended to pale by comparison as influential figures in their own right. They seemed virtually absent from Freud's theory and from his clinical narratives.

Plumbing the ontogenetic prehistory of the Oedipus complex, later analysts rediscovered the mother. She was a pre- or extraoedipal mother, as it were, the omnipotent mother of infancy and of self. Beginning with

Spitz [73, 74] and later spearheaded by the brilliant clinical and observational studies of Mahler [57, 58], analytic researchers began to scrutinize the interchanges transpiring within the mother-infant dyad. In so doing they further underscored the mother's real and distinctly personal contributions to her child's primary sense of self (see [11, 76]). From the very first weeks of life (see [83]), her personality left a distinct "imprint" on her baby [50, 77], shaping the "basic core" of his or her eventual identity and future character style. In this observational work on the mother-infant dyad, in contrast to the father of the clinical encounter, the roots of psychic life were found in the parent's explicit behavior and implicit and often unconscious communications with the child. Analytic observers began to reflect on the child's interpersonal environment and its internalization [8].

With the emphasis on identity and object relations in *statu nascendi,* there came in time the finding of a different sort of father. More or less explicitly, Loewald [51] and Jacobson [45] challenged the primacy of his image as tyrant and castrator, emphasizing instead the child's love for and attraction toward him. His was seen to be an instrumental presence [61], one which invited children out of the maternal orbit into an ever-widening and interpersonally differentiated universe [1, 2, 3, 30, 64, 65]. A father's own profound love for the child was further accented in this new awareness — that is, his deep-seated generativity and sex-specific expressions of nurturance [9, 38, 40, 44, 47, 48, 55, 62, 63, 70, 82]. His "paternal instincts," as it were, were seen to evolve epigenetically along a developmental line commencing in infancy.

But these theoretical fathers still lacked individuality. Except for the matter of their presence, their active and unique impact on the child's future adaptation or psychopathology still remained largely unaddressed (see [33]). Fathers still figured as ciphers and foils, and this was in contrast to the numerous studies that adumbrated the mother's inner life, character, and consequently her unique parental style. (Indeed, the mother had become the critical ingredient or set of complex variables in the environment, no longer merely "average" and/or "expectable" [35], into which the constitutionally partly "prewired" baby was thrust. Perhaps the theoretical omission of fathers' analogously distinctive inputs had to do with clinical and research artifacts — that is, with the relative absence of men, not so much from the home, but also from observational and clinical settings (see [13, 70]).

By the late 1970s, partly in response to the *Zeitgeist* of emerging feminism, analytic investigators had joined scores of researchers in examining fathering and fatherhood. Like their "empirical" counterparts, the clinicians tended to focus first of all on a father's absence — total and real as well as relative and emotional — and its deleterious corollaries. "Paternal deprivation" was how Biller [7], a pioneer in the field, put it. The consequences of this void were seen to include poor school performance, cognitive and intellectual deficits, deviations with respect to gender identity and sexual orientation, difficulties in controlling drives and affect modulation, and a variety of other demonstrable pathological phenomena [33, 68]. Sons were believed to be especially vulnerable, especially earlier on [39, 78, 81], while the impact of missing fathers on daughters during successive developmental eras remained a matter of uncertainty and debate [2, 3, 4, 28, 39]. In any event, researchers and clinicians at last found themselves in exquisite agreement, for their results converged and pointed to clear implications for all levels of prevention. Moreover, feminists could take heart: Men could and should share in the work of domesticity.

Biller himself had already understood the obvious, however. When present, fathers could serve as noxious agents, influencing development for the worse; even no father at all might be better than a bad one. When a consideration of the total family (e.g., the marital relationship) was brought to bear on the question of a father's either pathogenic or facilitative influence directly on different children as well as on their mother, the self-evident and oversimplified nature of existing propositions became inescapable. The transmuting impact of internalization also could not be ignored. The theorist thus found himself confronted with internal and external complexities governing a father's interaction with children, confounding him in his zealous efforts at generalization. One matter was becoming clear, however: Nothing could be understood without first considering the psychology and motivation of the individual adult father and his communication with the child.

The Erlkonig Syndrome and the Laius Complex

During nearly a decade of research and reflection on the unfolding and impact of fatherhood, both authors, Ross and Herzog, underscored a father's optimal or ideal functions and functioning. Each of us stressed the deep-seated parenthood of a man, with its childhood anlagen and evolution [62, 63] and the recapitulation of these during pregnancy and sociobiological paternity [34, 41].

Herzog was quicker than Ross to emphasize the pervasive impact of male aggressiveness and indeed to study clinically the pathological possibilities to which it might give rise. In one paper [39], he studied night-terrorlike phenomena observed in boys between the ages of 18 and 28 months. In each instance, the father had become absent within 4 months of the onset of the sleep disturbance. The boys were inconsolable, some of them calling out for their missing fathers. Although the boys ranged in age and level of development, they all seemed to struggle with similar pressures and problems: the establishment of a sense of identity, especially gender identity; intense oral- and anal-sadistic aggression; and various deficits in achieving separation-individuation, a task rendered all the more problematic by the absence of a parental object other than mother. The father, and only the father, seems to be able to help the boy modulate his aggression, Herzog asserted, and, in his absence, the boy suffers from "father hunger."

Herzog, inspired by Goethe's poem, called the presence of unmodulated aggression the *Erlkonig* syndrome. The poem describes the increasing terror of a little boy wrapped protectively in his father's arms as they ride through the night; the child tells his father he is being pursued by a monster—the Erlkonig. The father perceives no monster and reassures the child and reaches his destination with his child dead in his arms, a victim of his own and the child's disavowed aggression, according to Herzog. Boys seem most vulnerable, he added, especially during the preoedipal years, although girls also reveal the deleterious impact of insufficient fathering [2, 3].

Ross's emphasis had been on the father's relatively benign presence. The father's nurturance and durability act, he hypothesized, as a modulating or neutralizing force with regard to the rivalry leveled at him by sons and, to a certain extent, daughters. A father's libidinal availability and the reality of his caretaking offset a boy's positive Oedipus complex, relegating it to the increasingly demarcated realm of fantasy. Later, his mentorship helps effect the postoedipal son's rapprochement with him [63, 64, 65, 66]. In the process, a boy comes to identify with the procreative aspects of a father's masculinity, intimated during the oedipal era by way of his perceived role within the primal scene and proffered during middle childhood in the form of concrete teaching and guidance. Research also convinced Ross of the essential wisdon of Greenacre's [30], Kestenberg's [48], and Abelin's [1, 2] notions as to how the male parent's rather abrupt, angular body contours and interactive style encouraged muscular and locomotor development during the child's second year, enhancing the consolidation of body schemata, and thus promoting individuation. In the growing boy's struggle to disidentify [31] from the omnipotent mother, he discerns a central dilemma affecting a man's later capacity to tender paternal supplies. Phallic fixations, defending against feminine and maternal ambitions, seem to him particularly problematic, engendering a hypermasculinity in which hostile posturing compromises a man's capacity for sexual intimacy and fatherliness.

Beginning in 1982, Ross turned his attention more and more to the sex-specific rivalry besetting and potentially compromising a man's paternal capacity, matters he had previously simply alluded to [72]. These themes seemed to assert themselves in the analytic literature only then to elude attention [69], lapsing into obscurity and requiring repeated rediscovery [5, 10, 27]. Like his unrequited motherhood, a father's filicidal urges occasioned resistances to which analysts themselves proved to be vulnerable.

Scrutinizing the Oedipus myth, Ross [69] elaborated on the actual crime for which Oedipus's father, Laius, had been condemned to be murdered by his son and replaced by him in his wife's bed: pederasty, the kidnapping and rape of a boy, Chrysippus. Abstaining for a time from intercourse, Laius finally conceived with his wife Jocasta their fateful, avenging son, whom he had abandoned and mutilated in an effort to stave off the realization of the prophecy of patricide and incest. Later, Laius gratuitously and imperiously humiliated the adolescent Oedipus, who in being abandoned had become a stranger to him, exciting the boy's personal vengeance and thus acting to bring down doom on himself. For all his phallic narcissism, overwhelming rage, and arrogance, Oedipus himself, having killed his cruel father, did not inveigh against him, but succumbed instead to his own excruciating guilt, assuming total responsibility for the tragedy. Overdetermined as it was, oedipal guilt, Ross suggested, also served to obscure the crimes of the father, rendering Laius's sins as the child's own [43, 49, 53].

On the basis of this paradigm, Ross concluded that a whole constellation of paternal impulses and conflicts can become manifest in a variety of behaviors from storytelling and roughhousing to more blatant expressions of possession with regard to mother (wife) and to the outright neglect, abuse, and even murder of the children. The father's "Laius complex," including both filicidal and pederastic trends, is instigated partly in reaction to the child's own successive developmental demands. It represents a transfiguration of the adult father's childhood oedipal constellation, including both his competition with his father and his identification with the latter's felt or perceived paternal aggression, as well as an age-specific response to the succession of generations and his own predestined demise. It may be compounded by conflicts in sexual identity, hostile, sadistic, and phallic displays, serving to defend against bisexual and infantile trends. Thus, a father's history and "preparental" character structure figure in his capacity for child-rearing. But parenthood is further influenced by the child's unique characteristics and the marital and family context. Present to some degree in all fathers, the Laius complex can give rise to a variety of pathological phenomena, from an excessive, neurotic inhibition of impulses to quasi-transference psychoses, with the child as central object in the projection of unneutralized aggression [75].

Communications of these paternal impulses serve as dynamic preconditions for or releasers of the son's negative and positive Oedipus complex. The adult man's inevitable intrusion and domination invite a more or less sexualized submission, while his oppression and "interruptions of activity" [36, 37] (see also [8]) act to excite narcissistic and possessive hostility. Present in their own right, these constellations of impulses on the part of the child can themselves assume either a pathological or an adaptive form of expression, depending on a father's manifest actions as well as on the delicate balance between his empathy and mature love and his communications of unconscious hostility and selfish desire.

THE AGGRESSIVE DIALOGUE

Thus, the child's Erlkonig syndrome and its derivatives point to a void, the father's Laius complex to excesses. Both suggest that degrees of aggressive stimulation, overstimulation, or understimulation on the part of fathers may constitute important genetic factors in the etiology of numbers of psychopathological phenomena. Men, we argue, are inherently and behaviorally the more aggressive parents; they are, in any event, both exploited and perceived as such by their children. Hence, the father's "aggressivizing" function may parallel the more typical role of the mother with regard to early libidinal excitation: too little, early on, engenders apathy or even marasmus, as Spitz showed [74], whereas too much somewhat later can dispose the child to perversity and to severe psychoneuroses.

We are further reminded of Freud's reformulation of the pleasure principle in his paper "The Economic Problem of Masochism" [25], which followed his elaboration of both the early dual instinct theory and the structural hypotheses [20, 23]. At this juncture Freud did away with the crude absolutes governing his earlier economics. He now suggested that a rhythmicity, an ebb and flow of stimuli, endopsychic and external, rather than sheer quantities or constant levels, determined the phenomenology of pleasure and pain. Processes very similar to this may be involved in aggressive arousal and activity within the father-child dialogue. (Incidentally, by aggression we mean impelled sensorimotor schemata, involving the musculature as opposed to the mucosa, and its psychological correlates and diverging sequelae. We will discuss this further later.) Furthermore, because the drives are excited and organized within an object-relations context, as Loewald [52] and Kernberg [46] have argued, the doses are interpersonally titrated. They are meted out, received, and interpreted according to the caretaking object's attunement to the child and according to the child's own state of arousal. Such interchanges are further organized — stimulated or contained — by the nature of the father's relation to his wife and her capacity to empathize with his struggles and with the needs of her child. As Herzog [41] has stressed, adult-adult interaction can serve to predict, to shape, and potentially to safeguard childrearing. Before reflecting further on this oscillating aggressive interplay of father and child and its familial context, however, we would like to offer some clinical cases in point.

Cases: Too Much and Too Little

The two cases that ensue are gleaned from the author's supervisory work. They are presented in some detail in order to illustrate and partly explicate contrasting expressions of a father's aggressive and specifically filicidal urges and the pathogenic influence of these on children. In both instances, the father's inclinations are similar: to harm, murder, and/or abandon his child. (Abandonment and destructive violence seem to go hand in hand.) But a variety of mitigating factors have entered into the real-life manifestations of such murderousness, potential abuse, and neglect. In one instance, the father's hostility is given relatively free rein, overwhelming and overstimulating his son, whereas in the other case it is energetically inhibited, leaving the boy, on the contrary, aggressively deprived. Personal histories and consequent individual characteristics help determine these differences, of course — that is, each father's ability to draw on beneficent identifications and libidinal reservoirs with which to counter his envious hatred of and indifference to his child. To the psychoanalyst, such genetic and developmental factors have become self-evident.

But the pregnancy and early months of fatherhood also seem to constitute a time of crisis, with the potential for both regression and positive adaptation. Thus, perhaps more compelling, or more novel at least from our perspective, than individual dynamic and structural factors are the mothers' (the wives') parts in shaping the father-son dialogue.

In the first instance the wife, discarded and unprovided for by her husband, fails to act to help contain or mediate the adult man's impulses. She then succumbs herself to an almost affectless venting of her own urges, both sexual and aggressive. In the end she displaces onto the child what belongs in the marital relationship. In the second case, notwithstanding certain drawbacks of a different kind—an overriding fear of stimulating the child and a tendency altruistically to sacrifice the primacy of the couple's relationship for parenting of an overweening kind—the husband succeeds in adopting his proper place as provider for and protector of the mother-child dyad. His wife, in her turn, helps him to control the expression of his urges and thus to deflect his male aggression from the home.

Subjected to contrasting expressions of the father's Laius complex and to different failures in fatherliness, both boys, nonetheless, suffer to some measure from the Erlkonig syndrome. They are *hungry* for fathers to protect them from the press of their own instinctuality from within and from threats from without. In compromise formations aimed at drive control, they conjure up and fall prey to imaginary "monsters" who embody their own projected hostility; their father's real and imagined violence; their mother's unrequited and seemingly rapacious sexual desires; the dangers of the environment from which they have been insufficiently insulated; and self-emasculation as the only means available for the reduction of unbearable, unrelieved tension.

CASE ONE: BRAD, A "LATENCY" BOY

Brad was 7 when he was referred to the outpatient clinic. One might have questioned the referral even then, for the divorced father, a lawyer, was a wealthy man. True, there was the alimony and child support (even though Brad attended a parents' cooperative school with minimal tuition); Mr. P did have his expenses: mortgages to pay on a cooperative apartment and a country house, costs for these and the renovation of his law office, and an expensive and growing art collection. And Brad's mother, eking out a subsistence at her old job and taking courses during the evening for her M.B.A., could not contribute much financially to the boy's welfare.

It was the mother who, prompted by Brad's teachers, called for the first appointment. A woman in her mid 30s, Mrs. P described her son's life and current difficulties with measured concern. There was an eerie evenness to her speech, a cute little girl's voice hovering somewhere behind the studiedly professional demeanor. She loved her son, in a way, the young male therapist who was to treat the boy thought, or at least she *cared* for him. But where were the signs of empathic suffering? And those eyes, pale and immobile above her broad and again unmoving cheeks: When he met Brad he recognized that same impenetrable cast behind all the boy's obvious chaos.

The constellation of behavior problems was familiar enough. At school or at home, when in the throes of a temper tantrum, Brad could be neither consoled nor contained, but rather had to be isolated instead. When frustrated, he became unmanageable. Other children recoiled in terror from the fusilade of verbal epithets and hard blocks hurled at them by the boy whose face purpled with rage. From time to time Brad bit them—hard. There were mild developmental lags—in speech, articulation, and fine motor coordination—in a little boy of sound intelligence. Psychological tests picked up the faintest hints of minimal brain dysfunction. However, Brad showed a generally superior level of intellectual functioning. Brad's bouts of temper alternated with a glazed passivity at other times, especially in the morning when he demanded that his mother dress him and beseeched her not to leave him for so many hours. Most distressing to Mrs. P were Brad's confessions of self-loathing and despair, emotions that found a behavioral counterpart in Brad's proneness to injure himself.

Brad's parents, who married only a few months after they met, remained together for Brad's first 3 years. "We did not truly know each other," said Mrs. P, whose brother had died a year and a half before their meeting, leaving her depressed and longing to fill a void. The fighting grew with shouts, threats of physical violence, peccadilloes, and then a growing, cold, dull resentment. Finally came the abandonment. Returning from a visit to her parents shortly after Brad's third birthday, Mrs. P and her son found a nearly empty apartment. Mr. P had vanished, taking his most precious possesssions with him.

The typical court battles ensued, involving the financial settlement, sometimes cloaked in struggles over custody and visitation, but having much more to do with money. Brad and Mrs. P were abruptly thrust into relative poverty; Mrs. P's tightfisted parents refused to offer assistance. Mrs. P believed they had always preferred her brother anyway. Food was rationed, clothing sparse and cheap. Mrs. P was away from home many more hours than before, and a succession of baby-sitters and an occasional transient lover drifted in and out of the apartment. Mother and son did take some solace, as it were, in each other, cuddling a great deal and bathing together until Brad's fifth year. Mrs. P seemed unabashed about nakedness and later inquired of Brad's therapist whether her son should be allowed to pose nude for an anatomy textbook.

Brad's father, Mr. P, did not disappear completely from the boy's life. He visited with him for weekends and a week now and then during the summer. They went to a few baseball games, and Brad spent some time in his father's office. His father had girlfriends, serial live-ins, who showed a solicitous interest in the boy, at least for a few months. But it was all inconsistent, generally disappointing, and, occasionally, very strange.

Mrs. P heard vague talk of guns—of threats in the face of unrequited love. During one summer Brad stayed with his father and a girlfriend in the unfinished country home; his cot was separated from their well-used double bed by diaphanous curtains. From time to time Brad was left alone in the father's apartment without a baby-sitter. And, as a rule over weekends, he was granted an hour of Mr. P's time, only to be thrown to his own devices while his father played golf with friends.

On one occasion, Brad had slammed into a tree while skiing. Mr. P placed an ice pack on the swelling bruise between the boy's black eyes and tried to stop the nosebleed. But then his father left for a dinner party after returning the boy to his mother, who took the child to the hospital where he remained for several nights with a concussion. And, somewhat less dramatically but persistently, Mr. P was late. A 6:00 P.M. "date for dinner with Dad" typically turned into 2½ torturous hours of waiting, and sometimes a complete failure of his father to appear. For Mr. P to pick him up from school was out of the question. More than once Brad had been left to a deserted classroom and an exasperated, anxious teacher.

"I hate him," Mrs. P hissed, her generally colorless gaze reddening with anger. "And he scares me. . . . And the terrible thing is, Brad reminds me of him, the violence especially. I have this strange feeling sometimes that when he gets big he just might kill me. Isn't that odd?"

Mr. P jogged to his first consultation, 20 minutes late for an 8:30 P.M. hour, the only time he could "manage." Even in a T-shirt and gym shorts, which hugged his rather pudgy thighs as he did a final deep knee bend in the waiting room, this man seemed forbidding and overpowering despite his moderate stature. Perhaps it was his thick moustache or black eyes, the Apache headband or the bottomlessness of his voice, or the coiled-in tension of his body. In any event, he was frightening to the young therapist, who sensed immediately the self-absorption, the sadism, and the unpredictability and remembered the scandals of which the ex-wife had spoken: an alleged rape while he was in college, the accusations of sexual assault by a baby-sitter, and the gun. "He's sadistic," Mrs. P had said, "and I think he's really *gay*."

"Hi, I'm Stan," he said, extending a sweaty hand.

He sat, perspiration bleeding into the chair, and talked for a moment about Brad. He described the boy as a "good kid—what does he need treatment for?" They enjoyed the Mets, Rangers, and Knicks, and Brad hated to see them lose. He liked to have Brad visit. They did great things together, like having "peeing contests," their streams, large and little, crisscrossing into the toilet bowl. They boxed, though it sometimes got "out of hand." Ann, his newest girlfriend, liked Brad a lot. Brad's problem was that he did not understand what it meant to work hard and did not do his assigned chores. When he was frustrated, he got really obnoxious. Talking helped, but a whack of the hand or a smack across the face wasn't *so* terrible, was it? He himself had had to learn self-control. Explosions at subordinates in the office and at court had cost him employees and alienated judges. Women had left him. It had taken time, but his therapist, whom he now saw every other week, had helped.

Then he began. After the first few minutes of what remained of the hour, Mr. P left his son behind and talked about himself, *his* parents—the demanding mother and absent father—*his* money worries, and *his* health (he *had* to jog to stay lean and free of the diabetes that had killed his "old man"). The therapist realized that he feared this father at least in some measure because *he hated him.* The other hours, when they could be scheduled, were similar in spirit and content, with the additional problem of delayed payments. The obliviousness seemed almost willful underneath all the thin excuses and protestations to the contrary.

And Brad. At first he seemed a sweet boy, if not the "cute darling, with a lawyer's mind" his mother had portrayed. He left her easily enough for his first sessions, looking up expectantly and hopefully at the therapist, as if "father hungry," his lips parted slightly in a vague half smile, his speech lisping but not unintelligible. In this session, and those that followed over the next two or three months, he was generally happy to be there, it seemed. He ranged through the toys at his disposal, talking in the manner of early latency boys a little about himself. "Yes, he *was* sad," he said. He wanted more of his mother and his father, who was always late but who was "very rich and the best lawyer in the whole world." He hated his teachers and some of his classmates. School was a bore, and he got into fights. When angry there, he felt "all hot." He wanted to play with the "army men" and lay on the floor, turning away from the therapist as he marched the toy soldiers into battles punctuated with sibilant explosions. For a while at least, leave-takings from therapy sessions were somewhat protracted but still manageable.

At home and at school, little changed at first with the onset of therapy. Brad's teacher called to report periodic temper tantrums. His mother noted the intensity, the near violence of Brad's sexual curiosity: his bursting through the unlocked door into the bathroom, the convulsive snickering at her body. They still fought on the street, and once or twice she "blew" and hit him.

"Why was he so angry?" the therapist wondered aloud. "Was he mad at his mother and father? Was that scary to talk about?"

"Shut up, stupid," Brad rejoined. It was the first open display of protective rage, guarding his needed idealizations. "He makes a lot more money than you." Sometime after this the boy brought his terrible struggles more and more into the consulting room.

For the better part of a year, Brad made books with his therapist, dictating the stories with an increasing rapidity, which made them impossible to take down. When the therapist noted this and gingerly confronted the child about his anxious need to control the therapist, Brad burst into a rage, reviling the man's incompetence and failure to understand him.

The stories themselves were always the same, with slight variations on a consistent cast of characters and plot: Mr. and Mrs. P's children and family pets left for the wilderness, where they built a cabin and fed themselves opulent meals of ice cream and frankfurters. Then the army of the Big Foots came and attacked. Horrible things happened and there was a lot of blood. Then "Stanley" (Mr. P) and Mrs. P appeared, both very tall (especially Mr. P), flanked by family pets and by famous ballplayers. Together with the children and animals they defeated the Big Foots (Mr. P and Brad were the heroes of the hour); the occasional gorillas and snakes allied with them. The conquered foe suffered terrible fates, being drawn and quartered, decapitated, or hacked into hamburgers. Escapes through magic caves filled with danger and jewelry sometimes provided a further, quasi-oedipal denouement at the close of the battle.

The stories themselves might have been useful in the telling, even if they remained inaccessible to interpretation, because of Brad's stark resistance. The problem was that the narratives overflowed, spilling into the kind of action all too familiar to therapists of inadequately loved, angry, and aggressively overstimulated latency-age boys. Brad played an imperious and violent form of "baseball" with his therapist, abruptly hurling paper balls and curses point-blank at his face, altering the rules to ensure his victory, and winning most often by a hundred to one. He demanded food and exploded when denied. The appearance one day of another child at the close of a session prompted him to wail in rage and to empty the contents of a wastebasket onto the center of the floor en route to the door.

After this, all exits became a nightmare. There were provocations, spitting, and rages as Brad threw himself to the floor, legs flailing, as if demanding, in his wild defiance, intrusion and oppression—indeed emasculation—as a form of both violent control and violent love. And nothing, nothing changed this—not the tendering of precise understanding, controls, or even the gentlest word of support. Again and again, Brad forced his therapist, as he had his mother, father, and teachers, to actually constrain him. The shoes on his kicking feet had to be hastily removed and his arms had to be pinioned. Outside of the therapy hours, at least, there was improvement. School had become much more negotiable, and Brad and his mother had found the vicious circle of their interaction much abated.

One day the therapist told Brad that he believed Brad was furious because he really felt his father was mean and ignored him. But he was scared of his father's getting angry and hurting him or never showing up again. (He had said this often enough already.) And, as he had in the past, Brad, 9 years old now, spat back, "You're right, stupid. So what are *you* going to do about it? Nothing. I don't want to hear it." Another temper tantrum followed the clarity of that moment.

But this time Brad's message had struck a chord and was heard. Thereafter the therapist, like his supervisor more practiced in individual than other forms of treatment, shifted course. He had been, he realized, yet another baby-sitter, impotent and deeply resented. Brad's individual hours were now punctuated by family sessions involving mother, father, and child. For as long as they lasted, perhaps 6 months, these meetings saw a further and even more remarkable change in the boy's deportment. His eruptions, hitherto more physical than verbal, gave way to words and to a poignant disclosure of Brad's despair, muted until then by his chaotic, noisy anger. Lying beside the wall, glancing over his shoulder at his father while ignoring both mother and therapist, Brad told Mr. P:

You hate me, Daddy; you don't love me. It's all money, money. I never see you. . . . I'm scared of you. If you cared about me you'd be here. You hit me! [Again the father had been late, leaving mother, son, and therapist waiting through half of the time allotted for his arrival.]

The words and sentences were well formed, unlike the animalistic moans that marked Brad's stormy rages. They seemed to augur genuine structuralization.

But the arrangement did not last. Soon, when Mr. P's rationalizations failed, he revealed that the glimmers of dawning guilt were too great a blow to bear. Mr. P began missing hours altogether. And, after some time, battered and often ignored, the therapist himself conceded defeat for the time being. Brad and his family were referred to a family therapist who had even less luck. Brad finished his individual treatment, only symptomatically or behaviorally improved—a relative treatment failure.

There was not much he could have done, the therapist tried to tell himself. Most of all, it was the violence, the unmodulated destructiveness, that had proved so staggering. Efforts at the control or the avoidance of sadomasochistic confrontations met with an exacerbation of Brad's rage and abusiveness. And when, prompted by his supervisor, the therapist allowed himself a look into his own heart, he discovered something even more unsettling in the countertransference. He felt hated and feared by this little boy, and he hated and feared Brad. The impulses and emotions evoked in him threatened to undo the ties that secure and safeguard a therapeutic relation, the trust and moral commitment. They were terrible and surprising, starker and more inwardly unabashed than any countertransference feeling he had experienced toward an adult patient, as Glenn and Bernstein [29] have suggested. At least he could be comforted by the confession of the evaluating psychologist, a remarkably composed and experienced woman, that Brad was the first child she had ever wanted to strike. And, if he had at the time abstracted further, he might have discerned in the transference-countertransference tempests, which earmarked the treatment, a recapitulation of the stormy and, at the core, hollow interaction of a father and a virtually forgotten son. Brad found and made fathers like his own everywhere and let them know what it was like to be their son.

As in any clinical case, so with Brad it is not possible to isolate a single etiological determinant of his psychopathology. Mrs. P's own conflicts clearly helped determine the shape and intensity of both the mother-child and father-child dyad. Her air of blank withdrawal, her long absences, and the lack at times of sexual boundaries and sensible decorum on her part all contributed to Brad's overstimulation and intense anxiety. Yet even the quality of her mothering was itself very much a function of her former husband's treatment of her and, underlying this, his characteristics as a man and a father. Moved by selfishness and violence, he left her, deserting mother and child with singular suddenness and cruelty. She was, in turn, both prompted and forced to withdraw from the boy, who in her mind's eye resembled his frightening father. Indeed, Mrs. P calls up the specter of Jocasta, whose accession to filicide and later to incest doubly orphaned her son Oedipus. Yet, as with Oedipus's father

Laius and mother Jocasta, it was Mr. P, the father, who set in motion the sequence of terrible events that undid the proper bonds between mother and child.

Mr. P's direct relation with his son reflected similar traits, though their impact on the boy was different from the mother's responses to her husband. Self-absorption, constant displays of dominance, and rumored violence pervaded the brief and sporadic encounters of father and son. These were themselves woven into a single fabric, with destructive aggression as the red thread. The sadism of the father and, later, by way of identification and recompense, of the son served the end of self-enhancement. In addition, the aggressiveness in its purer form kept them pretty much apart, except for those moments—epitomized by the conjoining of their urinary streams—when they shared the illusion of supreme phallic power. (Brad won a sort of power by way of submission to pederastic invasion and by an idealization of his father's strength and perfection.)

Even this image of union conveyed the essential confounding of self-aggrandizement, violence, and object love. At other moments, Brad surrendered masochistically to an overwhelming onslaught, which he himself began increasingly to invite. For example, his rages culminated in his being restrained and overpowered. Self-emasculation seemed the only means available for alleviating the overwhelming tension induced by the aggressivity and sadistically toned erotic impulses welling up within him.

Thus, Brad and his father together created a mutual monster, a Big Foot representing the feared violence of the two of them. The Laius-like presentation of the father—the violence, narcissism, pederastic homosexuality, and abandonment, with the maternal failure and incestuous currents these invited or at least permitted—produced in the boy a caricature of oedipal ambition and strivings, which had less to do with any objects of desire than with the magnification and, indeed, the sustaining and shoring up of an uncertain self.

CASE TWO: LEE, A "PREMATURE GENIUS"

Lee, a 32-week premature infant, had suffered an apneic episode in the nursery but otherwise traversed a benign postnatal course. Upon his discharge, his parents were alerted to the possibility of subsequent apneic events and the specter of Sudden Infant Death Syndrome was raised. For the first 8 months of Lee's life, therefore, he slept in his parents' bedroom so that they could monitor his course at night. The parents abstained from intercourse during this period of time so that Lee would not be "overstimulated."

Assured by their pediatrician after this period that the danger of another prolonged incident was over, Mr. and Mrs. C moved Lee into his own room. The move did not proceed smoothly; Lee did not sleep well. He was irritable and soon seemed to develop nightmares and even occasional night terrors.

At 18 months of age, a behavioral pediatric consultation led to more consistent bedtime protocols and an apparent improvement in Lee's situation. By the time Lee was 2 years old he was for the most part sleeping through the night. He was also consummately verbal and had begun to express himself on a variety of topics. At about this time a sister was born. Lee voiced his dismay at this occurrence and suggested loudly that Felice be returned. He began to hit her and called her "The Creep."

Lee's parents tolerated and deferred to his imperious, aggressive behavior and did not limit these expressions of hostility. Lee's father did feel that perhaps " a good smack" was in order, but Lee had been so vulnerable as a child, and now he was so brilliant and verbal. How could one "smack a vulnerable genius?"

When Lee was born, his parents had been married for two years. Mrs. C, then 26, had worked as a nurse's aide. Her husband, 28, was a steelworker. Neither had attended college.

Mr. C portrayed himself as "easy going," just "one of the guys." He said that he had been glad that he and his wife were going to have a baby before Lee's arrival but became very scared when his son arrived so early. He was supportive of Mrs. C and did not manifest the superengrossed response displayed by some fathers of premature infants [38, 41].

Mr. C described his family of origin as traditional and very strict. His father had brooked no insubordination and had enforced his power with the strap. Mr. C grinned as he spoke about how effective this regimen had been. He said that this was the only circumstance in his life when he had been a quick learner. "God, did that sting!" he said, again grinning. He also told us that he knew from the beginning that he would never hit Lee. He did not feel this way about Felice, or about the baby who was en route later in the treatment, but how could one be strict with a boy who had stopped breathing? And then, "Lee was so smart. Why, he can run circles around me!"

Sometimes Mr. C would get "really angry" with Lee, he continued, especially when Lee interfered with disciplining Felice. Lee would look at his father as though to say, "What are you going to do about it?" Sometimes Mr. C's fury became so great that he would punch one hand with the other; on one occasion, he hit himself so hard that he cracked one of his phalanges. Lee looked frightened then, he said. Mr. and Mrs. C agreed about disciplining, or not disciplining, Lee.

Mrs. C thought that Lee was like her brother Sandy. He had been brilliant, too — and so nice, nice, that is, until he got cancer. Then he became "so angry and crazy that he had to see a psychiatrist" (just like Lee). But "it didn't do much good," for he died when he was 15. Mrs. C recognized that she often felt toward Lee the way she had felt toward Sandy. She used to love to hear Sandy talk. Now she would often find herself glued to Lee's "soliloquies."

There was one difference, however. Mrs. C used to only listen to Sandy, but she could talk and talk to Lee. He seemed fascinated, and she tried to teach him everything she knew. She would read both *Time* and *Newsweek,* cover to cover, and then impart what she had learned. Also, they would visit the library weekly so that she could learn new things in order to share them with Lee. Lee was usually adoring in these learning situations. The only thing wrong was that Mrs. C may have liked to share some of these discoveries with Mr. C as well. In some way she felt torn and pulled toward her precocious son. Mrs. C averred that he "didn't mind." They both felt that the care and feeding of a vulnerable genius was a most important undertaking.

Major problems arose as Lee continued his gibes at Felice. His sleep remained disturbed, and he had trouble relating to peers.

When Lee was 3½, his maternal grandfather died in an automobile accident. While he was alive, "Gramps" had taken an enormous interest in Lee; he could sometimes say no to the boy, and, to the parents' surprise, this did not precipitate a crisis. The grandfather had acknowledged how similar Lee and Sandy were and said that this rendered Lee especially dear to him. It was after Gramps's violent death that Lee really "came apart," Mrs. C thought.

Lee was inconsolable. He raged at God and at his parents for not saving Gramps. He even threatened suicide. His mother's grieving was itself significantly affected by Lee's display. His father also felt that he "couldn't really be angry" with his son because of the depth of his mourning. He said that some day Lee might be a writer or poet.

Within some six weeks of the death, Mrs. C felt that she had recovered — not Lee, however, who was once again having nightmares and cried out to God in fury and reproach during the day. Lee was finally brought to the clinic as an emergency when he was 3½; his mother said that he was threatening suicide.

Lee was a tall dark boy with huge and luminous eyes. During the critical segment of the diagnostic procedures, we watched him together with his parents. Lee ordered both Mr. and Mrs. C around, and they did his bidding. Father, a six-foot-tall man weighing some 190 pounds, seemed almost to cower as his son demanded this or that plaything. Mother seemed less subservient, but was certainly not assertive. When Lee, 3½, corrected his father's grammar, it did not appear to be in any way unusual to those concerned. It was also observed that, in his interactions with his parents, Lee often stated the same command three or four times.

When the interviewer engaged Lee alone and directly, the boy's tone changed markedly — it became decidedly conspiratorial. Lee said, "I have so much to tell you. I can't tell them. My father wouldn't understand." He began to speak of his bad dreams. He also began to play. The play focused on a boy by the name of Joey who had two cars, a bad Plymouth and a not-so-bad Buick. "I have much to tell you," Lee repeated. And, indeed, he did.

The adventures of Joey Jones were multidimensional and had mostly to do with cars. Joey was a driver, king of the road. He cruised to bars where men picked up women; he drank, swore, and hit women. But he could not be sent to jail because he was too powerful. Instead, terrible things happened in the play. The bad Plymouth, which he drove, would be hit by a truck and demolished. Joey would be dead, or he would be sentenced to death for his crimes against women or for reckless driving. There could be no mercy. Lee was very eager to have the diagnostic procedure continue and then expressed his precocious certainty that treatment was indicated.

The initial posture in the transference when treatment began very much resembled that seen in the evaluation. Lee was alternatively imperious and commanding and collusive and collegial. The play featured many examples of age-inappropriate adventures and peccadilloes, always accompanied by enormous guilt and fatal retaliation. These scenarios were repeated again and again, with virtually no mitigation of the outcome, an outcome that was black and white, all or nothing. Frequently Lee became terrified during the session. He heard knocks on the door and was sure that the angel of death had come to claim him.

Over a two-year period, it became progressively more possible to have the angel of death stay in the play sphere and direct activities toward Joey Jones, the protagonist, rather than toward Lee. Moreover, Joey learned ways in which the angel of death could be approached and even emulated. He discovered that indeed he could be an "angel" as well as a killer. Eventually Joey and the angel formed an alliance — they would work together. This was not possible, however, until the angel of death, now also called the guardian angel, dealt with some of his "hang-ups" about Joey's driving, which the angel felt was as good or better than his own. But as Joey finally realized, the guardian angel could also fly, which was not half bad and was an ability that Joey could only approximate when he grew up by learning to fly an airplane. The therapist then understood that Lee was struggling with issues of self-esteem and self-control that were directly related to his father's restraint and incapacity to interact with him, his inability in particular to engage and structure the boy's aggressive drive derivatives and phallic fantasies.

Mr. and Mrs. C's treatment paralleled Lee's. It focused on the multiple origins of their unique deference toward Lee. Mrs. C's intense involvement with her son was a salient feature of the parents' special deference toward him, further illustrating how the mother can mediate both directly and indirectly a father's access to his child [6]. She became the primary parent, abetting the child's frightening precocity while diminishing the father's stature in his eyes. In careful detail, it became clear how this special stance, which they had both agreed on, allowed Lee to get more of his mother and less of his father. This interactive patterning provided, on the one hand, a tremendous spur to the boy's intellectual development with a concomitant oedipal burden to his further psychosexual progression, and, on the other hand, a severe deprivation in terms of his masculine identification. With this, Lee also fell prey to the conviction that his own drive controls were as woefully inadequate as his father's seemed to be.

It became clear that Mrs. C was impelled to become intellectually enmeshed with her son because it was syntonic with her wish to expand her own intellectual scope. At the same time, it suited Mr. C to back off and to curtail his aggression because, at the very moment that he could feel his fury rise close to the surface in his dealings with Lee, he was aware of how his own father's corporal punishment had terrified, enraged, and inhibited him. Better to totally sheath his anger and aggressivity than try to set limits with the boy.

Both parents became aware that Lee could intuit these conflicts as well. As it became apparent that, in being concealed, his father's mounting hostility had become all the more terrifying to his son, Mr. C began to display aggression in manageable ways. By the time Lee was 4½, he was regularly sent to his room (he, "of course," went). At 5½, his father spanked him for the first time. Both parents reported that father had used his hand, that they had been very careful, and that Lee seemed almost relieved. Mrs. C spontaneously acted on her long-held belief that the one-to-one tutorials should be replaced by collective family hours, and this in fact occurred. An important by-product of this activity was that Mr. C, too, began to read and had much to contribute. Lee, the family, and both therapists observed that, as Lee's own psychological status improved and as the entire family continued to grow and develop, the boy's overwhelming interest continued to center on automobiles and auto mechanics — his father's avocation.

Discussion

Male aggressiveness, in its destructive, hurtful and in its nonhostile forms [60], plays an integral part of male caretaking. Fathers reveal a characteristic way of playing with their children — both boys and girls. Their play is proverbially "rough and tumble," pari passu exciting. The father's caretaking tends to be "disruptive" in contrast to the more homeostatic parenting provided by the mother.

Herzog [42] has dubbed this paternal style the "Kamikaze" mode of interaction. He stresses the contributions made to development by such large-motor play. It helps the child learn to "change gears" or states and to tolerate intense and shifting affects, providing her or him with an opportunity to exercise cognitive discrimination. Templates are thereby established for various accommodative modes of affective and cognitive functioning.

Fathers whose own conflicts within the aggressive realm are excessive cannot function in the Kamikaze mode in a modulated and growth-promoting fashion. They tend either to restrain themselves to the point of constriction, to absent themselves, or to become too overpowering and uncontrolled in such aggressive "play." Or else, rationalizing and moralizing their destructiveness, they become punitive. In some instances, concomitant obsessional defenses against aggression impinge on optimal fathering. In all these instances, they fail to attune to their child's rhythms or states of arousal. The range of these impingements is evident in the two fathers we have described, as are the disorders of aggressive-drive organization in their sons, which result from these difficulties in concert with other pathogenic factors.

Ross has elsewhere [65] described Kamikaze-like play as he observed it at Kestenberg's Child Development Research Project, further stressing its age specificity during the third year. In agreement with Herzog's recent [42] formulations, this early work stressed the manner in which the aggressive, phallic play of fathers tends to guide children toward the future, anticipating or releasing subsequent development. It is most often mothers (women) who must remind fathers of the limits of a child's immature drive and ego organization. In these cases, they act as and on external agents to reestablish homeostasis and, with it, the developmental status quo. Ross [65] wrote:

Jake and his son Richard, aged 2½, sit at the table where they and the other fathers and children in the observation center are in the midst of hammering sundry pieces of wood, plastic, and metal into objects. Like the other fathers, Jake does not face his son but sits to the side and slightly in back of him. Nor is this position a function of the seating arrangement alone, since it will be maintained throughout the morning, even while the pair are standing in the wide-open center of the room. Many fathers do not face their sons directly, rather moving beside or behind them. For that matter, they do not seem to say all that much to each other—with notable exceptions, of course—choosing to interrelate through various more inanimate media.

Richard wants his nail to protrude perpendicular to the side of his construction, and when his father affixes it in a less patently phallic manner, the boy yowls in disgusted rage, a yowl that culminates in half an obscenity hissed through pursed lips. With mock sternness and a transparent glee, Jake scolds the boy, who frowns coyly in retort. Momentarily, his father hoists him, end over end, heaving the compact little body up toward the ceiling, where he arcs barely short of it. Richard squeals and squeals, as the onlookers witness the ritual, silently aghast at all the near misses, until finally the boy is somersaulted and rolled across his father's chest and landed safely in his seat once again.

According to Judith Kestenberg [47], between 2 and 3 years a little boy may be seen to pass through his inner genital and urethral subphases of psychosexual development. . . . His relationship with his father will reflect the transitional stage between his earlier love affair with him, and the world in general, and the growing sense that they are both males who will become engaged in a rivalry for the mother's love. A father like Jake, sensitized at some level to the urges and fears abating and awakening in his boy, will respond in kind to his son's silent "ambitendencies" toward him. In addition, he will impose on his son certain of his own conflicts, left over from oedipal and postoedipal developmental phases, thus pointing the way toward the future.

In this instance, we might speculate that Jake's tendency not to position himself face-to-face with Richard spring from his sense of the boy's impetus toward increasingly autonomous functioning, which the father encourages as indicative of a budding masculinity. At the same time as he adjusts to his son's needs, Jake defends against his own more problematic temptations, avoiding face-to-face and thus genital-to-genital contact, with all its aggressive as well as increasingly homosexual implications. It is safer for the two males to communicate through impersonal if also rather phallic activities, which further assure both participants that they are acting as two males together. . . .

Paternal love, previously expressed more easily . . . , is not entirely submerged, of course. Rather it is left unstated, physicalized. Indeed, other fathers, who found it harder than Jake to talk with their boys or to participate in their activities, would nevertheless absently fondle them.

In this instance, too, Jake continued to love and stimulate Richard in characteristically fatherly fashion, tossing the boy up into the air. But this act now conveyed another opposing meaning. It was also a statement of limits, a demonstration of phallic power, exciting identification and affording pleasure to the son, if at the cost of a certain submission on his part, betrayed indeed by the boy's squeals of delight tinged with anxious and helpless defiance. Invited to be manly, a boy is enjoined by his father to go only so far, else he crash into the ceiling and fall to the floor. Remember, the father seems to say, ever so playfully, it was Icarus the son, not Daedalus the father, whose wings melted in the heat of their mutual overreaching, who plummeted to earth. One day you may fly like this, but on your own — one day, but not now. My love for and authority over you are one, a benevolent despotism. [See Weissman (84), on the meaning and impact of father-son play.]

Granted certain common trends, the variations were also striking among fathers in terms of which elements of this complex communication are to be exaggerated and which suppressed. One father simply ignores his son, four months older than Richard, letting the boy bump and thrust wildly about until his efforts end in a lonely crash, accompanied by screams of enraged pain. Another hovers about his son, watchful of his every move, both proud and cautious. A quiet, rather sad man, disappointed in his work life, retreats from the group with his son into corners where the two mumble together, intimate with each other and apart from others. Yet another man appears and disappears without notice, hardly greeting his 2½-year-old boy verbally, but simply settling in behind him, caressing the child while his gaze wanders off to spaces beyond the room. . . .

By the third year, indeed well before this point, the child has become the initiator of the playful interaction. He also acts to curtail it when the stimulation has become too great, indicating his distress. A father responds to these signals and to similar communications on the part of other adults. If the Kamikaze play tactics help to organize and modulate the child's aggressive repertoire, the reverse is also true. In such interactions, the child and the wife act to help the father modulate and organize his aggression toward the child, minimizing the possibility of his doing actual harm to his offspring.

There is considerable dispute as to the existence of or definition of the aggressive drive [60]. Many theorists who are uncomfortable with drive theory see the origins of aggression as reactive rather than innate (e.g., [79]. Our own perspective is a developmental one. We would choose to define aggression in terms of sensorimotor schemata in which the skeletal and muscular apparatuses are activated just as libidinal arousal involves visceral, proprioceptive, tactile, and mucosal – soft tissue sensations. Initial stimulation may involve both sets of drives, which are not as yet differentiated from each other. Libidinal and aggressive, these evolve or mature in the manner Freud and later Jacobson [45] suggested, differentiating from each other, only then to be variously integrated or fused (e.g., in the form of anal sadistic or phallic intrusive aims). As far as aggression itself is concerned, with affects increasingly organized in relation to objects and with growing representational capacities, a child's sensorimotor expressiveness gives way to subjective content. At this point, there is a bifurcation along the lines of constructive aggression on the one hand, and clearly hostile or destructive aims on the other hand. Such development coincides with the consolidation of object constancy and allows for ambivalence and, further, the dawning of intrapsychic conflict.

In any event, whatever aggression "is" and wherever it "comes from," ultimately, males of most primate species, including humans, do exhibit more *aggressivity* in their actions and disposition than their female counterparts [59]. According to Maccoby and Jacklin [54], these sex differences in the manifestation of aggression appear early on and continue throughout life. Differences in parental handling of boys as opposed to girls do not seem to have any long-lasting effect on the child's aggressiveness. Greater aggressivity in males has characterized all societies studied and, indeed, all primate species. According to Williams [85], behavioral aggression is associated with levels of sex hormones, though the direction of causality is by no means clear. For example, high levels of aggression can be both a cause and an effect of higher testosterone levels.

Under optimal circumstances, a man's greater aggressiveness finds avenues of expression in work, sex, sports, and stimulating activities with his children. It can be used to provide, protect, excite, discipline, and organize. The aggressive drive, like the libidinal, and its derivatives can be managed mutually within what one might call a "parentogenic alliance" of mother and father in contending with their young. The mother together with the father can contain, mete out, express, and explore within the caretaking dyad that which might, without the alliance, overflow or become fettered, in either event compromising development. Men who are deprived of issue-specific comanagement of their drives by their spouses are at an increased risk to actually harm or short-change their children.

The child's contributions to his or her interactions with the father determine to some degree the latter's drive expression. The relation is indeed best described as a developmental dialogue [64, 65]. The child's impact is typically limited, however, and he or she must respond to and at times suffer the level of integration and differentiation present in the adult. There is, of course, no linear correspondence between the father's actions and the child's imagery surrounding him. Constitutional factors, the influence of the mother, requisite idealizations, defensive distortions, and fantastical elaborations of various kinds all exert their effects on the internalization of the child's interactions with the parents.

Developmental shifts are perhaps most important. The competent father of the toddler may, for instance, fail his oedipal son by overexciting, angering, or scaring him. To return to the paradigm, one does not heave a 6-week-old infant into the air as one does a 2-year-old child. Nor for that matter does an attuned man subject his 4-year-old child to such an unwanted loss of control and tacit submission. Disturbances in the father impair his empathy with his growing child and may move him to mete out aggressive stimulation that is qualitatively and/or quantitatively out of phase. One is reminded of Stern's [76] studies of mother-infant play and of the caretaker's need to adjust to new plateaus, thresholds, and perceptual modalities in the baby's changing excitability, responsiveness, and capacity to maintain homeostasis.

Finally, the question of aggressive stimulation touches on the subject of sexual or pregenital seduction and its sadomasochistic underpinnings. *Over*stimulation of libidinal urges in children, who lack the capacity for orgastic discharge, inevitably arouses pain and, to borrow from Freud, "mental helplessness." Overstimulation can lead to destructuralization and regression. When these consequences are perceived by the father, who nonetheless persists in his provocativeness, the aims of his loving have clearly shifted from those of libidinal union to destruction and/or self-centered exploitation. Conversely, a man's severe inhibition of sensuality, like impotence, can also serve as a disguised, albeit highly defended, form of malice — a quintessential instance of passive aggression.

Girls, perhaps more than boys, are most subject to sadistic impulses in the strictest sense on the part of fathers — to their starker expression as well as defensive maneuvers against them. Seductive fathers are really cruel parents who make a mockery of a daughter's emerging sense of femininity and self. Conversely, constricted fathers, who have become withdrawn or withholding in order to restrain their more penetrating impulses toward daughters, are often experienced and internalized as rejecting or, at best, indifferent men who do not mirror the child's would-be womanhood. Clinicians are all too familiar with the narcissistic injuries and sexual identity conflicts that derive from excessively eroticized but also aggressivized fathering of a girl [28, 64, 65, 80] and from overzealous reaction formations against such impulses.

We will punctuate this discussion with a clinical vignette illustrating these pathogenic phenomena and the family constellations that help set them in motion.

MELODY

Melody was brought to the clinic at the age of 22 months by her worried parents with the chief complaint that she was pulling out the hair on the top of her head and eating it. A decided bald spot was visible.

Melody was the product of a full-term pregnancy and had a completely negative medical history. Her parents, Mr. and Mrs. T, had been married 18 months before her birth and wanted a family. They were now 27 and 29 years old. Mrs. T went to great extremes to fix Melody's hair in such a way as to conceal the baldness, and the child was beautifully attired in a matching bonnet and pinafore on the day of the initial clinic visit. Melody walked, had a little bit of speech, and presented as a pretty, but very shy little girl.

As is our protocol, the clinic staff watched behind the one-way screen as the family interacted. "We would like to see how Melody looks with you both being here," was the only instruction to the family. We immediately noticed that in addition to the usual nervousness that families experience when being observed, there was a pronounced tension in the room.

Mr. T began to play with Melody. He did not interact at all with his wife nor she with him. He took a doll and invited Melody to play with him. He seemed reserved, almost stiff. His wife simply looked on. Then he winked at Melody, seemed to relax, and reached over to tickle her. Mrs. T jumped up, took a hairbrush out of her pocketbook, interrupted the "play" between father and daughter in order to remove Melody's bonnet, and began to brush her hair vigorously. Melody at first looked a little startled but then smiled, patted her head, and said, "Br, Br" several times. Mr. T looked less pleased. He muttered, "Leave her alone, for Christ sake let her play." At that point, mother stopped brushing and started a kind of counting game with Melody.

Mr. T still looked disgruntled. He picked up the hairbrush that his wife had put down and began smacking his hand with it. It made a very loud noise. Melody looked up, flushed, became quite agitated, and said, "Br, Br, Br" again. She then assumed a faraway look in her eyes and began to play with her hair. Her father smacked his hand as her mother rose to her feet shouting: "Stop the observation: See she's going to pull out her hair and eat it. This is why we have to come to see you."

In the interview with the parents that followed, we were told that Melody had been very interested in the hairbrush for the past seven months. At about 15 months of age, she had become very irritated, no longer wanting her mother to brush her hair, which had been a previous practice. She turned to her Daddy and said at this time, "Br Br. Da Br Br Da." Neither parent had understood this to be a request for father to brush Melody's hair. Melody showed increasing interest in the hairbrush from this time on but seemed to prefer father's brush to mother's.

Melody would insist on being with Mr. T in the bathroom in the morning when he brushed his hair (see [28]). In fact, her wish to be with her father in the bathroom in the morning had preceded her preoccupation with the hairbrush. Mrs. T had disapproved, particularly when she noticed that Melody seemed interested in her husband's urinating. Mr. T initially did not mind Melody's presence, but as she grew more and more insistent and as his wife was more and more disapproving, he began to feel angry with Melody. Melody's pediatrician was consulted at this point and made the suggestion that she should be given a hairbrush of her own and a doll with hair to accompany it. For a week or two this seemed to suffice. Melody brushed the doll's hair with great vigor. This was replaced by her brushing her own hair from morning to night until the brush was discarded. She then began to play with her hair, pull it out, and eat it.

At around 20 months, Melody started to become very naughty. She would do nothing that her mother asked and always wanted her Daddy. We were told that the relationship between the parents was very poor. Mrs. T accused Mr. T of being too physical. "He always wants to make love and to touch me. I can't stand it," she said. She was aghast at her husband's behavior toward Melody. "He's too physical with her too. He always wants to play with her. The two of them would roughhouse all day if I didn't put a stop to it. Also, he wants to spank her. He suggested that she should get the hairbrush applied to her bottom when she was naughty. I told him that I would report him for child abuse."

Mr. T grinned and shrugged his shoulders as his wife spoke. "I believe in physical contact," he stated. "I would like a hell of a lot more of it with my wife, and I think it's fine for Melody for both play and punishment. Judy is so uptight. I feel like she has me in a straightjacket. I don't think that Melody or Judy is getting what she needs. I'm not either."

In the play episodes with Melody, the following scenario evolved. A teddy bear was on the rampage. He pushed over all the furniture. The therapist brought in a mommy teddy bear. He wondered what she would do. "No touch," Melody had the mother teddy bear say. Then she laughed. The little teddy bear continued to push everything over. "Oh, dear," the therapist said, "I hope it will be all right." "Broken," shrieked Melody, "broken." "What is the furniture?" "Ma Ma broken," said the little girl. She then reached for another teddy bear bigger than the others. "Daddy," she said. "What will he do?" he asked the little teddy bear. "Br, Br, Da, Da," she had the little teddy say. This vocalization was accompanied by two behaviors. Melody manipulated the little teddy bear close to the big bear. He smacked his hand. It could have been a spanking scene. Then she had the big bear go to the mother bear and bump into her several times. It could have been a lovemaking scene. Now the little teddy bear stopped pushing things over. "Good," said Melody, "now good." She was smiling broadly.

In following sessions, the same scene was repeated. When the daddy teddy bear could not be produced, the little teddy would push things over again and again and try to break them. Sometimes she would hit the mommy teddy. Sometimes, she would have the little teddy say "no, no," and sometimes "OK, OK." A garbled conversation of sorts would ensue, apparently "within" the teddy. Another variant involved putting the teddy to bed. The teddy would start to hit himself in the lower abdominal region and in the head. He would pull at his head and say, "Br Br Da Da." At the end of such sequences, Melody herself would be pulling at her hair with a faraway distant expression in her eyes.

The therapist introduced a Dr. Bear. He wanted to examine the little teddy after the self-abuse. "What happened?" the doctor asked. "Broken," replied little teddy, "all broken." "How can we fix it?" the doctor asked. "Daddy bear hairbrush," Melody had the little teddy say. These words were spoken very clearly — in contradistinction to her previous diction.

In this instance, the relationship between the father's display and stimulation of aggression and the development of sexual identity in his child are also illustrated. Melody, it seemed, deprived of contact with her father, directed toward herself a fusion of the aggressive and libidinal stimulation for which she yearned. Along with her sadomasochism, her early castration reaction was intensified with the hairbrush and hair pulling, which served as infantile fetishes. The whole symptomatic picture seemed, then, to bode ill for Melody's quickly evolving gender identity and future femininity. The mother's pathogenic influence on the father-daughter dyad is also telling, especially the way in which she herself confounded male sexuality and destructive aggression and then imparted this image to her toddler, entrenching her daughter's view of the sexual father as a "marauder" [30]. Finally, Melody's predicament may shed light on the genesis of sadomasochism within the preoedipal relationship of father and daughter, which is itself embedded in the parent-child triad.

Conclusion: Fathers and the Aggressive Line of Development

A father's envy, competitiveness, jealousy, and simple hostility are ubiquitous, it seems, but constitute only half of a dialectic. At the other pole lie paternal warmth, nurturance, pride, and love, as well as a father's positively toned object love for and narcissistic pleasure in his offspring. Yielding to one side of his ambivalence, as we have tried to demonstrate, an overzealously "loving" father does a potentially invasive disservice to the child, depriving a son or daughter and later burdening him or her with surplus guilt over hostile impulses toward so seemingly benevolent and controlled a caretaker. Resolving his aggressive conflicts neurotically (e.g., through obsessional ploys or by subsiding into depression), he may lapse into ironic sins of omission that rob a son or daughter of his emotional or even his actual masculine presence, as well as the recognition of the adult as a separate being with needs of his or her own. Such avoidances may be tantamount to a sort of mental murder: out of mind, out of sight, out of existence. The behavioral consequences include passivity on the father's part, deference to women's expertise, and a stilted, merely "instrumental" or self-consciously "adult" mode of dealing with a child, which is empty of pleasure and vitality.

To be aggressive with a child is not necessarily to abuse or injure. As we have suggested, aggression fuels the man's capacities for vigorous play, reasonable discipline (and the internal controls and protection it ultimately serves to provide), and an active, aggressive providing, which secures and protects the family and the home. It brings wit, humor, and reality to the child's life, sparking the sweet rebellion of mutually teasing mischief, and can make for those moments of childhood that are remembered throughout life as little family myths. And a father's aggressiveness and purposeful claims to his own dominion also breed tension of the kind that invites a child's more concerted, serious overreaching — his or her adaptive, purposeful development.

Both primary objects, mother and father, play roles in stimulating and inhibiting unfolding aggressiveness. But certainly by virtue of the representational capacities that begin to unfold in the second half of the child's second year, it is the latter, the father, who becomes most clearly associated with its activation. Yogman [86] has, in fact, traced this epigenetic progression to the first 6 months. In infancy, he asserts, a father's abrupt, intense stimulation may have begun to lay down sensorimotor precursors of later representations of fathers as specific male figures. From early on, aggressive excitation is associated in a variety of ways with masculinity (Abelin's "father principle" [2, 3, 4]). The father's precedence as the parental aggressor, good and bad, it seems, is a consequence of the child's private experience and his or her active eliciting or releasing of a father's gender-specific behavior, as well as the specific father's inherent makeup and those instinctive parental tendencies that override and sometimes contradict "preparental" characterological patterns.

The model, a veritable cliché, of father tossing the toddler into the air and then catching him or her, provides a metaphor for the arc of aggressive excitation around the time of practicing and transition into the second year. "Scary" games of chasing and playful teasing about being "such a bad boy (or girl)" earmark early representational development. During rapprochement, with these and other precursors to superego development, one sees a further laying down of relative object constancy and individuation (the latter in the sense of achieving a primary sense of oneself as a person and of others as individual human beings). The outright, often somewhat sadistic teasing of the oedipal child, a son especially, on the part of fathers and older males, and assertions of firm limits are characteristic of subsequent development. During latency, fathers and children, sons in particular, respond to the thrust of concrete operations more pragmatically. Men compete with children more realistically and join as wiser allies in the child's conquest of the widening world. The father, acting as mentor [68], enhances the child's skills of mastery and activity, which provides for more neutral expressions of aggression [71]. With adolescence [12], the struggles become real, presaging and embodying the succession of the generations. These battles reveal that the aggressive interplay of earlier years has served as a rehearsal for the real-life combat of life, for fending for oneself in an unprotected universe.

References

1. Abelin, E. The Role of the Father in the Separation-Individuation Process. In J. McDevitt and C. Settlage (Eds.), *Separation-Individuation*. New York: International Universities Press, 1971.
2. Abelin, E. Some further comments and observations on the earliest role of the father. *Int. J. Psychoanal.* 56:293, 1975.
3. Abelin, E. Panel. The role of the father in the preoedipal years, R. C. Prall, Reporter. *J. Am. Psychoanal. Assoc.* 26:143, 1978.
4. Abelin, E. Triangulation, the Role of the Father and the Origins of Core Gender Identity During the Rapprochement Subphase. In R. Lax, A. J.

Burland, and S. Back (Eds.), *Rapprochement: The Critical Subphase of Separation.* New York: Aronson, 1980.

5. Atkins, N. The Oedipus myth, adolescence, and the succession of generations. *J. Am. Psychoanal. Assoc.* 18:860, 1970.
6. Atkins, R. Discovering Daddy: The Mother's Role. In S. Cath, A. Gurwitt, and J. Ross (Eds.), *Father and Child.* Boston: Little, Brown, 1982.
7. Biller, H. Paternal Deprivation, Cognitive Functioning, and the Feminized Classroom. In A. Davids (Ed.), *Child Personality and Psychopathology.* New York: Wiley, 1974.
8. Burlingham, D. Child analysis and the mother. *Psychoanal. Q.* 4:69, 1935.
9. Demos, J. The Changing Faces of Fatherhood. In S. Cath, A. Gurwitt, and J. Ross (Eds.), *Father and Child.* Boston: Little, Brown, 1982.
10. Devereux, G. Why Oedipus killed Laius. *Int. J. Psychoanal.* 34:132, 1953.
11. Escalona, S. *The Roots of Individuality: Normal Patterns of Development in Infancy.* Chicago: Aldine Publishing Company, 1968.
12. Esman, A. Fathers and Adolescent Sons. In S. Cath, A. Gurwitt, and J. Ross (Eds.), *Father and Child.* Boston: Little, Brown, 1982.
13. Ferholt, J., and Gurwitt, A. Involving Fathers in Treatment. In S. Cath, A. Gurwitt, and J. Ross (Eds.), *Father and Child.* Boston: Little, Brown, 1982.
14. Freud, S. The Interpretation of Dreams (1900). In J. Strachey (Ed.), The Standard Edition of the Complete Psychological Works of Sigmund Freud. London: Hogarth, 1953. Vol. 4.
15. Freud, S. Fragment of an analysis of a case of hysteria (1905). *Standard Edition.* 1953. Vol. 7.
16. Freud, S. *The Origins of Psycho-Analysis* (1887–1892). New York: Basic Books, 1954.
17. Freud, S. Analysis of a phobia in a five-year-old boy (1909). *Standard Edition.* 1955. Vol. 10.
18. Freud, S. Notes upon a case of obsessional neurosis (1909). *Standard Edition.* 1955. Vol. 10.
19. Freud, S. From the history of an infantile neurosis (1918). *Standard Edition.* 1955. Vol. 17.
20. Freud, S. Beyond the pleasure principle (1920). *Standard Edition.* 1955. Vol. 18.
21. Freud, S. A special type of object choice made by men (1910). *Standard Edition.* 1957. Vol. 10.
22. Freud, S. Psychoanalytic notes upon an autobiographical account of a case of paranoia (1911). *Standard Edition.* 1958. Vol. 12.
23. Freud, S. The ego and the id (1923). *Standard Edition.* 1961. Vol. 19.
24. Freud, S. The dissolution of the Oedipus complex (1924). *Standard Edition.* 1961. Vol. 19.
25. Freud, S. The economic problem of masochism (1924). *Standard Edition.* 1961. Vol. 19.

26. Freud, S. Some psychical consequences of the anatomical distinction between the sexes (1925). *Standard Edition*. 1961. Vol. 19.
27. Freud, S. Civilization and its discontents (1930). *Standard Edition*. 1961. Vol. 21.
28. Galenson, E., and Roiphe, H. The Preoedipal Relationship of a Father, Mother and Daughter. In S. Cath, A. Gurwitt, and J. Ross (Eds.), *Father and Child*. Boston: Little, Brown, 1982.
29. Glenn, J., and Bernstein, I. The Child Analyst's Emotional Reactions to His Patients. In J. Glenn (Ed.), *Child Analysis and Child Psychotherapy*. New York: Aronson, 1978.
30. Greenacre, P. *Emotional Growth: Psychoanalytic Studies of the Gifted and a Great Variety of Other Individuals*. Vol. 1. New York: International Universities Press, 1971.
31. Greenson, R. *Explorations in Psychoanalysis*. New York: International Universities Press, 1978.
32. Grunberger, B. The oedipal conflicts of the analyst. *Psychoanal. Q*. 49:606, 1980.
33. Gunsberg, L. Selected Critical Review of Psychological Investigations of the Father-Infant Relationship. In S. Cath, A. Gurwitt, and J. Ross (Eds.), *Father and Child*. Boston: Little, Brown, 1982.
34. Gurwitt, A. Aspects of Prospective Fatherhood. In S. Cath, A. Gurwitt, and J. Ross (Eds.), *Father and Child*. Boston: Little, Brown, 1982.
35. Hartmann, H. *Ego Psychology and the Problem of Adaptation*. New York: International Universities Press, 1958.
36. Hartmann, H., Kris, E., and Loewenstein, R. Comments on the formation of psychic structure. *Psychoanal. Study Child* 2:11, 1946.
37. Hartmann, H., and Loewenstein, R. Notes on the superego. *Psychoanal. Study Child* 17:42, 1982.
38. Herzog, J. Attachment, Attunement, and Abuse, 1979, unpublished.
39. Herzog, J. Sleep disturbance and father hunger in 18-to-28-month-old boys: The Erlkonig syndrome. *Psychoanal. Study Child* 35:219, 1980.
40. Herzog, J. On Father Hunger. In S. Cath, A. Gurwitt, and J. Ross (Eds.), *Father and Child*. Boston: Little, Brown, 1982.
41. Herzog, J. Patterns of Expectant Fatherhood. In S. Cath, A. Gurwitt, and J. Ross (Eds.), *Father and Child*. Boston: Little, Brown, 1982.
42. Herzog, J. Plenary presentation. Second Congress, World Association for Infant Psychiatry. Cannes, France, April, 1983.
43. Hoffer, W. Defensive process and defensive organization. *Int. J. Psychoanal*. 35:194, 1954.
44. Jacobson, E. Development of the wish for a child in boys. *Psychoanal. Study Child* 5:139, 1950.
45. Jacobson, E. *The Self and the Object World*. New York: International Universities Press, 1964.

46. Kernberg, O. *Object Relations Theory and Clinical Psychoanalysis.* New York: Aronson, 1976.
47. Kestenberg, J. *Children and Parents.* New York: Aronson, 1975.
48. Kestenberg, J., Marcus, H., Sossin, K., and Stevenson, R., Jr. The Development of Paternal Attitudes. In S. Cath, A. Gurwitt, and J. Ross (Eds.), *Father and Child.* Boston: Little, Brown, 1982.
49. Kohut, H. *The Analysis of the Self.* New York: International Universities Press, 1971.
50. Lichtenstein, H. *The Dilemma of Human Identity.* New York: Aronson, 1977.
51. Loewald, H. Ego and reality. *Int. J. Psychoanal.* 32:10, 1951.
52. Loewald, H. The transference neurosis: Comments on the concept and the phenomenon. *J. Am. Psychoanal. Assoc.* 19:54, 1971.
53. Loewald, H. The waning of the Oedipus complex. *J. Am. Psychoanal. Assoc.* 27:751, 1979.
54. Maccoby, E., and Jacklin, C. *The Psychology of Sex Differences.* Stanford: Stanford University Press, 1974.
55. Machtlinger, V. The Father in Psychoanalytic Theory. In M. Lamb (Ed.), *The Role of the Father in Child Development.* New York: Wiley, 1981.
56. Mahl, G. Father-Son Themes in Freud's Self-Analysis. In S. Cath, A. Gurwitt, and J. Ross (Eds.), *Father and Child.* Boston: Little, Brown, 1982.
57. Mahler, M. Symbiosis and individuation: The psychological birth of the infant. *Psychoanal. Study Child* 29:89, 1974.
58. Mahler, M., Pine, F., and Bergman, A. *The Psychological Birth of the Human Infant.* New York: Basic Books, 1975.
59. Mitchell, G. *Human Sex Differences. A Primatologist's Perspective.* New York: Van Nostrand Reinhold, 1981.
60. Parens, H. *The Development of Aggression in Early Childhood.* New York: Aronson, 1979.
61. Parsons, T., and Bales, R. *Family, Socialization and Interaction Process.* Glencoe, Ill.: Free Press, 1955.
62. Ross, J. The development of paternal identity: A critical review of the literature on nurturance and generativity in boys and men. *J. Am. Psychoanal. Assoc.* 23:783, 1975.
63. Ross, J. Toward fatherhood: The epigenesis of paternal identity during a boy's first decade. *Int. J. Psychoanal.* 4:327, 1977.
64. Ross, J. Fathering: A review of some psychoanalytic contributions on paternity. *Int. J. Psychoanal.* 60:317, 1979.
65. Ross, J. The Forgotten Father. In M. Nelson and J. Ikenberry (Eds.), *Psychosexual Imperatives: Their Impact on Identity Formation.* New York: Human Sciences Press, 1979.
66. Ross, J. Paternal Identity: The Equations of Fatherhood and Manhood. In T. B. Krasu and C. Socarides (Eds.), *On Sexuality: Psychoanalytic Observations.* New York: International Universities Press, 1979.

67. Ross, J. From Mother to Father: The Boy's Search for a Generative Identity and the Oedipal Era. In S. Cath, A. Gurwitt, and J. Ross (Eds.), *Father and Child.* Boston: Little, Brown, 1982.
68. Ross, J. Mentorship in Middle Childhood. In S. Cath, A. Gurwitt, and J. Ross (Eds.), *Father and Child.* Boston: Little, Brown, 1982.
69. Ross, J. Oedipus revisited: Laius and the Laius complex. *Psychoanal. Study Child* 37:169, 1982.
70. Ross, J. In Search of Fathering. In S. Cath, A. Gurwitt, and J. Ross (Eds.), *Father and Child.* Boston: Little, Brown, Co., 1982.
71. Sarnoff, C. The Father's Role in Latency. In S. Cath, A. Gurwitt, and J. Ross (Eds.), *Father and Child.* Boston: Little, Brown, 1982.
72. Sheleff, L. *Generations Apart: Adult Hostility Toward Youth.* New York: McGraw-Hill, 1981.
73. Spitz, R. Hospitalism. *Psychoanal. Study Child* 1:53, 1945.
74. Spitz, R. *The First Year of Life.* New York: International Universities Press, 1965.
75. Steele, B. The Abusive Father. In S. Cath, A. Gurwitt, and J. Ross (Eds.), *Father and Child.* Boston: Little, Brown, 1982.
76. Stern, D. The goal and structure of mother-infant play. *J. Am. Acad. Child Psychiatry* 13:402, 1974.
77. Stoller, R. *Sex and Gender.* New York: Science House, 1968.
78. Stoller, R. Healthiest parental influences on the earlier development of masculinity in baby boys. *Psychoanal. Forum* 5:232, 1975.
79. Stone, L. Reflections on the psychoanalytic concept of aggression. *Psychoanal. Q.* 40:198, 1971.
80. Tessman, L. A Note on Father's Contributions to the Daughter's Ways of Loving and Working. In S. Cath, A. Gurwitt, and J. Ross (Eds.), *Father and Child.* Boston: Little, Brown, 1982.
81. Tyson, P. The Role of the Father in Gender Identity, Urethral Erotism, and Phallic Narcissism. In S. Cath, A. Gurwitt, and J. Ross (Eds.), *Father and Child.* Boston: Little, Brown, 1982.
82. Van der Leeuw, P. The preoedipal phase of the male. *Psychoanal. Study Child* 13:352, 1958.
83. Weil, A. The basic core. *Psychoanal. Study Child* 25:442, 1970.
84. Weissman, P. The effects of preoedipal paternal attitudes on development and character. *Int. J. Psychoanal.* 44:121, 1963.
85. Williams, J. H. *Psychology of Women: Behavior in a Biosocial Context.* New York: Norton, 1977.
86. Yogman, M. Observations on the Father-Infant Relationship. In S. Cath, A. Gurwitt, and J. Ross (Eds.), *Father and Child.* Boston: Little, Brown, 1982.

Epilogue

In this book, various authors have looked at parenthood and its human vicissitudes through psychoanalytic eyes from quite different perspectives. The book follows the nature and impact of parental influences as they emerge from early life and become sufficiently a part of the personal orientation of individuals and are used in the care of a new generation. In different parts of the book, attempts are made to trace the origins of both typical and atypical parental behavior. Although both conscious and unconscious learning influence development, as reflected in imitation, identification, and rehearsal, from an evolutionary point of view the perpetuation of the species is far too crucial to be left entirely to the hazards of psychologically induced inclinations. As we watch an animal mother in the process of caring for her newborn litter, we can empathize not only with the parental experience, but also with the quality of the nurturing. As a general rule, animal mothers convey the essence of what Winnicott had in mind when he spoke of the ordinary, devoted, "good-enough" mother, although this can be perverted by unnatural conditions of domestication and caging.

Clearly, we have come from a long line of parents reaching back on the evolutionary scale, and apparently these forebears did well through instinctual programming in conjunction with neuroendocrine concomitants. Primitive man followed along the same lines, although psychological and social complications were already beginning to complicate the issues of reproduction and muddying the waters of child care. As the study of the mind became paramount, instinctual behavior faded from the picture and the psychology and psychopathology of parenthood arose. The triumph of mind over instinct enhanced both the joys and sorrows of parenting, but it also led to perversions and distortions of the caring process. In becoming human parents, we depend less and less on what comes naturally and more and more on the extensive machinations of the hypertrophied cortex that we possess: We look to the mind to help us out—our own minds or the theories and ideas of other "expert" minds. Every now and then within our overcivilized culture, there are episodes characterized by a wish to revert to an earlier evolutionary status, and groups and individuals resort to "natural childbirth," breast-feeding, unscheduled feeding, "natural" foods, and the use of "natural" child-rearing procedures. This does not make human parenting any

511

more "instinctual," but it does permit the human mother to feel and behave more naturally and less bookishly.

On the positive side, human contributions to the cause of parenthood have not been inconsiderable. The psychoanalytic discovery of the unconscious led to an enrichment of the concept of parenting, making it more desirable to even the most intelligent members of the species, many of whom are turned away from propagation by the catastrophic self-destructive developments in the human condition. A second offering, almost peculiar to humankind (primates and midwife toads have not been remiss in this respect), has been the act of parenting. As indicated in several parts of this book, fathers have arrived on the scene preparing for birth along with their wives, participating in birth as eager and encouraging coaches, invading the nurseries, diapering and bathing the infants, and, during the early phase of life before the children come into their own at the level of the triadic Oedipus complex, acting as very good and often very efficient mother surrogates. As the child enters latency, the father becomes an integral part of the parental team. One sees the ordinary good-enough father at work and play with his offspring. So firmly are these relationships established, that even when divorced from his wife, he is continuing to play his fathering role and even to demand joint custody.

The business of this book, therefore, is to alert the professional world engaged in helping children that mothers need to be helped not only to get over their neuroses, psychoses, or even minor maladjustments, but also to overcome the psychological impediments that stand in the way of successful parental activity. We hope that parents will refer themselves spontaneously to the psychoanalyst and psychotherapist because of parental "complexes" that interfere with child rearing, and it is our hope that those who treat them will not dismiss these new types of referrals as mere rationalizations concealing other neurotic holdups, but will give them more sophisticated and knowledgeable consideration. Our wish would be to make poor parents into good-enough ones, and good-enough parents into even better ones; only thus will true generativity flourish.

Becoming a parent in this complex human world, however, is not to be taken lightly or impulsively. The wear and tear on the psyche, even under the most advantageous conditions, is appreciable, and there will be many occasions, as Winnicott reminded us, when ordinary devoted parents will hate their offspring—not only their babies, but their school children and especially their adolescents.

One should not be put off by the words of the Euripidean Medea when she questioned (and who better to do this) the worthwhileness of parenthood. First of all, Medea echoed the thoughts of many intelligent women today who feel that men want them to put their minds into cold storage and confine their activities to the nursery [1].

Through being considered clever I have suffered much. A person of sense ought never to have his children brought up to be more clever than the average. For, apart from cleverness bringing them no profit, it will make them objects of envy and ill-will. If you are thought superior to those who have some reputation for learning, you will become hated. I have some knowledge myself of how this happens; for being clever, I find that some will envy me, others object to me.

This is the predicament of the modern "liberated" mother voiced 2,500 years ago. But Medea asks herself if it is worthwhile and answers [1]:

This I say, that those who have never had children who know nothing of it in happiness have the advantage over those who are parents. The childless, who never discover whether children turn out as a good thing or as something to cause pain, are spared many troubles in lacking this knowledge. And those who have in their homes the sweet presence of children, I see that their lives are all wasted away by their worries. First they must think how to bring them up well and how to leave them something to live on. And then after this whether all their toil is for those who will turn out good or bad, is still an unanswered question.

And then, Medea concluded, there is the last and greatest trouble that even when you have successfully raised children, they can die, and this is "the most terrible grief of all."

To counteract this offsetting voice from the ancient past, there is Winnicott, the self-appointed spokesman for mothers (and occasionally for fathers). In response to Medea he says [2]:

Your thoughts come in the richness that may gradually appear in the personal potential of this or that boy or girl. And if you succeed you must be prepared to be jealous of your children who are getting better opportunities for personal development than you had yourselves. You will feel rewarded if one day your daughter asks you to do some baby-sitting for her, indicating thereby that she thinks you may be able to do this satisfactorily; or if your son wants to be like you in some way, or falls in love with a girl you would have liked yourself, had you been younger. Rewards come *indirectly*. And of course you know you will not be thanked.

The rewards do come mostly indirectly; there are so many of them in every developmental phase that even parents forget about them once that phase is over. However, they remain there among the unconscious memories of both parent and child to add to their ongoing relationship.

References

1. Euripides. *The Medea.*
2. Winnicott, D. W. Contemporary Concepts of Adolescent Development. In *Playing and Reality.* London: Tavistock, 1971.

Index

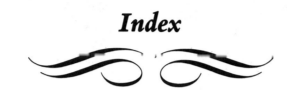

Index